NURSING
THEORIES

A FRAMEWORK
FOR PROFESSIONAL
PRACTICE

THE PEDAGOGY

Nursing Theories: A Framework for Professional Practice teaches students to understand nursing theory through a variety of strategies that meet the learning needs of students while generating enthusiasm about the application of popular theories. This interactive approach addresses different learning styles, making *Nursing Theories* the ideal text to ensure mastery of key concepts. The pedagogical aids that appear in most chapters include the following:

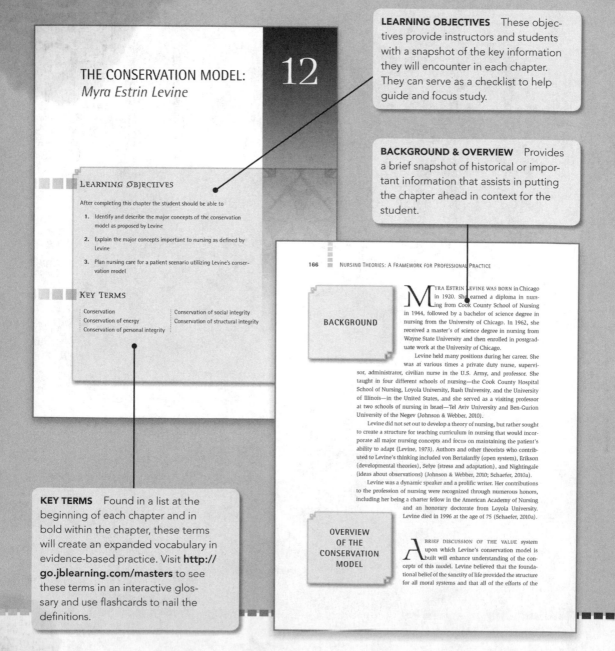

LEARNING OBJECTIVES These objectives provide instructors and students with a snapshot of the key information they will encounter in each chapter. They can serve as a checklist to help guide and focus study.

BACKGROUND & OVERVIEW Provides a brief snapshot of historical or important information that assists in putting the chapter ahead in context for the student.

KEY TERMS Found in a list at the beginning of each chapter and in bold within the chapter, these terms will create an expanded vocabulary in evidence-based practice. Visit **http://go.jblearning.com/masters** to see these terms in an interactive glossary and use flashcards to nail the definitions.

THE CONSERVATION MODEL:
Myra Estrin Levine

12

LEARNING OBJECTIVES

After completing this chapter the student should be able to

1. Identify and describe the major concepts of the conservation model as proposed by Levine
2. Explain the major concepts important to nursing as defined by Levine
3. Plan nursing care for a patient scenario utilizing Levine's conservation model

KEY TERMS

Conservation
Conservation of energy
Conservation of personal integrity
Conservation of social integrity
Conservation of structural integrity

---

166   NURSING THEORIES: A FRAMEWORK FOR PROFESSIONAL PRACTICE

BACKGROUND

MYRA ESTRIN LEVINE WAS BORN in Chicago in 1920. She earned a diploma in nursing from Cook County School of Nursing in 1944, followed by a bachelor of science degree in nursing from the University of Chicago. In 1962, she received a master's of science degree in nursing from Wayne State University and then enrolled in postgraduate work at the University of Chicago.

Levine held many positions during her career. She was at various times a private duty nurse, supervisor, administrator, civilian nurse in the U.S. Army, and professor. She taught in four different schools of nursing—the Cook County Hospital School of Nursing, Loyola University, Rush University, and the University of Illinois—in the United States, and she served as a visiting professor at two schools of nursing in Israel—Tel Aviv University and Ben-Gurion University of the Negev (Johnson & Webber, 2010).

Levine did not set out to develop a theory of nursing, but rather sought to create a structure for teaching curriculum in nursing that would incorporate all major nursing concepts and focus on maintaining the patient's ability to adapt (Levine, 1973). Authors and other theorists who contributed to Levine's thinking included von Bertalanffy (open system), Erikson (developmental theories), Selye (stress and adaptation), and Nightingale (ideas about observations) (Johnson & Webber, 2010; Schaefer, 2010a).

Levine was a dynamic speaker and a prolific writer. Her contributions to the profession of nursing were recognized through numerous honors, including her being a charter fellow in the American Academy of Nursing and an honorary doctorate from Loyola University. Levine died in 1996 at the age of 75 (Schaefer, 2010a).

OVERVIEW OF THE CONSERVATION MODEL

A BRIEF DISCUSSION OF THE VALUE system upon which Levine's conservation model is built will enhance understanding of the concepts of this model. Levine believed that the foundational belief of the sanctity of life provided the structure for all moral systems and that all of the efforts of the healing sciences were founded upon the holiness and wholeness of the human being (Levine, 1989a, p. 125). She also deliberately used the word "patient" in all of her publications rather than the word "client" to describe the recipient of care. She explained that the Latin root word for "client" means "follower"; given that this usage is reminiscent of a paternalistic relationship, she suggested, it ought to be forbidden in nursing on moral grounds. In contrast, the word "patient" comes from the Latin word for "suffering" (Levine, 1989a, p. 126). According to Levine (1990, p. 199), it is the condition of suffering that allows the patient to set independence aside and accept the services of another person.

Levine introduced the conservation principles in *Nursing Forum* (1967). Two years later, she published her textbook *Introduction to Clinical Nursing* (1969a), which was an application of the framework. She used the term **conservation** to label the framework because it was derived from the Latin word meaning "to keep together" (Pieper, 1989, p. 137).

The goals of the conservation model are achieved through interventions geared toward the four conservation principles:

❖ The principle of **conservation of energy** addresses the requirement of individuals in relation to a balance of energy and a constant renewal of energy to maintain life processes and activities.

❖ The principle of **conservation of structural integrity** addresses healing as a process of restoring structural and functional integrity through conservation and defense of wholeness, in which those individuals with permanent effects of illness or loss of structure are guided to a new level of adaptation (Levine, 1991, 1996).

❖ The principle of **conservation of personal integrity** recognizes the sanctity of life that is manifest in all persons and "includes recognition of the holiness of each person" (Levine, 1996, p. 40). This principle encompasses the ideas that self-worth and identity are important and, therefore, that nurses should show patients respect (Schaefer, 2010a, p. 229).

❖ The principle of **conservation of social integrity** reminds the nurse that life gains meaning through social communities and that the meaning of health is socially determined (Schaefer, 2010a, p. 229).

How does Levine's use of the word "patient" (and rejection of the term "client") compare with Neuman's preferred use of the word "client" to refer to the recipient of nursing care? Does this choice change nursing practice? If so, how?

CRITICAL THINKING   An integral part of the learning process, critical thinking questions are presented by the authors to spark thought and test the ability of the student to think critically about topics discussed in each chapter.

PULL QUOTES   Helpful tidbits pulled from the text to further highlight key content for the student.

BULLETED LISTS   Quick facts called out to highlight important aspects of topics within each chapter.

MAJOR CONCEPTS OF NURSING ACCORDING TO   A closer look at nursing concepts according to the individual theories and theorist being discussed in each chapter.

The four foundational principles of the conservation model are the conservation of energy, the conservation of structural integrity, the conservation of personal integrity and the conservation of social integrity.

Three major concepts form the basis of the conservation model and its assumptions: conservation, wholeness, and adaptation. *Conservation*, according to Levine, "describes the way complex systems are able to continue to function even when severely challenged" (1990, p. 192). It is through the process of conservation that persons are able to face challenges, adapt, and maintain their uniqueness. The primary focus of conservation is keeping together the wholeness of the person.

The second major concept in the conservation model is *wholeness* (or *holism*). Levine based her definition of wholeness on Erickson's description of wholeness of an open system because she believed that this definition provided the option of exploring the parts of the whole to understand the whole. Integrity refers to the oneness of the person (Schaefer, 2010a, p. 227).

The third major concept in the conservation model is *adaptation*. According to Levine, "adaptation is the process of change whereby the individual retains his integrity within the realities of his internal and external environment" (1973, p. 11). Conservation is the outcome of adaptation. Levine identified three characteristics of adaptation: historicity, specificity, and redundancy (1991). Levine believed that every person has "fixed patterns of responses uniquely designed to ensure success in essential life activities, and demonstrating that adaptation is both historical and specific" (1991, p. 5). Redundancy represents the fail-safe options available to persons to ensure adaptation. Loss of redundant choices through trauma, age, disease, or environmental changes may make it difficult for the person to maintain life (Schaefer, 2010a, p. 227).

The capacity of the person to adapt to the environmental condition is called the organismic response. There are four levels of organismic response integration: fight or flight, inflammatory response, response to stress, and perceptual awareness (Schaefer, 2010a, p. 228). Nursing care focuses on the management of these responses (Levine, 1969a).

MAJOR CONCEPTS OF NURSING ACCORDING TO THE CONSERVATION MODEL

IN ADDITION TO THE CONCEPTS already presented, the four metaparadigm concepts of nursing are identified in Levine's conservation model. These concepts are summarized in Table 12-1.

TABLE 12-1 Metaparadigm Concepts as Defined in Levine's Model	
Person	A "system of systems, [that] in its wholeness expresses the organization of all the contributing parts" (Levine, 1991, pp. 8–9); may be an individual, an individual in a group, or an individual in a community (Levine, 1973)
Environment	The context in which individuals live their lives; each individual has both internal and external environments
Health	Health and disease are patterns of adaptive changes; the concept of health implies wholeness and integrity, whereas disease represents the person's effort to protect self-integrity
Nursing	"Nursing is human interaction" (Levine, 1973, p. 1) and the goal of nursing is to promote adaptation and maintain wholeness (Levine, 1971a, p. 258)

Person

Levine views the person as a "system of systems, [that] in its wholeness expresses the organization of all the contributing parts" (1991, p. 8–9). Levine stresses the holistic nature of persons. She equates wholeness with integrity and integrity with concepts of freedom of choice, sense of identity, and self-worth (Levine, 1991)

Levine also views life as "a [...] Persons, as systems of systems, e[...] stant adaptation with the goal of c[...] as an individual; an individual in [...] vidual in a community (Levine, 19[...] the environment.

Environment

The environment is the context in [...] each individual has both internal a[...] environment includes physiologica[...] the patient that are challenged by [...] The external environment consist[...] lenge the person.

Levine acknowledges three le[...] ational, and conceptual (Levine,[...]

TABLES All tables are Metaparadigm Concepts as Defined for each theory covered in their respective chapters.

CASE STUDIES Found in select chapters, these studies are designed to enhance the student's learning experience by teaching how theory applies to practice.

THE FOLLOWING SCENARIO ILLUSTRATES NURSING care of the patient relative to one identified nursing problem framed by Levine's conservation model. This scenario is not intended to cover all aspects of care, but rather to stimulate thinking about how specific care might be approached using this theory as a framework for practice.

Mrs. C. is an 85-year-old recent widow who has been discharged from the acute care setting after an exacerbation of congestive heart failure. The nurse who visits Mrs. C. will collect data through interview and observation related to the conservation principles—including conservation of energy, conservation of structural integrity, conservation of personal integrity, and conservation of social integrity—in an effort to promote adaptation and maintain wholeness. The assessment reveals that Mrs. C. is specifically struggling with wholeness to in relation to conservation of structural integrity as she adapts to a new lifestyle, specifically in relation to the dieta[...]

Trophicognosis for Mrs. C. m[...] validates the problem with Mrs. C[...] interventions will be designed to [...] ciple, the intervention for Mrs. C.[...] level of adaptation in relation to [...] based on observations of Mrs. C.'s [...] ment as to whether the hypothes[...] apply the model simultaneously [...] other identified problems as indi[...] current best practices.

SCENARIO ILLUSTRATING NURSING CARE FRAMED BY THE CONSERVATION MODEL UTILIZING THE NURSING PROCESS

CLASSROOM ACTIVITY 12-1

Form small groups. Each group should add to the plan of care for Mrs. C. in the preceding scenario based on other potential or actual nursing problems typical for a patient with the same medical diagnosis or symptoms and demographics. Each group should develop a plan for one additional nursing problem using Levine's conservation theory as the basis for practice. Each group should then share its plan with the class.

CLASSROOM ACTIVITY 12-2

Form small groups. Using a case study provided by the instructor, develop a plan of care using Levine's nursing theory as the basis for practice. Each group should then share its plan of care with the class.

CLASSROOM ACTIVITY 12-3

Form small groups. Using a case study provided by the instructor, develop a plan of care using one of the theories as the basis for practice; each group should select a different nursing theory. Each group should then share its plan of care with the class and discuss the similarities and differences in care.

CLASSROOM ACTIVITIES Suggested activities for the classroom to stimulate and engage the student in interactive learning.

NURSING
THEORIES

A FRAMEWORK
FOR PROFESSIONAL
PRACTICE

Kathleen Masters, DNS, RN

Associate Director and Associate Professor
University of Southern Mississippi
School of Nursing
Hattiesburg, Mississippi

JONES & BARTLETT
LEARNING

World Headquarters

Jones & Bartlett Learning
40 Tall Pine Drive
Sudbury, MA 01776
978-443-5000
info@jblearning.com
www.jblearning.com

Jones & Bartlett Learning Canada
6339 Ormindale Way
Mississauga, Ontario L5V 1J2
Canada

Jones & Bartlett Learning International
Barb House, Barb Mews
London W6 7PA
United Kingdom

Jones & Bartlett Learning books and products are available through most bookstores and online booksellers. To contact Jones & Bartlett Learning directly, call 800-832-0034, fax 978-443-8000, or visit our website www.jblearning.com.

Substantial discounts on bulk quantities of Jones & Bartlett Learning publications are available to corporations, professional associations, and other qualified organizations. For details and specific discount information, contact the special sales department at Jones & Bartlett Learning via the above contact information or send an email to specialsales@jblearning.com.

The author, editor, and publisher have made every effort to provide accurate information. However, they are not responsible for errors, omissions, or for any outcomes related to the use of the contents of this book and take no responsibility for the use of the products and procedures described. Treatments and side effects described in this book may not be applicable to all people; likewise, some people may require a dose or experience a side effect that is not described herein. Drugs and medical devices are discussed that may have limited availability controlled by the Food and Drug Administration (FDA) for use only in a research study or clinical trial. Research, clinical practice, and government regulations often change the accepted standard in this field. When consideration is being given to use of any drug in the clinical setting, the health care provider or reader is responsible for determining FDA status of the drug, reading the package insert, and reviewing prescribing information for the most up-to-date recommendations on dose, precautions, and contraindications, and determining the appropriate usage for the product. This is especially important in the case of drugs that are new or seldom used.

Production Credits

Publisher: Kevin Sullivan
Acquisitions Editor: Amy Sibley
Editorial Assistant: Rachel Shuster
Production Assistant: Sara Fowles
Marketing Manager: Meagan Norlund
V.P., Manufacturing and Inventory Control:
  Therese Connell

Text Design and Composition: Shawn Girsberger
Cover Design: Kristin E. Parker
Cover Image: © Mirka Moksha/ShutterStock, Inc.
Printing and Binding: Malloy, Inc.
Cover Printing: Malloy, Inc.

To order this product, use ISBN: 9781449626013

Library of Congress Cataloging-in-Publication Data
Masters, Kathleen.
  Nursing theories : a framework for professional practice / Kathleen Masters.
  p. ; cm.
Includes bibliographical references and index.
ISBN 978-0-7637-7237-6 (pbk.)
1. Nursing models. 2. Nursing—Philosophy. I. Title.
[DNLM: 1. Nursing Theory. 2. Models, Nursing. WY 86]
RT84.5.M364 2011
610.7301—dc22
           2010038293

6048
Printed in the United States of America
15 14 13 12 11   10 9 8 7 6 5 4 3 2 1

This book is dedicated to my Heavenly Father and to my loving family:
my husband Eddie and my two daughters Rebecca and Rachel.
Words cannot express my appreciation
for their continuous encouragement and support.

CONTENTS

UNIT II | PHILOSOPHIES OF NURSING 23

CHAPTER 3 | ENVIRONMENTAL MODEL OF NURSING: *Florence Nightingale* 25

CHAPTER 4 | FOURTEEN COMPONENTS OF BASIC NURSING CARE: *Virginia Henderson* 37

UNIT III | CONCEPTUAL MODELS 89

CHAPTER 7 | BEHAVIORAL SYSTEM MODEL: *Dorothy Johnson* 91

CHAPTER 8 | INTERACTING SYSTEMS FRAMEWORK AND THEORY OF GOAL ATTAINMENT: *Imogene King* 105

CHAPTER 9 | SCIENCE OF UNITARY HUMAN BEINGS:
Martha Rogers **121**

CHAPTER 10 | ROY ADAPTATION MODEL: *Sister Callista Roy* **133**

CHAPTER 11 | THE NEUMAN SYSTEMS MODEL: *Betty Neuman* **149**

UNIT IV | NURSING THEORIES   195

CHAPTER 14 | THEORY OF INTERPERSONAL RELATIONS: *Hildegard Peplau* **197**

CHAPTER 15 | THEORY OF CULTURE CARE DIVERSITY AND UNIVERSALITY: *Madeleine Leininger* **211**

CHAPTER 16 | NURSING PROCESS THEORY: *Ida Jean Orlando (Pelletier)* 225

CHAPTER 17 | HEALTH AS EXPANDING CONSCIOUSNESS: *Margaret Newman* 237

CHAPTER 27 | THEORY OF COMFORT: *Katharine Kolcaba*   377

CHAPTER 28 | THEORY OF BUREAUCRATIC CARING: *Marilyn Anne Ray*   389

CHAPTER 29 | SYNERGY MODEL FOR PATIENT CARE: *The American Association of Critical-Care Nurses* **401**

PREFACE

WHILE MANY BOOKS HAVE BEEN published about nursing theory and nursing theorists, the focus of this book is unique in many ways. Many theory books target the nurse who is pursuing graduate-level nursing education; in contrast, this book targets the undergraduate nursing student and the practicing nurse. Some theory books focus on only the works of nursing theorists who have historically been associated with nursing theory; while this book includes the work of those theorists who have been central to nursing theory for decades, it also includes the work of many newer theorists. Finally, many books on nursing theory address the philosophies, conceptual models, and theories of nursing, whereas other books deal with only middle-range theories of nursing. This book, while not all inclusive, covers all four of these levels of theory. Although it was developed using the original works of the theorists as available, references throughout the text identify the published books and journal articles of many well-known experts in nursing theory.

This book is divided into five units. The first unit provides a general overview of nursing theory and the application of nursing theory as a framework for professional practice. Unit II addresses some of the philosophies of nursing. Unit III explores seven of the major theoretical models of nursing. Unit IV introduces several of the major theories of nursing, and Unit V discusses selected middle-range theories of nursing. Each chapter in Units II through V provides information related to the background of the theorist, an overview of the theory, a brief analysis of the theory, and information related to application of the theory in nursing practice.

The purpose of this book is to assist the undergraduate-level nursing student and the practicing nurse in gaining an understanding of the relationship between nursing theory and nursing practice that is both evidence based and guided by the nursing process—in other words, an understanding of nursing theory as a framework for professional nursing practice. Whether one believes that theory emerges from practice or that practice emerges from theory, most will agree that if nursing theory is not incorporated into practice by the nurses who actually provide care for patients, then it is merely an academic exercise that does not advance the discipline of nursing but rather creates a further disconnect between theory and practice. To build a culture in which nursing theory becomes the framework for practice, it is necessary to expose nursing students and practicing nurses to theories in a manner that is uncomplicated and practical, and that allows for exploration of multiple theories so that nurses can find those models that best fit their practice. Once a nurse finds that fit, then exploration beyond the scope of this book is in order, including the reading of both the theorist's original works and experts' critiques of the theory.

—*Kathleen Masters*

THEORETICAL NURSING KNOWLEDGE AS THE FRAMEWORK FOR PRACTICE

INTRODUCTION TO THEORETICAL NURSING KNOWLEDGE

1

LEARNING OBJECTIVES

After completing this chapter the student should be able to

1. Identify and define terminology related to theoretical thinking

2. Identify and describe several types of theoretical works in nursing

3. Identify and explain the four metaparadigm concepts of nursing

KEY TERMS

Assumptions	Health
Clarity	Human being (person)
Concept	Metaparadigm
Conceptual model	Nursing
Derivable consequences	Philosophies of nursing
Empirical precision	Proposition
Environment	Simplicity
Generality	Theory

BACKGROUND AND OVERVIEW

ALTHOUGH THE BEGINNING OF NURSING theory development can be traced to Florence Nightingale, it was not until the second half of the twentieth century that nursing theory caught the attention of nursing as a discipline. During the decades of the 1960s and 1970s, theory development was a major topic of discussion and publication. During the 1970s, much of this discussion related to the development of a single global theory for nursing. However, in the 1980s, attention turned away from the development of a global theory for nursing as scholars began to recognize the validity of multiple approaches to theory development in nursing.

Because of the plurality in nursing theory, this information must be organized to be meaningful for practice, research, and further knowledge development. The goal of this chapter is to present an organized and practical overview of the major concepts that are essential to understanding theoretical perspective in professional nursing practice. Definitions of key terms are included throughout the discussion.

STRUCTURE OF NURSING KNOWLEDGE

TO APPLY NURSING THEORY IN practice, the nurse must have some knowledge of the theoretical works of the nursing profession. Theoretical works in nursing are generally categorized either as philosophies, conceptual models, theories, or middle-range theories, depending on the level of abstraction. The most abstract of these theoretical works are the philosophies of nursing, followed by the conceptual models, theories, and middle-range theories. However, the metaparadigm of the discipline is considered the highest level of abstraction.

Metaparadigm of Nursing

Before discussing the metaparadigm concepts that are important to nursing, it is important to define the term "concept." A **concept** is a term or label that describes a phenomenon or group of phenomena (Meleis, 2007). The label may be a word or phrase that summarizes ideas, observations, and experiences so as to provide a mental image for the purpose of facilitating communication and understanding about the phenomenon (Fawcett, 2005). The phenomenon described by a concept may be either empirical or abstract. An empirical concept is one that can be either observed or experienced through the senses. An abstract concept is one that is not observable, such as hope or caring (Hickman, 2002).

A metaparadigm is the most global perspective of a discipline. A **metaparadigm** is defined by Fawcett (2005, p. 4) "as the global concepts that identify the phenomenon of central interest to a discipline, the global propositions that describe the concepts, and the global propositions that state the relations between or among the concepts." Each discipline singles out phenomena of interest that it will deal with in a unique manner. The concepts and propositions that identify and interrelate these phenomena are even more abstract in the metaparadigm than those found in the conceptual models, yet identification of these metaparadigm concepts allows members of the discipline to identify and communicate the boundaries of the subject matter specific to the discipline (Kim, 2000). Most disciplines have a single metaparadigm but multiple conceptual models. Multiple conceptual models allow the members of the discipline to view the phenomena of interest in different ways (Fawcett, 2005).

Most disciplines have a single metaparadigm but multiple conceptual models. Multiple conceptual models allow the members of the discipline to view the phenomena of interest in different ways.

While several proposals have sought to define what should be included as the metaparadigm concepts for the discipline of nursing, most scholars accept the central concepts of the discipline of nursing as person (human being), environment, health, and nursing:

❖ **Human being or person:** individuals, families, communities, and other groups who are participants in nursing

❖ **Environment:** human beings' significant others and physical surroundings as well as local, regional, national, and worldwide cultural, social, political, and economic conditions that are associated with human beings' health

❖ **Health:** human processes of living and dying

❖ **Nursing:** the definition of nursing, the actions taken by nurses on behalf of or in conjunction with human beings, and the goals or outcomes of nursing actions; the process of which encompasses activities that are referred to as assessment, diagnosis (labeling), planning, intervention, and evaluation (Fawcett, 2005, p. 6)

Because concepts are so abstract at the metaparadigm level, many conceptual models have developed from the metaparadigm of nursing. Subsequently, multiple theories have been developed from each conceptual model in an effort to describe, explain, and predict the phenomena within the model. These conceptual models and theories of nursing represent various paradigms derived from the metaparadigm of the discipline of nursing. Therefore, although each of the conceptual models and nursing theories may link and define the four metaparadigm concepts somewhat differently, the four metaparadigm concepts are generally present and defined either implicitly or explicitly in each of the models and theories.

Philosophies of Nursing

Philosophies of nursing set forth the general meaning of nursing and nursing phenomena through reasoning and the logical presentation of ideas. Philosophies are broad and address general ideas about nursing. Because of their breadth, nursing philosophies contribute to the discipline by providing direction, clarifying values, and forming a foundation for theory development (Alligood, 2006). Four theoretical works that have been categorized as philosophies of nursing will be presented in Chapters 3 through 6 of this book.

Conceptual Models of Nursing

Conceptual models are composed of abstract and general concepts and propositions that provide a frame of reference for members of a discipline. This frame of reference determines how the world is viewed by members of a discipline and guides the members as they propose questions and make observations relevant to the discipline (Fawcett, 1994). A **conceptual model** is specifically defined as a set of concepts and statements that integrate the concepts into a meaningful configuration (Lippitt, 1973; as cited in Fawcett, 1994). **Assumptions** are accepted as truth and represent the values and beliefs of the theory or conceptual framework.

Assumptions form the basis for defining concepts and framing propositions (Meleis, 2007). A **proposition** is a statement about a concept or a statement of the relation between two or more concepts (Fawcett, 2005).

Conceptual models of nursing are models containing abstract concepts that are not directly observable and that are not limited to a particular type of patient, situation, or event (Fawcett, 2005, p. 16). At the level of the conceptual model, each metaparadigm concept is defined and described in a manner unique to the model, with the model providing an alternative way to view the concepts considered important to the discipline. The definitions and overall framework presented in a conceptual model are formal and explicit. Thus they identify the purpose and scope of nursing for nurses, for other healthcare providers, and for the public. In addition, they provide a framework for recording the effects of nursing. Using a conceptual model or framework also helps to provide consistency in nursing practice by facilitating communication and provides a mechanism for engaging in a systematic approach to nursing research, education, and practice (Fawcett, 2005, p. 17–18).

Nursing Theories

A nursing **theory** is more specific than a conceptual model (Alligood, 2010). A "theory is an organized, coherent, and systematic articulation of a set of statements related to significant questions in a discipline that are communicated in a meaningful whole . . . discovered or invented for describing, predicting, or prescribing events, situations, conditions, or relationships" (Meleis, 2007, p. 37). More specifically, nursing theory is defined by Meleis (p. 41) as "a conceptualization of some aspect of reality (invented or discovered) that pertains to nursing. The conceptualization is articulated for the purpose of describing, explaining, predicting, or prescribing nursing care." According to Fawcett (1994), "The primary distinction between a conceptual model and a theory is the level of abstraction. A conceptual model is a highly abstract system of global concepts and linking statements. A theory, in contrast, deals with one or more specific, concrete concepts and propositions."

Theories vary in their scope and level of abstraction. The theory that is broad in scope and highly abstract conceptually may be referred to

The primary distinction between a conceptual model and a theory is the level of abstraction.

as a grand theory, whereas the theory that has a narrow scope and is more concrete or practical may be referred to as a middle-range theory (Fawcett, 2005, p. 19). Middle-range theories also generally include fewer concepts and propositions (Fawcett, 2005), represent a limited or partial view of nursing reality and are more appropriate for empirical testing (Liehr & Smith, 1999), and are more applicable to practice (Smith, 2008).

Nursing theories may be derived from existing conceptual models of nursing. Such theories evolve from nursing reality as perceived by the theorist. Nurse theorists, like other nurses, are affected by both historical events and philosophical influences in their lives. Nursing theories may also evolve from a perception of ideal nursing practice. As a consequence, various nursing theories represent different realities and address different aspects of nursing (Meleis, 2007). For this reason, the multiplicity of nursing theories presented in the following chapters should not be viewed as competing theories, but rather as complementary theories that may provide insight into different ways to describe, explain, and predict nursing concepts and/or prescribe nursing care.

Curley (2007, p. 3) describes this understanding in an interesting way by comparing the multiplicity of nursing theories to a collection of maps of the same region. Each map may display a different characteristic of the region, such as rainfall, topography, or air currents. Although all of the maps are accurate, the best map for use depends on the information needed or the question being asked. This is precisely the case with the nurse's choice of nursing theories for practice.

ANALYSIS AND EVALUATION OF THEORETICAL KNOWLEDGE IN NURSING

SEVERAL AUTHORS HAVE DEVISED CRITERIA for the analysis and evaluation of nursing conceptual models and theories. In general, the criteria that are used for analysis include examination of the origins of the model relative to logic and reasoning as well as the work of other scholars who have influenced the thinking of the theorist, the unique focus of the model, and the definitions of the metaparadigm concepts (Fawcett, 2005, p. 52–53). Other authors suggest that the criteria for analysis should include clarity, simplicity, generality, empirical precision, and derivable consequences (Chinn & Kramer, 2008, p. 237). **Clarity** refers to consistency in terms of terminology and structure—or put simply, "How clear is the theory?" (p. 237). **Simplicity** is highly valued in nursing model and theory development: "How simple is this theory?" (p. 237). **Generality** refers to the scope of the concepts and the purpose of the theory (Alligood, 2010, p. 12) and is reflected in the question, "How general is this theory?" (Chinn & Kramer, 2008, p. 237). The fourth criterion in analytic schema is **empirical precision**, which is linked to the testability and usability of the theory (Alligood, 2010, p. 13). Chinn and Kramer (2008, p. 237) express this notion by asking, "How accessible is this theory?" Finally, the last criterion is "How important is this theory?" (p.237)—that is, the **derivable consequences** of the theory.

Suggested evaluation criteria include an explanation of the origins of the model and an examination of statements of values and philosophical claims of the theorist. This step is followed by an exploration of the comprehensiveness of the content of the model, which entails looking at the depth and the breadth of the model to ascertain, for example, if definitions of the metaparadigm concepts of the discipline are included. The third step considers whether the structure of the model is logical.

Step 4 considers whether the model will lead to further theory generation, and step 5 of the evaluative process focuses on the credibility of the model for use in practice. As a part of the criterion for step 5, attention is also paid to the factors of social utility, social congruence, and social significance. The criterion of social utility considers whether special education is required to use the model in practice. The criterion of social congruence considers whether the model will lead to nursing activities that meet the expectations of the public. The criterion of social significance considers whether the model makes differences in the health conditions of the public.

Finally, in step 6 of the evaluation process, a determination is made as to the contributions of the model to the discipline of nursing. This determination reflects the findings from a review of literature, where the expectation is that the model will enhance understanding of the phenomena of interest rather than being based up any type of comparison of one model to another (Fawcett, 2005, p. 54–57).

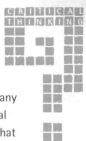

CRITICAL THINKING

Can you think of any additional criteria that should be added to the list for analysis and evaluation of models and theories? If so, what are they? Share your rationale for adding these criteria.

A combination of these criteria will be used in the brief analysis of each nursing model and theory in the chapters that follow in this book. While some of the theories will fare better than others based on the way they satisfy these criteria, in the final analysis all of the theorists whose work is included in the subsequent chapters of this book have made substantial contributions to the discipline of nursing.

CLASSROOM ACTIVITY 1-1

Select one nursing model or theory for review. Review the chapter in this book that pertains to this model or theory, and conduct an analysis and evaluation of the theory using the criteria presented in this chapter, based on the information in the model- or theory-specific chapter. Compare your evaluation with the evaluations made by your fellow students, and discuss areas of agreement and disagreement.

REFERENCES

Alligood, M. R. (2006). Philosophies, models, and theories: Critical thinking structures. In M. R. Alligood & A. M. Tomey (Eds.), *Nursing theory: Utilization and application* (3rd ed., pp. 43–65). St. Louis, MO: Mosby.

Alligood, M. R. (2010). Introduction to nursing theory: Its history, significance, and analysis. In M. R. Alligood & A. M. Tomey (Eds.), *Nursing theorists and their work* (7th ed., pp. 3–15). Maryland Heights, MO: Mosby.

Chinn, P. L., & Kramer, M. K. (2008). *Integrated knowledge development in nursing* (7th ed.). St. Louis, MO: Elsevier-Mosby.

Curley, M. A. Q. (2007). *Synergy: The unique relationship between nursing and patients.* Indianapolis, IN: Sigma Theta Tau International.

Fawcett, J. (1994). *Analysis and evaluation conceptual models of nursing.* Philadelphia: F. A. Davis.

Fawcett, J. (2005). *Contemporary nursing knowledge: Analysis and evaluation nursing models and theories* (2nd ed.). Philadelphia: F. A. Davis.

Hickman, J. S. (2002). An introduction to nursing theory. In J. B. George (Ed.), *Nursing theories: A base for professional nursing practice* (5th ed., pp. 1–20). Upper Saddle River, NJ: Prentice Hall.

Kim, H. S. (2000). *The nature of theoretical thinking in nursing* (2nd ed.). New York: Springer.

Liehr, P., & Smith, M. J. (1999). Middle range theory: Spinning research and practice to create knowledge for the new millennium. *Advances in Nursing Science, 21*(4), 81–91.

Lippitt, G. L. (1973). *Visualizing change: Model building and the change process.* Fairfax, VA: NTL Learning Resources.

Meleis, A. I. (2007). *Theoretical nursing: Development and progress* (4th ed.). Philadelphia: J. B. Lippincott.

Smith, M. C. (2008). Disciplinary perspectives linked to middle range theory. In M. J. Smith & P. R. Liehr (Eds.), *Middle range theory for nursing* (2nd ed., pp. 1–11). New York: Springer.

NURSING THEORY AS A FRAMEWORK FOR PROFESSIONAL PRACTICE

2

RELATIONSHIP OF THEORY TO PROFESSIONAL NURSING PRACTICE

How will theory affect your nursing practice? Using a theoretical framework to guide your nursing practice will assist you as you organize patient data, understand and analyze patient data, make decisions related to nursing interventions, plan patient care, predict outcomes of care, and evaluate patient outcomes (Alligood & Tomey, 2002). Why? The use of a theoretical framework provides a systematic and knowledgeable approach to your nursing practice. The framework also becomes a tool that will assist you in thinking critically as you plan and provide nursing care. This tool provides a paradigm within which to view the process of nursing and the patient care scenario.

CHOOSING A THEORETICAL FRAMEWORK FOR NURSING PRACTICE

How do you begin? Now that you know why nursing theory is important to your nursing practice, you will want to identify a theoretical framework that fits you and your practice. The first step to determine a fit is to identify your personal worldview. Next you must consider the worldview upon which the theoretical framework you have identified is based and determine if there is congruence between the worldviews.

Sire (2004) defines a **worldview** as "a commitment, a fundamental orientation of the heart, that can be expressed as a story or in a set of presuppositions (assumptions which may be true, partially true or entirely true) which we hold (consciously or subconsciously, consistently or inconsistently) about the basic constitution of reality, and that provides the foundation on which we live and move and have our being" (p. 122). According to Shelly and Miller (2006), because a worldview is so overarching, it can integrate many theories from various aspects of life and assist us to see how different theories complement one another. However, when theories reflect different worldviews, upon close examination the theories are likely to conflict with one another. Ultimately, differing worldviews cannot be reconciled (p. 35).

The use of a theoretical framework provides a systematic and knowledgeable approach to your nursing practice.

Sire (2004, p. 20) identifies seven questions that must be answered to understand the concept of a worldview. Answering these seven questions will assist you in identifying your own worldview as well as the underlying worldview of theoretical frameworks:

- ❖ What is prime reality?
- ❖ What is the nature of the world around us?
- ❖ What is a human being?
- ❖ What happens to a person at death?
- ❖ Why is it possible to know anything at all?
- ❖ How do we know what is right and wrong?
- ❖ What is the meaning of human history?

After considering these general questions, you are ready to consider some questions more specific to nursing that will assist you in determining which theories of nursing are congruent with your personal values and beliefs. Alligood (2006) presents guidelines for the individual nurse who is selecting a framework for theory-based nursing practice:

- ❖ Consider the values and beliefs that you truly hold in nursing.
- ❖ Write a philosophy of nursing that clarifies your beliefs related to person, environment, health, and nursing.
- ❖ Survey definitions of person, environment, health, and nursing in the various nursing models.
- ❖ Select two or three frameworks that best fit with your beliefs related to the concepts of person, environment, health, and nursing.
- ❖ Review the assumptions of the frameworks that you have selected.
- ❖ Apply those frameworks in a selected area of nursing practice.
- ❖ Compare the frameworks in terms of client focus, nursing action, and client outcome.
- ❖ Review the nursing literature written by persons who have used the frameworks.
- ❖ Select a framework and develop its use in your nursing practice.

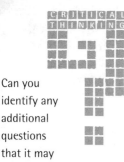

Can you identify any additional questions that it may be helpful to think about as you consider a theoretical framework for practice?

In addition to determining whether a theory is congruent with your belief system, it is important to identify whether a theory is congruent with your area of practice within the discipline of nursing. Miller (1989, p. 47) states that relevance to practice is the central issue when selecting a theory for use in practice and that you should ask the following questions when choosing a theory:

❖ Does the theory have direct relevance for the way that nursing is practiced?

❖ Does the theory describe real or ideal care?

❖ Have the assumptions and propositions been tested?

❖ Does the theory deal with the resources that are necessary for care?

❖ Does the theory guide the use of the nursing process?

❖ Does the theory provide practicing nurses with good direction for clinical actions?

❖ Are the concepts within the theory too abstract to be applied in practice?

❖ Is the language in the theory easy to understand?

❖ Does the theory correspond with the practicing nurses' knowledge?

Finally, as we move beyond the individual nurse and consider a group of nurses on a unit or within an entire organization, the level of complexity related to theory selection is compounded. Several issues arise if all of the individual nurses on a unit or in an organization select a model or theory for use in practice without making some effort to provide a framework for their choices. The use of multiple theories of nursing within the same organization or nursing unit will lead to issues with communication between nurses, between nursing units, and between disciplines within an organization; it will also complicate the training necessary to prepare staff for the sophisticated level of understanding required to function using multiple theories (McKenna & Slevin, 2008). While the selection of nursing theories based on the nurses' preference and patient population fit may be desirable, the successful implementation projects reported in the literature describe the incorporation of only one nursing theory—rather than multiple nursing theories—in practice at the organizational level (Fawcett, 2005). Therefore, while the criteria presented earlier in this chapter are important in determining the preferences of individual nurses, it is necessary to go beyond these criteria when selecting a nursing model or theory for incorporation into practice.

Fawcett (2005, p. 40) suggests four steps for the process of selecting a conceptual model of nursing or nursing theory for practice for a nursing unit or organization:

❖ Analyze and evaluate several nursing models and nursing theories.

❖ Compare the content of each of the nursing models and nursing theories to the mission statement of the healthcare organization to determine if the model or theory is appropriate.

❖ Determine whether the philosophy of the model or theory is congruent with the philosophy of the nursing department.

❖ Select the nursing model or theory that most closely matches the mission of the organization and the philosophy of the nursing department.

As one can see from these steps, this schema applies to the adoption of theoretically based nursing practice throughout an organization. According to Fawcett (2005), the implementation of a theoretical framework in a healthcare organization is a process that would take 27 to 36 months and would include 10 phases: the initial vision, feasibility study, planning for a long-range plan, review of the organization's philosophy, selection of the conceptual model or nursing theory, education of the nursing staff, designation of specific nursing units as demonstration sites, institution-wide implementation, evaluation of outcomes, and dissemination of project outcomes.

I F USING NURSING THEORY IN practice is so important, then why don't all nurses practice using a theoretical framework? This question is best answered by looking at the history of theory development in nursing. The earliest nurse theorists did not plan to develop theories of nursing, but rather sought to explicate guidelines for practicing nursing care. Among those who followed in their footsteps,

PAST CHALLENGES AND FUTURE DIRECTIONS

however, were nurse educators who were interested in developing guidelines for nursing curricula. Because nursing as a discipline was relatively new, these later theorists relied heavily on borrowed knowledge from other related disciplines.

Relying on borrowed theoretical knowledge was not seen as congruent with nursing being a strong and free-standing discipline. In response to this perception, a determination developed within the nursing profession that, looking back, makes it seem as though nursing as a discipline was on a mission to build the theoretical knowledge base to prove itself worthy of being called a separate discipline. Research and theory development was done primarily in university settings, primarily within the context of graduate nursing education. Many of the early theories were grand and complex, as the discipline struggled to find a theory that fit the entire discipline. This process occurred mostly in isolation in research and education pockets within academic settings, and most graduates of these programs taught in academic settings after graduation or practiced in advanced roles in the service arena. As a consequence of this pattern, nursing theory has not yet been incorporated fully into the practice of nursing care at the level of the bedside nurse. It is important for the profession of nursing to close this gap so that nursing theory is interwoven into nursing practice as intended, rather than continuing the pretense that currently exists.

In addition to the historical issues that have impeded the incorporation of theory into nursing practice, many nurses believe that the trend in more recently developed nursing theories is more about "being with the person" and less about "doing for the patient" (Shelly & Miller, 2006). Thus many nurses who have had only superficial exposure to nursing theory do not see nursing theory as practical or relevant to their very busy nursing practice, which is filled with doing for patients. In addressing this point, it is important to understand that even though a particular theory might focus on one aspect of care, the professional nurse is responsible for providing *all* aspects of required care for the patient. Providing care within a theoretical framework does not excuse the nurse from providing care that is evidence based and that meets the current standards for professional nursing care as described by the American Nurses Association (2004) within the context of the nursing process.

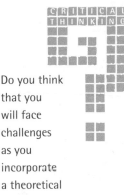

In an effort to illustrate the relationship of nursing theory to evidence-based practice as well as the incorporation of the nursing process, each of the subsequent chapters includes a case study that will be analyzed using the identified theory as a framework for practice. The nursing process in a format congruent with the nursing theory presented in the chapter will also be integrated into the scenario for one identified nursing problem. In addition, the scenario will illustrate the inclusion of evidence-based practice in the plan of care so that the relationship between all three of these components—the theoretical framework, the evidence, and the nursing process—is apparent.

As the descriptions of the philosophies, conceptual models, and theories presented in the following chapters make clear, there are a wide variety of perspectives and choices of frameworks from which to practice nursing. There is no one right or wrong answer. Begin with whichever one seems to "fit" your situation, and then practice using it as you provide nursing care. According to Cody (2006, p. 119), "The full realization of nursing theory-guided practice is perhaps the greatest challenge that nursing as a scholarly discipline has ever faced." So be patient, because developing a nursing practice that is driven by nursing theory will take time and practice. All nursing theories require in-depth study over time to master fully, but the incorporation of theory into your practice will most assuredly transform your nursing practice. The end result of this process will be evidenced in the excellent nursing care that you are able to provide to patients over the course of your professional nursing career. Today, when you frame your practice within the perspective of nursing theory, you may be the exception and an exemplar. As a discipline, however, nursing is approaching a time when practice guided by a theoretical framework will be expected of the professional nurse, just as practice based on evidence and formulated within the context of the nursing process is the current standard.

CRITICAL THINKING

Do you think that you will face challenges as you incorporate a theoretical framework into your own nursing practice? Who or what do you see as the biggest challenge related to the incorporation of a theoretical framework into your nursing care?

The full realization of nursing theory-guided practice is perhaps the greatest challenge that nursing as a scholarly discipline has ever faced.

CLASSROOM ACTIVITY 2-1

Reflect on the questions posed in this chapter, and then begin to draft a philosophy of nursing paper that expresses your individual values and beliefs about the concepts important to nursing. Using your philosophy of nursing paper, compare your own values and beliefs to those of the theorists discussed in the subsequent chapters.

REFERENCES

Alligood, M. R. (2006). Philosophies, models, and theories: Critical thinking structures. In M. R. Alligood & A. M. Tomey (Eds.), *Nursing theory: Utilization & application* (3rd ed., pp. 43–65). St. Louis, MO: Mosby.

Alligood, M. R., & Tomey, A. M. (2002). Significance of theory for nursing as a discipline and profession. In A. M. Tomey & M. R. Alligood (Eds.), *Nursing theorists and their work* (5th ed., pp. 14–31) St. Louis, MO: Mosby.

American Nurses Association. (2004). *Nursing: Scope and standards of practice.* Washington, DC: Author.

Cody, W. K. (2006). Nursing theory-guided practice: What it is and what it is not. In W. K. Cody (Ed.), *Philosophical and theoretical perspectives for advanced nursing practice* (4th ed., pp. 119–121). Sudbury, MA: Jones and Bartlett.

Fawcett, J. (2005). *Contemporary nursing knowledge: Analysis and evaluation of nursing models and theories* (2nd ed.). Philadelphia: F. A. Davis.

McKenna, H. P., & Slevin, O. D. (2008). *Nursing models, theories and practice.* Oxford, United Kingdom: Blackwell.

Miller, A. (1989). Theory to practice: Implementation in the clinical setting. In M. Jolley & P. Allen (Eds.), *Current issues in nursing* (pp. 47–65). London: Chapman & Hall.

Shelly, J. A., & Miller, A. B. (2006). *Called to care: A Christian worldview for nursing* (2nd ed.). Downers Grove, IL: InterVarsity Press.

Sire, J. W. (2004). *Naming the elephant: Worldview as a concept.* Downers Grove, IL: InterVarsity Press.

PHILOSOPHIES OF NURSING

ENVIRONMENTAL MODEL OF NURSING:
Florence Nightingale

LEARNING OBJECTIVES

After completing this chapter the student should be able to

1. Identify the 13 canons of nursing as proposed by Nightingale

2. Explain the major concepts important to nursing as defined by Nightingale

3. Plan nursing care for a patient scenario utilizing Nightingale's 13 canons of nursing care

KEY TERM

: Canon

BACKGROUND

FLORENCE NIGHTINGALE WAS BORN ON May 12, 1820, the second child of an affluent English family. As a child, she displayed exceptional intellectual ability and was well educated for a female in the Victorian era, having been tutored by her father in math, philosophy, languages, and religion. Nightingale was active in aristocratic society but believed that her life could be more useful. She was obsessed with the poverty, disease, and suffering of the masses. To the dismay of her family, she believed that she was called of God to be a nurse (Woodham-Smith, 1951). At the age of 25, Nightingale expressed a desire to become a nurse but her parents refused her request. During the next seven years she continued her study of math, science, hospitals, and public health and made repeated attempts to change the minds of her parents (Dietz & Lehozky, 1963).

During a trip to Egypt with family and friends in 1849, Nightingale spent time with the Sisters of Charity of St. Vincent de Paul, where her conviction to study nursing was reinforced (Tooley, 1910). The next year, Nightingale traveled to the Kaiserwerth Institute in Germany. She spent only two weeks at Kaiserwerth, but vowed that she would return to study nursing. In 1851, Nightingale announced to her family that she planned to return to Kaiserwerth to study nursing. Finally, at the age of 31, Nightingale was permitted to travel back to Kaiserwerth where she learned about the care of the sick and the importance of discipline and commitment to God (Donahue, 1985).

In 1853, after receiving an endowment from her father, Nightingale moved to London, where she became the Superintendent of the Hospital for Invalid Gentlewomen, thereby realizing her goal of working as a nurse (Cook, 1913). During the Crimean War, Nightingale traveled to the Scutari, Turkey, along with 38 other nurses. When they arrived, the nurses were faced with overcrowded barracks and atrocious sanitary conditions. Nightingale focused her efforts on organized nursing services and eliminating sanitation problems in the hospital. Her work proved successful in decreasing the mortality rate in the Crimean War, and upon her return home she eventually began the Nightingale School of Nursing at St. Thomas. Its founding marked the beginning of professional nursing (Donahue, 1985).

Nightingale expressed her views about nursing in many formats. She wrote many letters, pamphlets, and government reports. In 1859, she published *Notes on Nursing: What It Is and What It Is Not*, which represented her first effort at putting her philosophy and description of nursing into one document (Reed & Zurakowski, 1996).

During the last 50 years of her life, although she suffered from poor health, Nightingale spent much time writing letters, books, reports, and meeting with friends and colleagues from within the confines of her home. Florence Nightingale died on August 13, 1910, in London.

NIGHTINGALE DID NOT PLAN TO develop a theory, but rather sought to describe nursing and delineate general rules for nursing practice. Thus her model is both descriptive and practical. Nightingale's philosophy includes the four metaparadigm concepts of nursing, but the focus is primarily on the patient and the environment, with nursing interventions aimed at manipulating the environment to enhance patient recovery. Nursing interventions using Nightingale's philosophy are centered on her 13 **canons**, which include the following (Nightingale, 1860/1969):

> *Nightingale's*
> **THIRTEEN CANONS CENTRAL TO ENVIRONMENTAL MODEL OF NURSING**

❖ **Ventilation and warmth:** The interventions subsumed in this canon include keeping the patient and the patient's room warm and keeping the patient's room well ventilated and free of odors. Specific instructions included to "keep the air within as pure as the air without" (p. 10).

❖ **Health of houses:** This canon includes the five essentials of pure air, pure water, efficient drainage, cleanliness, and light.

❖ **Petty management:** Continuity of care for the patient when the nurse is absent is the essence of this canon.

❖ **Noise:** Instructions include the avoidance of sudden noises that startle or awaken patients and keeping noise in general to a minimum.

Nightingale's focus is primarily on the patient and the environment, with nursing interventions aimed at manipulating the environment to enhance patient recovery.

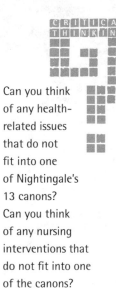

Can you think of any health-related issues that do not fit into one of Nightingale's 13 canons? Can you think of any nursing interventions that do not fit into one of the canons?

❖ **Variety:** This canon refers to an attempt to provide variety in the patient's room, so as to help the patient avoid boredom and depression.

❖ **Food intake:** Interventions include documentation of the amount of food and liquids that the patient ingests.

❖ **Food:** Instructions include trying to include patient food preferences.

❖ **Bed and bedding:** The interventions in this canon include comfort measures related to keeping the bed dry and wrinkle-free.

❖ **Light:** The instructions contained in this canon relate to adequate light in the patient's room.

❖ **Cleanliness of rooms and walls:** This canon focuses on keeping the environment clean.

❖ **Personal cleanliness:** This canon includes measures such as keeping the patient clean and dry.

❖ **Chattering hopes and advises:** Instructions in this canon include the avoidance of talking without reason or giving advice that is without fact.

❖ **Observation of the sick:** This canon includes instructions related to making observations and documenting observations.

The 13 canons were central to Nightingale's theory but were not all-inclusive. Nightingale believed that nursing was a calling and that the recipients of nursing care were holistic individuals with a spiritual dimension; thus the nurse was expected to care for the spiritual needs of the patients in spiritual distress. Nightingale also believed that nurses should be involved in health promotion and health teaching both with the sick and with persons who were well (Bolton, 2006).

MAJOR CONCEPTS OF NURSING ACCORDING TO *Nightingale*

NIGHTINGALE'S ENVIRONMENTAL MODEL OF NURSING was a landmark in the development of nursing science and provided the foundation for the metaparadigm concepts of the discipline of nursing. Although this model includes all four metaparadigm concepts of nursing (Table 3-1), its focus is primarily on the patient and the environment. According to Nightingale's model, the primary function of the nurse is to manipulate the physical and social factors that affect health and illness so as to enhance patient recovery.

Person

While not specifically defined, the person in the Nightingale's environmental model is quite simply the recipient of care of nursing care. The person is viewed in relationship to the environment and the impact of the environment on his or her health status.

Environment

The physical environment was stressed in Nightingale's model, although she did acknowledge the potential impact of the social environment upon the health of the patient. Components of the environment discussed by Nightingale include both the external environment (e.g., temperature, bedding, ventilation) and the internal environment (e.g., food, water, medications).

Health

Nightingale did not specifically define the concept of health, but believed that nature alone could cure disease. She described health as "not only to be well, but to be able to use well every power we have to use" (Nightingale, 1860/1969, p. 24).

TABLE 3-1 Metaparadigm Concepts as Defined in Nightingale's Model

Person	Recipient of nursing care
Environment	External (temperature, bedding, ventilation) and internal (food, water, and medications)
Health	"Not only to be well, but to be able to use well every power we have to use" (Nightingale, 1969, p. 24)
Nursing	To alter or manage the environment to implement the natural laws of health

Nursing

Nursing to Nightingale was, above all, "service to God in the relief of man" (Nightingale, 1858, p. 2). The nurse's function, according to Nightingale, was to alter or manage the environment so as to put the patient in the best possible situation for the natural laws of health to act upon him or her (Johnson & Webber, 2010); thus the ultimate goal of nursing activities was patient health. Nightingale also believed that nursing should provide care to both the healthy and the ill and discussed health promotion activities as part of the role of the nurse (Lobo, 2002).

ANALYSIS OF *Nightingale's* ENVIRONMENTAL MODEL OF NURSING

THE ANALYSIS PRESENTED HERE CONSISTS of an examination of Nightingale's assumptions and propositions as well as a brief critique of her environmental model of nursing.

Assumptions of Nightingale's Environmental Model of Nursing

While Nightingale did not explicitly state any theoretical assumptions, a number of assumptions can be extracted from her work. Philosophical assumptions that can be extracted include the following:

❖ Nursing is a calling.

❖ Nursing is both an art and a science.

❖ People can control the outcomes of their lives and, therefore, can pursue perfect health.

❖ Nursing requires a specific educational base.

❖ Nursing is distinct and separate from medicine (Selanders, 1998).

Additional assumptions that can be extracted from Nightingale's work include these ideas:

❖ Maintaining a clean room, bedding, and clothes aids in patient recovery.

❖ Noise can be harmful to patients.

❖ Managing the environment improves the health of the patient
(Johnson & Webber, 2010).

Propositions of Nightingale's Environmental Model of Nursing

The primary relationship statements that can be extracted from the writings of Nightingale include the following:

❖ The person is desirous of health, so that the nurse, nature, and the person will cooperate so that all reparative processes to occur.

❖ The nurse's role is to prevent the reparative process from being interrupted and to provide conditions to optimized the reparative process (Pfettscher, 2010).

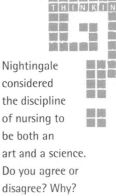

Nightingale considered the discipline of nursing to be both an art and a science. Do you agree or disagree? Why?

Brief Critique of Nightingale's Environmental Model of Nursing

Nightingale's model emphasizes relationships that are not regarded as either revolutionary or complex by current standards. Even so, her model provides a broad framework for organizing observations about a large number of nursing phenomena, making the model broad in scope and giving it generality (Reed & Zurakowski, 1989). The components of the model are clearly articulated. The model is a simple one, characterized by only three major relationships: (1) environment to patient, (2) nurse to environment, and (3) nurse to patient. Despite this simplicity, an attempt is to provide guidelines for all nurses in all times. While some of the specific directives may no longer be applicable, the general concepts—including the relationships between the nurse, the patient, and the environment—are still relevant (Pfettscher, 2010).

Nightingale's model was developed inductively, based on the laws of health and nursing gleaned from her observations and experiences, with many of the principles originating from observations made during wartime experiences (Pfettscher, 2010). The major concepts are clearly defined and the relationships among the concepts flow logically based on the definitions of the concepts, giving the model internal consistency (Reed & Zurakowski, 1989). At the same time, concepts and relationships are presented as truths rather than as testable statements (Pfettscher, 2010).

The writings of Nightingale remain important to the profession of nursing. Indeed, her basic principles of environmental manipulation and psychological patient care continue to be applied in modern nursing situations (Pfettscher, 2010). While Nightingale probably would not have described her work as theoretical, today it is recognized as a scholarly effort that continues to give credibility to basic ideas related to nursing theory. Nightingale's model was developed long ago in response to a need for environmental reform. Although some of Nightingale's rationales have been modified or disproved by advances in medicine and science, many of the concepts in her theory have not only endured, but have been used to provide general guidelines for nurses for more than 150 years (Pfettscher, 2010). In particular, her model remains relevant to illness prevention and health restoration (Johnson & Webber, 2010).

Nightingale's ENVIRONMENTAL MODEL AS A FRAMEWORK FOR NURSING PRACTICE

NIGHTINGALE EXPECTED NURSES TO USE their skills of observation in caring for patients. That expectation is evidenced by an entire section of her book (1860/1969) being devoted to observation of the sick and the documentation of observations. It follows that nursing observations and documentation should focus on the assessment of the patient in relation to the 13 canons identified by Nightingale when nursing care is provided that is framed by Nightingale's environmental model.

THE NURSING PROCESS AND Nightingale's ENVIRONMENTAL MODEL

THE NURSING PROCESS AS IT is now known did not exist in the time of Florence Nightingale. Nevertheless, for the sake of discussion, consistency, and comparison, Nightingale's environmental model will be discussed here in the context of the steps of the nursing process.

Assessment and Planning

Using Nightingale's 13 canons, the nursing assessment of the patient includes questioning and observation. Questions the nurse asks would, for example, relate to food preferences as well as food and fluid intake. Observations are focused on the effects of the environment on the patient. Nursing observations would, for example, include the presence of odors, noise, and light in the patient's room. Observations would also include the amounts of food and drink ingested by the patient.

Implementation

The Nightingale model involves manipulation of the environmental factors that are affecting the patient's health status. Environmental factors that might be the focus of manipulation include noise, light, cleanliness, bedding, and ventilation in the patient's room.

Evaluation

Evaluation is based on the effects of changes in the environment on the patient's health. Observation with documentation is the primary method of data collection and evaluation of outcomes (Nightingale, 1860/1969).

THE FOLLOWING SCENARIO ILLUSTRATES NURSING care of the patient related to one identified nursing problem framed by Nightingale's 13 canons. This scenario is not intended to cover all aspects of care, but rather is meant to stimulate your thinking about how specific care might be approached using this theory as a framework for practice.

Mrs. L. is a 78-year-old Caucasian who was came to the emergency room two nights ago with a fractured hip. She was admitted to the medical–surgical unit yesterday status post hip repair. This morning Mrs. L.

SCENARIO ILLUSTRATING NURSING CARE FRAMED BY *Nightingale's* THIRTEEN CANONS complains to the nurse that she has not been able to sleep since she was hospitalized.

Nursing care for Mrs. L. using Nightingale's environmental model will begin with an assessment of environmental factors that are affecting the ability of Mrs. L. to sleep. The nurse, after conducting this assessment, determines the appropriate nursing diagnosis is sleep pattern disturbance related to environmental factors. Interventions in this case will include the manipulation of the environment to promote sleep; other interventions will include measures that decrease the patient's pain, promote her mobility, promote wound healing, prevent infection at the surgical site, and manage any other actual or potential problems identified by the nurse from the assessment of the patient. Manipulation of the environment might include elimination of noise and unnecessary lights during the hours that Mrs. L. normally sleeps. In addition, nursing interventions might include comfort and relaxation measures such as clean, wrinkle-free linens and maintenance of a room temperature conducive to sleeping as well as other best practice interventions for which evidence substantiates their effectiveness in promotion of rest and sleep for elderly post-surgical patients. Evaluation will be based on the quantity and quality of sleep experienced by Mrs. L. (as reported by the patient and observed and documented by the nurse) as well as her subsequent restoration of health.

CLASSROOM ACTIVITY 3-1

Form small groups. Each group should add recommendations to the plan of care for Mrs. L. in the preceding scenario, based on other potential or actual nursing diagnoses typical for a patient with same medical condition or symptoms and demographics. Each group should develop a plan for one additional nursing problem using Nightingale's nursing theory as the basis for practice. Each group should then share its plan with the class.

CLASSROOM ACTIVITY 3-2

Form small groups. Using a case study provided by your instructor, develop a plan of care using Nightingale's nursing theory as the basis for practice. Each group should then share its plan of care with the class.

CLASSROOM ACTIVITY 3-3

Form small groups. Using a case study provided by your instructor, develop a plan of care using one of the theories as the basis for practice; each group should select a different nursing theory. Each group should then share its plan of care with the class and discuss the similarities and differences in care.

REFERENCES

Bolton, K. (2006). Nightingale's philosophy in nursing practice. In M. R. Alligood & A. M. Tomey (Eds.), *Nursing theory: Utilization and application* (3rd ed., pp. 89–102). St. Louis, MO: Mosby.

Cook, E. (1913). *The life of Florence Nightingale* (Vols. 1 & 2). London: Macmillan.

Dietz, D. D., & Lehozky, A. R. (1963). *History and modern nursing.* Philadelphia: F. A. Davis.

Donahue, M. P. (1985). *Nursing: The finest art.* St. Louis, MO: Mosby.

Johnson, B. M., & Webber, P. B. (2010). *An introduction to theory and reasoning in nursing* (3rd ed.). New York: Lippincott Williams & Wilkins.

Lobo, M. (2002). Florence Nightingale. In J. B. George (Ed.), *Nursing theories: The base for professional nursing practice* (5th ed., pp. 43-60). Upper Saddle River, NJ: Pearson Education, Inc.

Nightingale, F. (1858). *Subsidiary notes as to the introduction of female nursing into military hospitals in peace and in war.* London: Harrison and Sons.

Nightingale, F. (1860/1969). *Notes on nursing: What it is and what it is not.* New York: Dover.

Pfettscher, S. A. (2010). Florence Nightingale: Modern nursing. In A. M. Tomey & M. R. Alligood (Eds.), *Nursing theorists and their work* (7th ed., pp. 71–90). St. Louis, MO: Mosby.

Reed, P., & Zurakowski, T. (1996). Nightingale: Foundations of nursing. In J. Fitzpatrick & A. Whall (Eds.), *Conceptual models of nursing: Analysis and application* (3rd ed., ppl 27-54). Stamford, CT: Appleton & Lange.

Selanders, (1998). The power of environmental adaptation: Florence Nightingale's original theory for nursing practice. *Journal of Holistic Nursing, 16*(2), 247–263.

Tooley, S. A. (1910). *The life of Florence Nightingale.* London: Cassell.

Woodham-Smith, C. (1951). *Florence Nightingale.* New York: McGraw-Hill.

FOURTEEN COMPONENTS OF BASIC NURSING CARE:
Virginia Henderson

4

LEARNING OBJECTIVES

After completing this chapter the student should be able to

1. Identify the 14 components of basic nursing care proposed by Henderson

2. Explain the major concepts important to nursing as defined by Henderson

3. Plan nursing care for a patient scenario utilizing Henderson's 14 components of nursing care

KEY TERM

Components of nursing care

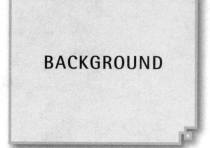

BACKGROUND

VIRGINIA AVENEL HENDERSON WAS BORN on March 19, 1897, in Kansas City, Missouri; she died on November 30, 1996, when she was 98 years old. During her lifetime and more than 60-year career as a nurse, teacher, author, and researcher, Henderson made such significant contributions to the discipline of nursing that she has been referred to by some as the "Florence Nightingale of the twentieth century" (Tomey, 2006).

Henderson's interest in nursing began during World War I and grew out of her desire to help the sick and wounded in the military. She graduated from the Army School of Nursing in 1921 and began practice at Henry Street Visiting Nurse Service in New York. In 1926, Henderson returned to school at Columbia University Teachers College, where she completed her bachelors of science and master of arts degrees in nursing education. Henderson taught nursing at Teachers College and Yale University. In her faculty role, she worked with Harmer on the revision of *The Principles and Practice of Nursing* (1939). In the next edition, published in 1955, Henderson introduced her now-famous definition of nursing. Some of Henderson's other scholarly endeavors included the Nursing Studies Index Project; *Basic Principles of Nursing Care* (1960, 1997), which was translated into more than 20 languages; *The Nature of Nursing* (1966); and *The Nature of Nursing: Reflections After 25 Years* (1991). At the age of 75, Henderson began to focus on international teaching and speaking.

Virginia Henderson authored one of the most accurate definitions of nursing, promoted nursing research as the basis for nursing knowledge, advocated for humane and holistic care for patients internationally, and represented nursing with dignity, honor, and grace throughout her career, which spanned most of the twentieth century. She was awarded 12 honorary doctoral degrees as well as the International Council of Nursing's prestigious Christianne Reimann Prize during her exemplary career (American Nurses Association, n.d.).

HENDERSON ELABORATED ON HER DEFINI-
TION of nursing by identifying 14 basic needs
upon which nursing care is based. Eight of
these needs pertain directly to bodily functions, while
the remaining six relate to safety and finding meaning
in life (Shelly & Miller, 2006). It follows that the fundamentals of nursing, or 14 **components of nursing care**,
include helping others provide for their basic needs.
The 14 basic needs are outlined here:

Henderson's
**FOURTEEN
COMPONENTS OF
NURSING CARE**

1. Breathe normally.

2. Eat and drink adequately.

3. Eliminate bodily wastes.

4. Move and maintain desirable postures.

5. Sleep and rest.

6. Select suitable clothes; dress and undress.

7. Maintain body temperature within normal range by adjusting
clothing and modifying the environment.

8. Keep the body clean and well groomed and protect the
integument.

9. Avoid dangers in the environment and avoid injuring others.

10. Communicate with others in expressing emotions, needs, fears,
or opinions.

11. Worship according to one's faith.

12. Work in such a way that there is a sense of accomplishment.

13. Play or participate in various forms of recreation.

14. Learn, discover, or satisfy the curiosity that leads to normal
development and health and use the available health facilities
(Henderson, 1966, 1991).

MAJOR
CONCEPTS
OF NURSING
ACCORDING TO
Henderson

WHILE HENDERSON DID NOT CONSIDER her work to be a theory of nursing, and she did not explicitly state assumptions or define all of the domains of nursing, it is possible to identify and describe the metaparadigm concepts of nursing (Furukawa & Howe, 2002) in her work (Table 4-1).

Person

Henderson viewed the person as the patient, who is considered to be composed of biological, psychological, sociological, and spiritual components (although these components are inseparable), and who requires assistance to achieve independence in relation to the 14 basic needs that correspond to the 14 identified components of nursing care. The patient and his or her family are viewed as a unit (Henderson, 1964).

Environment

Henderson broadly defined environment as "the aggregate of all the external conditions and influences affecting the life and development of an organism," using the definition from the 1961 edition of *Webster's New Collegiate Dictionary* (Henderson & Nite, 1978). She considered the environment to be composed of biological, physical, and behavioral components. Biological components of the environment include all living

TABLE 4-1 Metaparadigm Concepts as Defined in Henderson's Model	
Person	Recipient of nursing care, who is composed of biological, psychological, sociological, and spiritual components
Environment	External environment (biologic, physical, and behavioral); some discussion of the impact of community on the individual and family
Health	Based on the patient's ability to function independently (as outlined in the 14 components of basic nursing care)
Nursing	Assist the person, sick or well, in performance of activities (14 components of basic nursing care) and help the person gain independence as rapidly as possible (Henderson, 1966, p. 15)

things, such as plants, animals and microorganisms. The physical components of the environment consist of sunlight, water, oxygen, carbon dioxide, organic compounds, and nutrients used by plants for growth; collectively, they provide a sphere "in which all living things operate" (Henderson & Nite, 1978, p. 829). According to Henderson, biologic and physical components together form an ecosystem with a delicate balance. An interdependent relationship exists between living organisms and their surroundings, such that changes in one component result in changes in other parts of the ecosystem.

There is also a third environmental component: the behavioral component. For humans, this component includes social interactions, customs, economic, legal, political, and religious systems, all of which affect human health (Henderson & Nite, 1978).

Health

While Henderson did not explicitly state a definition of health, she implied that health is equivalent to independence. The level of health is directly related to the patient's ability to independently satisfy his or her basic needs (Henderson & Nite, 1978).

Nursing

Henderson is perhaps best known for her definition of nursing, which was first published in 1955 (Harmer & Henderson, 1955) and then published in 1966 with minor revisions. According to Henderson,

> The unique function of the nurse is to assist the individual, sick or well, in the performance of those activities contributing to health or its recovery (or to a peaceful death) that he would perform unaided if he had the necessary strength, will, or knowledge and to do this in such a way as to help him gain independence as rapidly as possible. (Henderson, 1966, p.15)

While Henderson defined nursing in functional terms, she emphasized the art of nursing as well as empathetic understanding, stating that the nurse must "get inside the skin of each of her patients in order to know what he needs" (Henderson, 1964, p. 63). She believed that "the

"The unique function of the nurse is to assist the individual, sick or well, in the performance of those activities contributing to health or its recovery (or to a peaceful death) that he would perform unaided if he had the necessary strength, will, or knowledge and to do this in such a way as to help him gain independence as rapidly as possible."

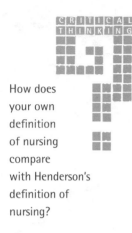

How does your own definition of nursing compare with Henderson's definition of nursing?

beauty of . . . nursing is the combination of your heart, your head and your hands and where you separate them, you diminish them" (McBride, 1997; as cited by Gordon, 2001).

Henderson went on to say:

The nurse is, and should be an independent practitioner and able to make independent judgments as long as he, or she, is not diagnosing, prescribing treatment for disease, or making a prognosis, for these are the physicians functions. But the nurse is viewed as the authority on basic nursing care. (Henderson, 1991)

ANALYSIS OF *Henderson's* DEFINITION OF NURSING AND FOURTEEN COMPONENTS OF NURSING

THE ANALYSIS PRESENTED HERE CONSISTS of an examination of Henderson's assumptions and propositions as well as a brief critique of the definition of nursing and 14 components of nursing as proposed by Henderson.

Assumptions of Henderson's Definition and Fourteen Components of Nursing Care

Henderson did not explicitly state assumptions; however, it is possible to identify assumptions form her publications. The primary assumptions include the following ideas:

- ❖ The nurse has a unique function to help well or sick persons.
- ❖ The nurse functions as a member of the medical team but functions independently of the physician.
- ❖ The patient's needs are covered by the 14 components of nursing.
- ❖ The 14 components of nursing care encompass all possible functions of nursing.
- ❖ The nurse and the patient are always working toward a goal, whether it be independence or a peaceful death.
- ❖ Health promotion is an important goal of the nurse.

- ❖ The patient and the family are a unit.
- ❖ The mind and the body of the person are inseparable.
- ❖ The patient requires assistance toward independence.
- ❖ The person must maintain physiological and emotional balance.
- ❖ Health is basic to human functioning.
- ❖ Health requires independence and interdependence.
- ❖ Persons will achieve or maintain health if they have the strength, will, and knowledge.
- ❖ Illness may interfere with the ability of persons to control their environment.
- ❖ Nurses should protect persons from environmental injury.
- ❖ Nurses should know about social customs and religious practices.
- ❖ Professional practice is generated from research-based knowledge (Henderson, 1966, 1991; Runk & Muth Quillin, 1989; Tomey, 2002, p. 102).

Propositions of Henderson's Definition and Fourteen Components of Nursing Care

The primary relationship statements that can be gleaned from Henderson's work are as related to the nurse–patient relationship:

- ❖ The nurse as a substitute for the patient
- ❖ The nurse as a helper to the patient
- ❖ The nurse as a partner with the patient (Tomey, 2002)

In times of serious illness, the nurse is seen as the substitute for what the patient lacks due to lack of strength, will, or knowledge. Henderson reinforced this view when she stated that the nurse "is temporarily the consciousness of the unconscious, the love of life for the suicidal, the leg of the amputee, the eyes of the newly blind, a means of locomotion for the infant, knowledge and confidence for the young mother, and the mouthpiece for those too weak or withdrawn to speak and so on" (Henderson, 1966, p. 16; 1991, p. 22).

During convalescence, the nurse assists the patient to regain his or her independence. Working as partners, the nurse and the patient together formulate the plan of care. Henderson asserted that the "nurse must get inside the skin" of each patient to know what the patient needs, and then the identified needs must be validated with the patient (Henderson, 1966, p. 16; 1991, p. 22; Tomey, 2002).

Brief Critique of Henderson's Definition and Fourteen Components of Nursing Care

Henderson seems to have used deduction to develop her definition of nursing and 14 needs from physiological and psychological principles. The assumptions of Henderson's definition are logical and have a high level of agreement with literature and research conclusions of scientists in other fields. For example, her 14 basic needs correspond closely to Maslow's hierarchy of human needs, even though Henderson had no knowledge of Maslow's work at the time she identified needs in her work (Tomey, 2002).

Henderson's definition of nursing and the basic needs are simply stated and clear, yet broad in scope, attempting to include the function of all nurses and all patients. Her work is of sufficient scope to affect both nursing theory and practice. Moreover, her definition has the potential to include the whole person, even though the definition is derived primarily from the physiological perspective (Runk & Muth Quillin, 1989).

The concept of nursing in Henderson's work contains many variables and relationships. Indeed, while the 14 needs might appear simple, they can become complex when an alteration in need occurs and all of the parameters relating to the need are considered. Even with this increased level of complexity, the conceptual definitions and relationships demonstrate internal consistency. Because Henderson did not intend to develop a theory of nursing, she did not develop the interrelated theoretical statements or operational definitions necessary to provide theory testability. As Tomey (2002) points out, however, this can be done.

Henderson's work is viewed as a philosophy of the purpose and function of nursing (Pokorny, 2010). Her textbook *Principles and Practices of Nursing*, in which the definition of nursing and 14 nursing functions were explicated, was widely used in schools of nursing over several decades.

As a consequence, her definition of nursing has significantly influenced the practice of nursing. Henderson's definition of nursing and 14 nursing functions were aimed at explaining the totality of nursing behavior rather than the development of a nursing theory; however, her ideas have continued to be useful in promoting further conceptual development among nurse theorists. Henderson's work has also been influential in nursing curriculum development, in clinical nursing practice, and in the promotion of clinical nursing research.

D ELIVERY OF NURSING CARE BASED on the 14 basic needs and corresponding 14 components of nursing care identified by Henderson is not difficult to conceptualize—especially given that Henderson and Nite used the 14 components as a framework for the 1978 edition of their textbook, *Principles and Practice of Nursing*. Nursing care utilizing Henderson's theory will revolve around meeting patient needs in the areas of respiration, nutrition, elimination, body mechanics, rest and sleep, keeping clean and well groomed, controlling the environment, communication, human relations, work, play, and worship.

Henderson's
FOURTEEN COMPONENTS OF NURSING AS A FRAMEWORK FOR NURSING PRACTICE

According to Henderson and Nite (1978), meeting basic needs involving patient respiration includes considering the following areas:

❖ Pulmonary ventilation

❖ Diffusion and transport of gases

❖ Regulation of respiration

❖ Factors affecting normal respiration (e.g., smoking, age, obesity, emotions, environmental pollution, anesthesia and surgery)

Providing nursing care to meet basic needs involving nutrition will consider the following areas:

❖ Nutrition and quality of life

❖ Dietary essentials

- ❖ Fluid balance

- ❖ Food selection and the optimal diet

- ❖ Conditions that favor digestion and assimilation

- ❖ Diet in sickness

- ❖ Nursing measures in oral feedings

Providing nursing care to meet basic needs involving elimination will include these areas:

- ❖ Elimination of waste from the intestines

- ❖ Elimination of waste from the kidneys

- ❖ Elimination of waste by the skin and lungs

- ❖ Measuring and recording elimination

Meeting basic needs involving patient movement and posture requires consideration of the following areas:

- ❖ Body mechanics and posture

- ❖ Exercise in health and sickness

- ❖ Helping the sick and handicapped to move

- ❖ Transportation in illness and traveling with patients

- ❖ Prevention and treatment of pressure ulcers

Meeting basic needs involving patient rest and sleep focuses on these areas:

- ❖ Rest in health and illness

- ❖ Inducing sleep

- ❖ Preparation of the patient for the night

- ❖ Selecting and making beds

Providing nursing care to meet basic needs involving keeping the patient clean and well groomed and maintaining temperature will include the following areas:

- ❖ Personal cleanliness and morning care: care of skin and nails; shaving; care of the mouth, teeth, and dentures; care of the nose; hygiene of the eyes; care of the hair; making the patient's bed

❖ Providing the patient with suitable clothing and conditions to maintain body temperature

Nursing care involved in controlling the environment will focus on meeting the patient's basic needs related to these areas:

❖ Lighting: natural light, artificial light, psychology of lighting

❖ Atmospheric conditions: humidity, temperature, purity of air, air pressure, altitude

❖ Water supply and waste disposal

❖ Esthetics

❖ Controlling pests: insects and rodents

❖ Preventing mechanical injury, burns, poisoning, and electric shock

❖ Providing and maintaining a sanitary environment

❖ Providing and maintaining a sanitary food service and maintaining a sanitary laundry service

❖ Disinfection and sterilization

❖ Preventing and controlling infection

Nursing care that affects the basic needs of communication, human relations, and learning include factors associated with the following concerns:

❖ Ways of communication: being as communication, use of the senses in communication, speech and language, nonlanguage communication, communication technology

❖ Communication: strengthening bonds and reducing barriers (mental states and sensory defects as barriers; language, culture, age-related and gender-related communication bonds and barriers; and hospitalization and illness effects upon communication)

❖ Therapeutic communication and relationships: nurse–patient interaction, family and groups, communication through touch, music, art, role-playing, reading and writing, and creating a therapeutic environment

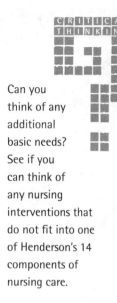

Can you think of any additional basic needs? See if you can think of any nursing interventions that do not fit into one of Henderson's 14 components of nursing care.

❖ Learning and perception through the life cycle

❖ Health goals (national and international health goals, individual health goals, health education for health promotion and prevention of illness) and health guidance or health teaching

Basic needs and nursing care involving work and play include the following areas:

❖ The meaning and nature of work and leisure

❖ Retirement and leisure time

❖ Adult play and recreation

❖ Children's play

❖ The nurse's role in providing opportunities for work and play

Providing nursing care to meet basic needs involving worship will include these areas:

❖ The search for meaning in life

❖ Knowledge of major living religions

❖ Religious leaders as member of health teams

❖ Ways in which nurses help those they serve meet their spiritual needs

Finally, the involvement of the nurse will vary depending on the setting of care and the level dependence of the patient. Henderson illustrated this concept by using a series of circles divided into segments to depict the levels of involvement of the nurse, physician, other healthcare team members, and family members and to illustrate how that involvement changes over time as the patient's condition changes. For example, on the first day postoperatively, a patient will require more nursing care as compared to the nursing care required when the patient is ready for discharge to the home setting; these differences demonstrate the impact of the dimensions of time and space on human behavior and health.

THE NURSING PROCESS AS IT is now known did not exist when Henderson initially developed her definition of nursing and 14 components of care. Nevertheless, for the sake of discussion, consistency, and comparison, Henderson's components of care will be discussed here within the context of the steps of the nursing process.

> THE NURSING
> PROCESS
> FRAMED BY
> *Henderson's*
> FOURTEEN
> COMPONENTS OF
> CARE

Assessment

The assessment phase of the nursing process includes assessing the patient relative to the 14 basic needs identified by Henderson. During the assessment phase of care, the nurse will assess the patient's respiratory status; nutritional status; elimination; movement; activities of daily living; sleep; maintenance of body temperature; hygiene; environment; ability to communicate; needs related to work, recreation, and learning; and spiritual needs. Based on the assessment data and considering the strength, will, and knowledge of the patient, the nurse will determine if the patient requires assistance to meet his or her basic needs. If assistance is required, then a plan will be designed so that the appropriate nursing care can be provided.

> Based on the assessment data and considering the strength, will, and knowledge of the patient, the nurse will determine if the patient requires assistance to meet his or her basic needs.

Planning

The goal of the planning phase of the nursing process is to design a plan to meet patient needs based on the deficits that were identified in the assessment phase of the process. At the same time, care focuses on helping the patient gain independence as rapidly as possible so that the nurse becomes dispensable (rather than indispensable).

Implementation

The implementation phase of the nursing process includes assisting the patient with the performance of activities that contribute to the maintenance of health, recovery from illness, or peaceful death. Interventions in this phase of the nursing process are based on physiological principles as well as on individual characteristics such as age, culture, and physical, intellectual, and emotional capabilities.

Evaluation

Evaluation is based on the ability of the patient to meet his or her basic human needs without or with decreasing assistance of the nurse.

> ### SCENARIO ILLUSTRATING NURSING CARE FRAMED BY *Henderson's* FOURTEEN COMPONENTS OF NURSING

THE FOLLOWING SCENARIO ILLUSTRATES NURS-ING care of the patient relative to one identified nursing problem, as framed by Henderson's 14 components of nursing. This scenario is not intended to cover all aspects of care, but rather is intended to stimulate thinking about how specific care might be approached using this theory as a framework for practice.

Mrs. M. is an 84-year-old, recently widowed, African American woman who lives alone in a rural community. Mrs. M. has been discharged to the home setting after a two-day hospital stay due to dehydration and weight loss. The home health nurse has been assigned to visit Mrs. M. post hospital discharge and will care for her using the framework provided by Henderson's 14 components of nursing and the nursing process.

The nurse will assess Mrs. M.'s respiratory status; nutritional status; elimination; movement; activities of daily living; sleep; maintenance of body temperature; hygiene; environment; ability to communicate; needs related to work, recreation, and learning; and spiritual needs. Based on her assessment data, which includes a recent history of a lack of appetite and lack of transportation to the grocery store in town, the nurse determines that an appropriate nursing diagnosis is as follows: nutrition, less than body requirements related to a decrease in appetite and lack of access to adequate food. Planning will include the patient as well as her family and community resources in an effort to make the patient independent, rather than dependent on the nurse. Implementation will include evidence-based interventions that have been shown to increase appetite in elderly patients as well as interventions to connect the patient with local community resources and networks to address her lack of access to food. Evaluation of this particular problem for Mrs. M. will be based on evidence of increasing appetite with no further weight loss and the adequacy of access to food without dependency on the nurse for arrangements.

CLASSROOM ACTIVITY 4-1

Form small groups. Each group should add to the plan of care for Mrs. M. in the preceding scenario based on other potential or actual nursing diagnoses typical for a patient with same medical diagnosis or symptoms and demographics. Each group should develop a plan for one additional nursing problem using Henderson's nursing theory as the basis for practice. Each group should then share its plan with the class.

CLASSROOM ACTIVITY 4-2

Form small groups. Using a case study provided by the instructor, develop a plan of care using Henderson's nursing theory as the basis for practice. Each group should then share its plan of care with the class.

CLASSROOM ACTIVITY 4-3

Form small groups. Using a case study provided by the instructor, develop a plan of care using one of the theories as the basis for practice; each group should select a different nursing theory. Each group should then share its plan of care with the class and discuss the similarities and differences in care.

REFERENCES

American Nurses Association. (n.d.). Hall of fame: Virginia A. Henderson (1897–1996) 1996 inductee. http://www.nursingworld.org/Functional MenuCategories/AboutANA/WhereWeComeFrom_1/HallofFame/ 19962000Inductees/hendva5545.aspx

Furukawa, C. Y., & Howe, J. S. (2002). Definition and components of nursing: Virginia Henderson. In J. B. George (Ed.), *Nursing theories: The base for professional nursing practice* (5th ed., pp. 83–109). Upper Saddle River, NJ: Prentice Hall.

Gordon, S. C. (2001). Virginia Avenel Henderson: Definition of nursing. In M. Parker (Ed.), *Nursing theories and nursing practice* (pp. 143–149). Philadelphia: F. A. Davis.

Harmer, B., & Henderson, V. (1939). *Textbook of the principles and practice of nursing* (4th ed.). New York: Macmillan.

Harmer, B., & Henderson, V. (1955). *Textbook of the principles and practice of nursing* (5th ed.). New York: Macmillan.

Henderson, V. (1960). *Basic principles of nursing care.* New York: American Nurses Publishing.

Henderson, V. (1964). The nature of nursing. *American Journal of Nursing, 64,* 62–68.

Henderson, V. (1966). *The nature of nursing: A definition and its implications for practice, research, and education.* New York: Macmillan.

Henderson, V. (1991). *The nature of nursing: Reflections after 25 years.* New York: National League for Nursing Press.

Henderson, V., & Nite, G. (1978). *Principles and practice of nursing* (6th ed.). New York: Macmillan.

Pokorny, M. E. (2010). Nursing theorists of historical significance. In A. M. Tomey & M. R. Alligood (Eds.), *Nursing theorists and their work* (7th ed., pp. 54–68). St. Louis, MO: Mosby.

Runk, J. A., & Muth Quillin, S. I. (1989). Henderson's definition of nursing. In J.J. Fitzpatrick & A. L. Whall (Eds.), *Conceptual models of nursing: Analysis and application* (2nd ed., pp. 68–82). Stamford, CT: Appleton & Lange.

Shelly, J. A., & Miller, A. B. (2006). *Called to care: A Christian worldview for nursing* (2nd ed.). Downers Grove, IL: InterVarsity Press.

Tomey, A. M. (2002). Virginia Henderson: Definition of nursing. In A. M. Tomey & M. R. Alligood (Eds.), *Nursing theorists and their work* (5th ed., pp. 98–111). St. Louis, MO: Mosby.

Tomey, A. M. (2006). Nursing theorists of historical significance. In A. M. Tomey & M. R. Alligood (Eds.), *Nursing theorists and their work* (6th ed., pp. 54–67). St. Louis, MO: Mosby.

PHILOSOPHY AND THEORY OF TRANSPERSONAL CARING:
Jean Watson

5

BACKGROUND

JEAN HARMAN WATSON WAS BORN in 1940 in the Appalachian Mountains of West Virginia. After graduation from the Lewis-Gale School of Nursing, she married her husband and moved to Colorado where she continued her nursing education at the University of Colorado. Since completing her PhD, Watson has held both faculty and administrative positions in the School of Nursing at the University of Colorado Health Sciences Center.

During her career, Watson has worked to restructure nursing education through the development of nursing curriculum in human caring, health, and healing. She has also worked to establish the Center for Human Caring at the University of Colorado, which has a commitment to develop and use knowledge of human caring and healing as the basis of clinical practice and nursing scholarship.

Watson's work has been influenced by the work of Nightingale, Henderson, Leininger, Peplau, Maslow, Whitehead, Heidegger, Erikson, Seyle, Lazarus, and Hegel, among others. Her work also has been influenced by her spiritual and cultural encounters in as she traveled in New Zealand, Australia, Indonesia, Malaysia, China, Thailand, India, and Egypt. Watson attributes her emphasis on interpersonal and transpersonal qualities of congruence, empathy, and warmth to Carl Rogers (Watson, 1985) and gives credit to Yalom's work on the 11 curative factors for stimulating her thinking and leading to her own development of the 10 carative factors in nursing (Watson, 1979).

OVERVIEW OF *Watson's* TEN CARATIVE FACTORS AND CARITAS PROCESSES

ACCORDING TO WATSON'S THEORY (1996a), the goal of nursing is to facilitate individuals in gaining a higher degree of harmony within the mind–body–spirit; such harmony generates self-knowledge, self-reverence, self-healing, and self-care processes through human-to-human caring process and caring transactions. Attainment of that goal can potentiate healing and health. This goal is pursued through transpersonal caring guided by carative factors and corresponding caritas processes.

Watson's (1979) theory for nursing practice is based on 10 carative factors. The original carative factors, as revised by Watson, are as follows:

1. The formation of a humanistic–altruistic system of values

2. The instillation of faith–hope

3. The cultivation of sensitivity to oneself and to others

4. Development of a helping–trusting, human caring relation

5. The promotion and acceptance of the expression of positive and negative feelings

6. Systematic use of a creative problem-solving caring process

7. The promotion of transpersonal teaching–learning

8. The provision of a supportive, protective, and corrective mental, physical, societal, and spiritual environment

9. The assistance with gratification of human needs

10. Allowance for existential–phenomenological–spiritual forces

Watson proposed what are known as caritas processes that correspond with each of these carative factors. As her work evolved, she renamed what she had previously called carative factors into what she termed clinical caritas processes (Fawcett, 2005). **Caritas** means to cherish, to appreciate, and to give special attention; it conveys the concept of love (Watson, 2001). The 10 caritas processes are summarized here:

1. Practicing loving kindness and equanimity for oneself and other

2. Being authentically present and enabling, sustaining, and honoring the deep belief system and subjective life world of oneself and the one being cared for

3. Cultivating one's own spiritual practices; deepening of self-awareness, going beyond the ego self

4. Developing and sustaining a helping–trusting, authentic caring relationship

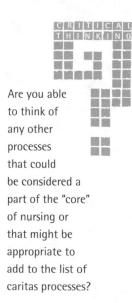

5. Being present to, and supportive of, the expression of positive and negative feelings as a connection with a deeper spirit of oneself and the one being cared for

6. Creatively using oneself and all ways of knowing as part of the caring process and engagement in the artistry of caring–healing practices

7. Engaging in a genuine teaching–learning experience within the context of a caring relationship, while attending to the whole person and subjective meaning; attempting to stay within the other's frame of reference

8. Creating a healing environment at all levels (physical, nonphysical), subtle environment of energy and consciousness whereby wholeness, beauty, comfort, dignity, and peace are potentiated

9. Reverentially and respectfully assisting with basic needs, with an intentional caring consciousness of touching and working with the embodied spirit of another, honoring the unity of being; allowing for a spirit-filled connection while administering human care essentials, which potentiate alignment of the mind–body–spirit, wholeness, and unity of being in all aspects of care; attending to both the embodied spirit and evolving emergence

10. Opening and attending to spiritual, mysterious, and unknown existential dimensions of life, death, suffering; "allowing for a miracle" (Watson, 2008, p. 31)

Watson (2001) referred to the clinical caritas processes as the "core" of nursing, which is grounded in the philosophy, science, and art of caring. She contrasts this core of nursing with what she terms the "trim," a term she used to refer to the practice setting, procedures, functional tasks, clinical disease focus, technology, and techniques of nursing. The "trim," Watson explained, was not expendable, but it cannot be the center of professional nursing practice (Watson, 1997, p. 50).

The carative factors and caritas processes described by Watson provide guidelines for nurse–patient interactions; however, her theory does not furnish instructions about what to do to achieve authentic

Watson's model "does not consider caring as a soft nice thing for nurses to do, or a nice way to be, in some romantic premodern sense," but rather "it posits caring knowledge and actions as a serious ontological, ethical, and pragmatic concern for the discipline."

caring–healing relationships. Although Watson's theory focuses more on being than on doing, it provides a useful framework for the delivery of caring, patient-centered, nursing care (Neil & Tomey, 2006). According to Watson, "the model does not consider caring as a soft nice thing for nurses to do, or a nice way to be, in some romantic pre-modern sense," but rather "it posits caring knowledge and actions as a serious ontological, ethical, and pragmatic concern for the discipline" (1996b, p. 146).

I N ADDITION TO THE CONCEPTS already presented, the four metaparadigm concepts of nursing are identified by Watson. These concepts are summarized in Table 5-1.

MAJOR CONCEPTS OF NURSING ACCORDING TO *Watson*

Person

In Watson's theory, the person is viewed holistically as a "unity of mind–body–spirit–nature" (Watson, 1996a, p. 147), in which each part is a reflection of the whole, yet the whole is greater than, and different from, the sum of the parts (Watson, 1979). According to Watson, a person is neither simply an organism nor simply a spiritual being, but rather is embodied in experience in nature and in the physical work; a person is also able to transcend the physical world by controlling it, changing it, or living in harmony with it (Jesse, 2010b).

TABLE 5-1 Metaparadigm Concepts as Defined in Watson's Philosophy and Science of Caring	
Person (human)	A "unity of mind–body–spirit–nature" (Watson, 1996a, p. 147); embodied spirit (Watson, 1989)
Healing space and environment	A nonphysical energetic environment; a vibrational field integral with the person where the nurse is not only in the environment but "the nurse IS the environment" (Watson, 2008, p. 26)
Health (healing)	Harmony, wholeness, and comfort
Nursing	Reciprocal transpersonal relationship in caring moments guided by carative factors and caritas processes

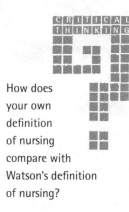

How does your own definition of nursing compare with Watson's definition of nursing?

Watson's notions of personhood are based on the concept that human beings are "embodied spirit"; thus human life is defined as being-in-the-world, which is continuous in time and space (Watson, 1989). Both the nurse and the patient enter into a relationship as persons who participate and grow from the nurse–patient encounter (Boyd & Mast, 1989).

Environment

Watson's definition of the environment has evolved over time. Her early definitions included references to "supportive, protective, and corrective mental, physical, societal, and spiritual environments" (Watson, 1979, p. 10). She has also identified the environment as a "field of connectedness" at all levels (Watson, 1996a, p. 147). More recently, Watson's definition of healing space and environment has expanded to a nonphysical energetic environment, a vibrational field integral with the person where the nurse is not simply in the environment but "the nurse IS the environment" (Watson, 2008, p. 26). Watson also addresses the nurse's role in the environment as creating a healing environment at all levels (2008, p. 129).

Health

Health is defined as unity and harmony within the body, mind, and soul; a harmony between the self and others, and between the self and nature; and openness to increased possibility (Jesse, 2010b). According to Watson, illness is not necessarily disease, but rather a subjective disharmony within the spheres of the person. Disease, in turn, creates more disharmony (Jesse, 2010a).

Nursing

The goal of nursing care is to promote growth and find meaning in one's existence and experience.

Nursing is viewed by Watson as both a human science and an art. She describes the concept of nursing as a reciprocal transpersonal relationship in caring moments guided by carative factors and caritas processes—a human-to-human connection in which both persons are influenced though the relationship and being together in the moment (Watson, 1999). The goal of nursing care is to promote growth and find meaning in one's existence and experience.

T HE ANALYSIS PRESENTED HERE CONSISTS of an examination of Watson's assumptions and propositions as well as a brief critique of the philosophy and theory of transpersonal caring as proposed by Watson.

> **ANALYSIS OF *Watson's* PHILOSOPHY AND THEORY OF TRANSPERSONAL CARING**

Assumptions of Watson's Philosophy and Theory of Transpersonal Caring

The major assumptions of the philosophy and theory of transpersonal caring include the following ideas:

❖ Moral commitment, intentionality, and caritas consciousness by the nurse protect, enhance, and potentiate human dignity, wholeness, and healing, allowing a person to create his or her own meaning for existence, healing, wholeness, and living and dying.

❖ The conscious will of the nurse affirms the subjective and spiritual significance of the patient, while seeking to sustain caring in the midst of threat and despair.

❖ The nurse seeks to recognize, accurately detect, and connect with the inner condition of spirit of another person through genuine presencing and by being centered in the caring moment. Actions, words, behaviors, cognition, body language, feelings, intuition, thoughts, senses, and the energy field all contribute to this transpersonal caring connection.

❖ The nurse's ability to connect with another at this transpersonal, spirit-to-spirit level is translated via movements, gestures, facial expressions, procedures, information, touch, sound, verbal expressions, and other means of communication into intentional caring–healing modalities.

❖ The caring–healing modalities within the context of transpersonal caring/caritas consciousness potentiate harmony, wholeness, and unity of being by releasing some of the disharmony or blocked energy that interferes with healing processes.

❖ Ongoing personal and professional development and spiritual growth assist the nurse in entering into this deeper level of professional healing practice (Watson, 2001, p. 348).

Propositions of Watson's Philosophy and Theory of Transpersonal Caring

Primary relationship statements seen in the philosophy and theory of transpersonal caring are included in the following premises:

❖ Nursing care can be and is physical, procedural, objective, and factual. Nevertheless, at the highest level of nursing, the nurse's human care responses, the human care transactions, and the nurse's presence in the relationship transcend the physical and material world, bound in time and space, and make contact with the person's emotional and subjective world as a route to the inner self and the higher sense of self.

❖ A person's body is confined in time and space, but the mind and soul are not confined to the physical universe.

❖ A nurse may have access to a person's mind, emotions, and inner self indirectly though the spheres of the mind, body, or soul, provided the body is not perceived or treated as separate from the mind and emotions and higher sense of self.

❖ The spirit, inner self, or soul of a person exists in and for itself. The spiritual essence of the person is related to the human ability to be free. The destiny of one's being is to develop the spiritual essence of self and in the highest sense to become more Godlike. However, each person has to question his or her own essence and moral behavior toward others, because if people are dehumanized at a basic level, that dehumanizing process is not capable of reflecting humanity back upon itself.

❖ Persons need one another in a caring, loving way. Love and caring are two universal givens.

❖ A person's human condition may not be related to the external world as much as to the person's inner world as it is being experienced (Watson, 1985, p. 50).

Brief Critique of Watson's Philosophy and Theory of Transpersonal Caring

Watson seeks to address the core of nursing and provide a moral and philosophical basis for nursing through her philosophy and theory of transpersonal caring. As such, her framework is general and addresses all aspects of the health–illness phenomenon. Most of the concepts within the theory are simple but abstract and, therefore, are difficult to measure (Jesse, 2010a). Despite this abstraction, according to Fawcett (2005, p. 580), evidence of the theory's empirical adequacy is emerging. Watson uses metaphors, artwork, poetry, and personal reflections to make the complex concepts more tangible for her readers across disciplines who utilize the theory (Jesse, 2010a). She continues to refine her work, stating that it is an evolving work in progress "geared toward a paradigmatic structure for the whole of nursing and its emergence as a distinct caring–healing–health discipline and profession" (Watson, 1996b, p. 142).

THE PRACTICE OF NURSING AS driven by Watson's philosophy and theory differs from biomedical-based nursing practice. While the body is certainly cared for by the nurse using Watson's framework, nursing care is never separated from the context of the unity of the mind–body–spirit–nature of the patient.

WHILE THE NURSING PROCESS is not explicitly mentioned in Watson's theory, the various phases known as the nursing process can be identified for the sake of discussion, consistency, and comparison.

Watson's PHILOSOPHY AND THEORY OF TRANSPERSONAL CARING AS A FRAMEWORK FOR NURSING PRACTICE

THE NURSING PROCESS AND Watson's PHILOSOPHY AND THEORY OF TRANSPERSONAL CARING

Assessment

Assessment using Watson's theory involves the mutual engagement of the nurse and the patient as well as the identification of problems, whether physical or psychosocial in nature. Analysis and nursing diagnosis follow the gathering of assessment data.

Planning

Planning will include discussion and establishment of goals. The goals of Watson's theory relate to growth of oneself and others.

Implementation

The list of the caritas is presented by Watson as a series of interventions intended to achieve goals appropriate to her philosophy and theory of transpersonal caring. These interventions reflect interactions—and interactions require intention, will, relationship, and actions. All interactions presuppose the appropriate professional knowledge and clinical competence.

Evaluation

Effective interventions are related to achieving the goals of the interventions. The evaluation process is enhanced through mutual reflection.

SCENARIO ILLUSTRATING NURSING CARE FRAMED BY *Watson's* **PHILOSOPHY AND THEORY OF TRANSPERSONAL CARING UTILIZING THE NURSING PROCESS**

THE FOLLOWING SCENARIO ILLUSTRATES NURSING care of the patient relative to one identified nursing problem framed by Watson's philosophy and theory of transpersonal caring. This scenario is not intended to cover all aspects of care, but rather is intended to stimulate thinking about how specific care might be approached using this theory as a framework for practice.

Ms. W. is a 42-year-old single mother who has been diagnosed with lung cancer. She has two daughters, who are currently in high school. Since her admission to the hospital unit, diagnosis, and treatment initiation, Ms. W. has been tearful and spent most of her time alone. Upon preparation for the initiation of the nurse–patient relationship, the nurse is mindful of the first three caritas: practicing loving kindness and equanimity for self and other; being authentically present and enabling, sustaining, and honoring the deep belief system and subjective life world of self and the one being cared for; and cultivating one's own spiritual practices, including deepening of self-awareness and going beyond the ego self as necessary before the initiation of the assessment phase of nursing care.

As the nurse–patient relationship is established and the assessment and planning phase of the process begins, it is important that the relationship that is developed and sustained is a helping trusting, authentic caring relationship and that the plan developed allows for growth. As the nurse engages in the assessment and planning process with Ms. W., she is cognizant that she is in a professional caring relationship, and she makes a conscious effort to see the mind–spirit–body–nature person—in other words, the whole person for whom she is caring.

At this point in the patient's care, assessment data indicate that nausea and vomiting with weight loss are of some concern. Nevertheless, Ms. W.'s primary concern is her daughters' future if she does not survive. The nurse uses current best practices to administer the prescribed medication and other comfort measures to alleviate the nausea and vomiting associated with her treatment. During this process, the nurse also uses the caritas principles to allow for meeting the primary, deeper concern of the patient and to address the core of her current distress—that is, the issues of her ultimate survival and the well-being of her daughters if she does not survive.

The nurse uses the caritas principles of being present to, and supportive of, the expression of positive and negative feelings as a connection with a deeper spirit of self and the one being cared for, and creative use of self and all ways of knowing as part of the caring process. In this way, she creates a healing environment whereby wholeness, beauty, comfort, dignity, and peace are potentiated. She reverentially and respectfully assists with Ms. W.'s basic needs, with an intentional caring conscious-ness of touching and working with the embodied spirit of another, hon-oring the unity of being. She allows for a spirit-filled connection while administering human care essentials, which potentiate alignment of the mind–body–spirit, wholeness, and unity of being in all aspects of care. She attends to both Ms. W.'s embodied spirit and evolving emergence, and opens and attends to the spiritual, mysterious, and unknown existential dimensions of life, death, and suffering (Watson, 2008, p. 31) to create interactions as she provides for the care of the whole patient, including the physical realm. Evaluation is based on the effectiveness of interac-tions and mutual reflection by the nurse and the patient.

CLASSROOM ACTIVITY 5-1

Form small groups. Each group should add to the plan of care for Ms. W. in the preceding scenario based on other potential or actual nursing diagnoses typical for a patient with same medical diagnosis or symptoms and demographics. Each group should develop a plan for one additional nursing problem using Watson's theory as the basis for practice. Each group should then share its plan with the class.

CLASSROOM ACTIVITY 5-2

Form small groups. Using a case study provided by the instructor, develop a plan of care using Watson's nursing theory of transpersonal caring as the basis for practice. Each group should then share its plan of care with the class. It may be helpful to play the CD-ROM of *Caritas Meditations* that comes with the 2008 edition of Watson's book during this activity.

CLASSROOM ACTIVITY 5-3

Form small groups. Using a case study provided by the instructor, develop a plan of care using one of the theories as the basis for practice; each group should select a different nursing theory. Each group should then share its plan of care with the class and discuss the similarities and differences in care.

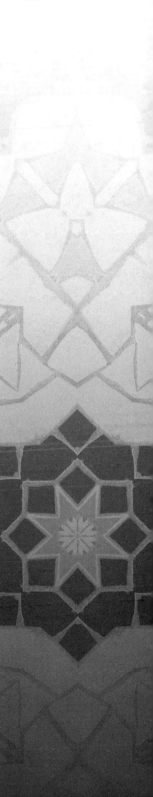

REFERENCES

Boyd, C., & Mast, D. (1989). Watson's model of human care. In J. J. Fitzpatrick & A. L. Whall (Eds.), *Conceptual models of nursing: Analysis and application* (2nd ed., pp. 371–383). Norwalk, CT: Appleton & Lange.

Fawcett, J. (2005). *Contemporary nursing knowledge: Analysis and evaluation of nursing models and theories* (2nd ed., pp. 553–585). Philadelphia: F. A. Davis.

Jesse, D. E. (2010a). Jean Watson: Watson's philosophy and theory of transpersonal caring. In A. M. Tomey & M. R. Alligood (Eds.), *Nursing theorists and their work* (7th ed., pp. 91–112). St. Louis, MO: Mosby.

Jesse, D. E. (2010b). Watson's philosophy and science of caring in nursing practice. In M. R. Alligood (Ed.), *Nursing theory: Application and practice* (4th ed., pp.111–136). St. Louis, MO: Mosby.

Neil, R. M., & Tomey, A. M. (2006). Jean Watson: Philosophy and science of caring. In A. M. Tomey & M. R. Alligood (Eds.), *Nursing theorists and their work* (6th ed., pp. 91–115). St. Louis, MO: Mosby.

Watson, J. (1979). *Nursing: The philosophy and science of caring.* Boston: Little, Brown.

Watson, J. (1985). *Nursing: Human science and human care: A theory of nursing.* Sudbury, MA: Jones and Bartlett.

Watson, J. (1989). Watson's philosophy and theory of human caring in nursing. In J. P. Riehl-Sisca (Ed.), *Conceptual model for nursing practice* (3rd ed., pp. 219–236). Norwalk, CT: Appleton & Lange.

Watson, J. (1996a). Watson's philosophy and theory of human caring in nursing. In J. P. Riehl-Sisca (Ed.), *Conceptual models for nursing practice* (4th ed., pp. 219–235). Norwalk, CT: Appleton & Lange.

Watson, J. (1996b). Watson's theory of transpersonal caring. In P. H. Walker & B. Neuman (Eds.), *Blueprint for use of nursing models: Education, research, practice and administration* (pp. 141–184). New York: National League for Nursing Press.

Watson, J. (1997). The theory of human caring: Retrospective and prospective. *Nursing Science Quarterly, 10,* 49–52.

Watson, J. (1999). *Postmodern nursing and beyond.* Edinburgh: Churchill Livingstone Saunders.

Watson, J. (2001). Jean Watson: Theory of human caring. In M. E. Parker (Ed.), *Nursing theories and nursing practice* (pp. 343–354). Philadelphia: F. A. Davis.

Watson, J. (2008). *Nursing: The philosophy and science of caring* (revised edition). Boulder, CO: University Press of Colorado.

CLINICAL WISDOM IN NURSING PRACTICE:
Patricia Benner

6

BACKGROUND

PATRICIA BENNER WAS BORN IN Virginia but moved to California as a child. As a young woman, she earned a bachelor of arts degree, with a major in nursing, in 1964 from Pasadena College. During her years prior to entering nursing research and education, Benner gained clinical experience in acute medical–surgical, critical care, and home health care, in both staff nurse and head nurse positions. She obtained a master's degree in nursing with an emphasis in medical–surgical nursing from the University of California, San Francisco (UCSF), School of Nursing in 1970. Following her completion of this degree, Benner accepted a position as a postgraduate nurse researcher at UCSF. In 1982, she received a PhD from the University of California, Berkeley. Upon completion of the PhD program, Benner accepted a position as nursing professor at UCSF. She retired from full-time teaching in 2008 but continues to be involved in research, consultation, presentations, and writing (Brykczynski, 2010a, p. 137–138).

Benner's thinking was influenced by the work of Virginia Henderson. Benner's work has also been influenced to a large degree by the work of Hubert Dreyfus, a professor at the University of California at Berkeley who introduced her to pheonomenology. Stuart Dreyfus, a researcher and also professor at the University of California at Berkeley, and Hubert Dreyfus developed the Dreyfus model of skill acquisition, which Benner later adapted to clinical nursing practice (Benner, 1984/2001). Benner's thinking has also been influenced by many philosophers, though she specifically credits Jane Rubin's scholarship, teaching, and collegiality as an influence; Richard Lazarus, who mentored her in the field of stress and coping; and Jane Wrubel, who has been her collaborating author in the areas of caring practices for many years (Brykczynski, 2010a, p. 140).

Throughout her career, Benner has published extensively. Some of her most notable publications include *From Novice to Expert: Excellence and Power in Clinical Nursing Practice* (1984/2001), *Expertise in Nursing Practice: Caring, Clinical Judgment, and Ethics* (1996, 2009), and *Clinical Wisdom and Interventions in Critical Care* (1999). For her contributions to the profession of nursing, Benner has received numerous honors and awards, including induction into the American Academy of Nurses, the American Association of Colleges of Nursing Pioneering Spirit Award, and a National Council State Boards of Nursing Award. Benner's contributions to the nursing profession have continued past her retirement from academia, with her most recent endeavor being her role as the Nursing Education Study Director for the Carnegie Foundation's Preparation for the Professions Program. The results of this study were published in 2010 in a widely acclaimed book, *Educating Nurses: A Call for Radical Transformation.*

Overview of Benner's Philosophy of Clinical Wisdom in Nursing

Benner's work over several decades has focused on the understanding of perceptual acuity, clinical judgment, skilled know-how, ethical comportment, and ongoing experiential learning (Brykczynski, 2010b, p. 141). According to Benner's model, clinical nursing expertise is embodied; in other words, "through experience, skilled performance is transformed from the halting, stepwise performance of the beginner . . . to the smooth, intuitive performance of the expert" (Brykczynski, 1998, p. 352). Related and also important in the study of Benner's philosophy is an understanding of ethical comportment. According to Day and Benner (2002), good conduct is a product of an individual relationship with the patient that involves engagement in a situation combined with a sense of membership in a profession. Professional conduct is socially embedded, lived, and embodied in the practices, ways of being, and responses to clinical situations that promote patient well-being, where clinical and ethical judgments are inseparable.

Benner's original domains and competencies of nursing practice were derived inductively from clinical situation interviews and observations of nurses in actual practice. From these interviews and observations, 31 competencies and seven domains were identified and described (Benner, 1984/2001). Later, in an extension of her original work, Benner and her colleagues identified nine domains of critical care nursing (Benner, Hooper-Kyriakidis, & Stannard, 1999). Along with the identification of the competencies and domains of nursing, Benner identified five stages of skill acquisition based on the Dreyfus model of skill acquisition as applied to nursing along with characteristics of each stage (Benner, 1984/2001).

The five stages of skill acquisition identified by Benner include novice, advanced beginner, competent, proficient, and expert. In the **novice stage of skill acquisition**, the person has no background experience of the situation. The novice stage is characterized by the person requiring rules to govern performance. Typically, he or she has difficulty discerning between relevant and irrelevant features of a situation (Benner, 1984/2001). Through instruction, the novice learns rules for drawing conclusions or for determining actions based on the features of the situation that are recognizable, without the benefit of experience in the skill domain begin learned. This stage most often applies to nursing students but can be applicable to more experienced nurses when they are placed in an unfamiliar situation (Benner, Tanner, & Chesla, 1996; 2009).

A person in the **advanced beginner stage of skill acquisition** demonstrates a marginally acceptable level of performance after now having considerable experience coping with real situations. Nurses functioning at the advanced beginner stage are still guided by rules and are oriented toward task completion, and will continue to rely on the assistance of more experienced nurses to manage patient care (Benner, 1984/2001; Benner, Tanner, & Chesla, 1996; 2009). At this stage, clinical situations are viewed in terms of the nurse's abilities and the demands that the situation places on the nurse rather than in terms of the needs of patients (Benner, Tanner, & Chesla, 1992).

The nurse who reaches the **competent stage of skill acquisition** begins to recognize patterns and is able to discern which features of a situation require attention. Because the competent nurse must devise new rules and reasoning procedures while applying learned rules for action based on the relevant features of the situation, the competent nurse feels a great sense of responsibility for his or her actions; by comparison, the novice and advanced beginner are simply applying rules. The competent nurse also displays a focus on time management and organization because planning and predictability are required to achieve a sense of mastery (Benner, Tanner, & Chesla, 1996; 2009).

At the **proficient stage of skill acquisition**, the nurse perceives the situation as a whole, plans can be formulated intuitively, and certain features of the situation stand out as important without the nurse having to stand back and choose to adopt a perspective or a plan. At this stage, the nurse demonstrates increased confidence in his or her abilities and has the ability to turn the focus away from self and toward the patient. The proficient stage can be seen as a transition into expertise (Benner, Tanner, & Chesla, 1996; 2009).

In the fifth stage, the nurse is classified as an **expert**. The expert nurse no longer relies on rules to connect his or her understanding of the situation to the appropriate action, but rather has an intuitive grasp of the situation (Benner, 1984/2001). The expert nurse has the ability to recognize patterns owing to his or her deep experiential background. The expert nurse's practice is characterized by demonstration of a clinical grasp and resource-based practice, possessing embodied know-how, seeing the big picture, and seeing the unexpected (Benner, Tanner, & Chesla, 1996; 2009).

The seven domains were identified inductively from Benner's 31 competencies. These domains, which are outlined here, were set apart based on similarity of function and intent:

- ❖ The helping role
- ❖ The teaching–coaching function
- ❖ The diagnostic and patient monitoring function
- ❖ Effective management of rapidly changing situations
- ❖ Administering and monitoring therapeutic interventions and regimens
- ❖ Monitoring and ensuring the quality of healthcare practices
- ❖ Organizational work role competencies (Benner, 1984/2001)

The eight competencies within the domain of the helping role include (1) creating a climate for and establishing a commitment to healing, (2) providing comfort measures and preserving personhood in the face of pain and extreme breakdown, (3) presencing (being with the patient), (4) maximizing the patient's participation and control in his or her own recovery, (5) interpreting kinds of pain and selecting appropriate strategies for pain management and control, (6) providing comfort and communication through touch, (7) providing emotional and informational

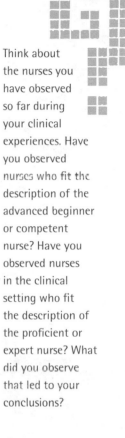

CRITICAL THINKING 6

Think about the nurses you have observed so far during your clinical experiences. Have you observed nurses who fit the description of the advanced beginner or competent nurse? Have you observed nurses in the clinical setting who fit the description of the proficient or expert nurse? What did you observe that led to your conclusions?

The expert nurse no longer relies on rules to connect his or her understanding of the situation to the appropriate action, but rather has an intuitive grasp of the situation.

support to patients families, and (8) guiding a patient through emotional and developmental change (Benner, 1984/2001, p. 50). The five competencies within the domain of the teaching–coaching function include (1) capturing a patient's readiness to learn (timing), (2) assisting patients to integrate the implications of illness and recovery into their lifestyles, (3) eliciting and understanding the patient's interpretation of his or her illness, (4) providing an interpretation of the patient's condition and giving a rationale for procedures, and (5) making culturally avoided aspects of an illness approachable and understandable (Benner, 1984/2001, p. 79).

The five competencies within the domain of diagnostic and monitoring function include (1) detecting and documentating significant changes in a patient's condition, (2) anticipating breakdown and deterioration prior to explicit confirming diagnostic signs, (3) anticipating problems, (4) understanding particular demands and experiences of an illness, and (5) assessing the patient's potential for wellness and for responding to various treatment strategies (Benner, 1984/2001, p. 97). The three competencies within the domain of effective management of rapidly changing situations include (1) skilled performing in extreme life-threatening emergencies, (2) rapid matching of demands and resources in emergency situations, and (3) identifying and managing a patient crisis until physician assistance is available (Benner, 1984/2001, p. 111).

The four competencies within the domain of administering and monitoring therapeutic interventions and regimens include (1) starting and maintaining intravenous therapy with minimal risks and complications; (2) administering medications accurately and safely, including monitoring untoward effects, reactions, therapeutic responses, toxicity, and incompatibilities; (3) combating the hazards of immobility, including preventing and intervening with skin breakdown, ambulating and exercising patients to maximize mobility and rehabilitation, and preventing respiratory complications; and (4) creating a wound management strategy that fosters healing, comfort, and appropriate drainage (Benner, 1984/2001, p. 123). The three competencies within the domain of monitoring and ensuring the quality of healthcare practices include (1) providing a backup system to ensure safe medical and nursing care, (2) assessing what can safely omitted from or added to medical orders, and (3) getting appropriate and timely responses from physicians (Benner, 1984/2001, p. 137). The final three competencies include those related to the organizational and work-role domain: (1) coordinating, ordering, and meeting multiple patient needs and requests—in other words, setting priorities; (2) building and maintaining a therapeutic team to provide optimal therapy; and (3) coping with staff shortages and high turnover (Benner, 1984/2001, p. 147).

The nine domains of critical care nursing practice were also identified inductively using similar techniques:

- ❖ Diagnosing and managing life-sustaining physiological functions in unstable patients
- ❖ Using skilled know-how to manage a crisis
- ❖ Providing comfort measures for the critically ill
- ❖ Caring for patients' families
- ❖ Preventing hazards in a technological environment
- ❖ Facing death: end-of-life care and decision making
- ❖ Communicating and negotiating multiple perspectives
- ❖ Monitoring quality and managing breakdown
- ❖ Using the skilled know-how of clinical leadership and the coaching and mentoring of others (Benner, Hooper-Kyriakidis, & Stannard, 1999)

In their 1999 publication, Benner, Hooper Kyriakidis, and Stannard provide readers with an entire chapter of narrative that explains and provides exemplars for each of the identified domains of critical care nursing practice. In addition, the nine domains of critical care nursing practice are used as broad themes in data interpretation for the identification and description of six aspects of clinical judgment and skilled comportment. These six aspects are summarized here:

- ❖ **Reasoning-in-transition**: practical reasoning in an ongoing clinical situation
- ❖ **Skilled know-how**: also known as embodied intelligent performance; knowing what to do, when to do it, and how to do it
- ❖ **Response-based practice**: adapting interventions to meet the changing needs and expectations of patients

❖ **Agency**: one's sense of and ability to act upon or influence a situation

❖ **Perceptual acuity and the skill of involvement**: the ability to tune into a situation and hone in on the salient issues by engaging with the problem and the person

❖ **Links between clinical and ethical reasoning**: the understanding that good clinical practice cannot be separated from ethical notions of good outcomes for patients and families (Benner, Hooper-Kyriakidis, & Stannard, 1999)

Major Concepts of Nursing Based upon Benner's Philosophy

In addition to the concepts already presented, Benner identifies and defines the four metaparadigm concepts of nursing. These concepts are summarized in Table 6-1.

Person

The concept of person is defined by Benner as a "self-interpreting being, that is, the person does not come into the world pre-defined but gets defined in the course of living a life" (Benner & Wrubel, 1989, p. 41). An additional important component of the definition of person is the notion that the person is embodied. Benner and Wrubel (1989) define the term

TABLE 6-1 Metaparadigm Concepts as Defined in Benner's Philosophy	
Person	Embodied person living in the world who is a "self-interpreting being, that is, the person does not come into the world pre-defined but gets defined in the course of living a life" (Benner & Wrubel, 1989, p. 41)
Environment (situation)	A social environment with social definition and meaningfulness
Health	The human experience of health or wholeness
Nursing	A caring relationship that includes the care and study of the lived experience of health, illness, and disease

"embodiment" as the capacity of the body to respond to meaningful situations. Thus understanding the embodied person as living in the world requires understanding the role of the situation, the role of the body, the role of personal concerns, and the role of temporality.

According to Benner and Wrubel (1989, p. 71), there are five dimensions of the body that nurses attend to and seek to understand the role of embodiment in situations of health and illness:

- ❖ The unborn complex, unacculturated body of the fetus and newborn baby

- ❖ The habitual skilled body, complete with socially learned postures, gestures, customs, and skills, evident in bodily skills such as sense perception and body language that are learned over time

- ❖ The projective body, which is set to act in specific situations

- ❖ The actual projected body, indicating an individual's current bodily orientation or projection in a situation that is flexible and varied to fit the situation

- ❖ The phenomenal body—the body that is aware of itself and that has the ability to imagine and describe kinesthetic sensations

Environment

Benner and Wrubel (1989) use the term "situation" to address the concept of environment. This term conveys the notion of a social environment with social definition and meaningfulness, which is congruent with the phenomenological perspective and terminology used in the descriptors of the concept. Benner and Wrubel (1989, p. 84) use the words "being situated" and "situated meaning" to describe the person's engaged interaction, interpretation, and understanding of the situation, meaning that each person's past, present, and future, which include the individual's own personal meanings and perspectives, influence each situation (Brykczynski, 2010a, p. 149).

Health

Health and disease are defined based on what can be assessed at the physical level. Benner and Wrubel (1989) focus their definitions on well-being and illness rather than on health and disease. Health is defined as the human experience of health or wholeness. As such, a person may have a disease and not experience illness because illness is the human experience of loss (Brykczynski, 2010a, p. 149).

Nursing

According to Benner, nursing is a caring practice that includes a relationship between nurses and patients; this caring practice includes the care and study of the lived experience of health, illness, and disease and the relationships among these elements (Benner & Wrubel, 1989). For Benner, "caring is primary because it sets up the possibility of giving help and receiving help" (Benner & Wrubel, 1989, p. 4) and the science of the caring practice of nursing "is guided by the moral art and ethics of care and responsibility" (Benner & Wrubel, 1989, p. xi).

The science of the caring practice of nursing "is guided by the moral art and ethics of care and responsibility."

ANALYSIS OF *Benner's* PHILOSOPHY

THE ANALYSIS PRESENTED HERE CONSISTS of an examination of Benner's assumptions and propositions as well as a brief critique of her philosophy.

Assumptions of Benner's Philosophy

According to Brykczynski (2010a, p. 147–148), assumptions included in Benner's ongoing research related to her philosophy include the following:

❖ Meanings are embedded in skills, practices, intentions, expectations, and outcomes. They are taken for granted and often are not recognized as knowledge.

❖ People who share a common cultural history and language have a background of common meanings that allows for understanding and interpretation.

❖ The meanings embedded in skills, practices, intentions, expectations, and outcomes cannot be made completely explicit; however, they can be interpreted by someone who shares a similar background and can be validated by participants and practitioners.

❖ Humans are integrated, holistic beings; the Cartesian notion of the mind–body split is abandoned. Embodied intelligence enables skilled activity that is transformed through experience and mastery.

Propositions of Benner's Philosophy

Benner (1984/2001, p. 178) asserts that there is always more to any situation than theory predicts and that the skilled practice of nursing exceeds the bounds of formal theory. Specific theoretical relationship statements embedded in the philosophy include the following:

❖ Discovering assumptions, expectations, and sets can uncover an unexamined area of practical knowledge, which can then be systematically studied and extended or refuted (Benner, 1984/2001, p. 8).

❖ Clinical knowledge is embedded in perceptions rather than precepts.

❖ Perceptual awareness is central to good nursing judgment (Benner, 1984/2001).

❖ "Expertise develops when the clinician tests and refines propositions, hypotheses, and principle based expectations in actual practice situations" (Benner, 1984/2001, p. 3).

❖ Formal rules are limited and discretionary judgment is needed in actual clinical situations.

❖ Clinical knowledge develops over time, and each clinician develops a personal inventory of practice knowledge that can be shared with other clinicians (Brykczynski, 2010a, p. 149).

Brief Critique of Benner's Philosophy

Benner's concepts in describing the novice to expert levels of practice are easy to understand and are readily generalized across practice settings and varying demographics. Terminology is used consistently throughout the various components of the philosophy. In fact, Virginia Henderson (1989), after reviewing Benner's *From Novice to Expert: Excellence and Power in Clinical Nursing Practice* (1984/2001), stated that Benner's work had the potential to affect the practice of nursing and the preparation of nurses for practice. The competencies and domains in the model were derived inductively and have been tested. The framework remains useful for practice and for further knowledge development within nursing (Brykczynski, 2010a, p. 152–153).

Benner's PHILOSOPHY AS A FRAMEWORK FOR NURSING PRACTICE

IT IS IMPORTANT TO POINT out that the competencies and domains for nursing practice as defined by Benner are not linear concepts that have clear beginning and ending points; rather, the nurse enters the circle of caring for the patient through whichever competency is needed at the time. Patient needs may dictate that one competency in a particular domain is more pronounced at a certain point in time; yet, in the context of the patient's unique situation, there may be significant overlap in domains and competency requirements during the process of caring for the patient and family. The nurse using Benner's philosophy as a framework for practice will consider each of the domains of practice and the corresponding competencies. In addition, the nurse will remain cognizant of the need to practice with salience and ethical comportment.

THE NURSING PROCESS AND *Benner's* PHILOSOPHY

WHILE NOT SPECIFICALLY ADDRESSED, USE of the nursing process is easily incorporated into the structure of Benner's philosophy.

Assessment and Planning

During the assessment phase of the nursing process, the nurse meets with the patient to discover the patient's concerns, thereby enabling the pair to develop a shared under-standing of how to proceed. The nurse observes, describes, and studies the patient in the current situation, while remaining free of preconceived assumptions, so as to interpret the nursing care required by the patient (Brykczyński, 2010a, p. 145; 2010b, p. 150). Assessment within the help-ing domain will include assessment learning about the patient's unique situation. Another variable in this domain is the nurse's experience and background in situations similar to those of the patient. Assessment will also include those needs in the teaching–coaching domain, such as readi-ness to learn. In the diagnostic and monitoring domain, the nurse will anticipate the future needs of the patient and assess the patient's potential for wellness as well as the ongoing response to current treatment strate-gies. The nurse and the patient will jointly plan for care based on the results of the assessment.

Implementation

The implementation phase can be easily viewed through the lens of Benner's domains, given that the competencies from which the domains were derived were identified inductively through the study of actual nurs-ing practice. Nursing care in the helping role will include those competen-cies listed earlier in the chapter, such as presencing, providing comfort and pain management and providing emotional support to the patient's family. Nursing care interventions related to the teaching role will include explaining rationales for procedures, teaching, and assisting patients to integrate illness and recovery issues into their lifestyles.

As a part of the diagnostic function domain, nursing interventions might include documentation of changes in patient condition and antici-pating patient care needs. Skilled performance and grasp of a problem, along with identification and management of a patient crisis, are interven-tions included in the domain of effective management of rapidly changing situations. This domain may or may not be applicable depending on the particular patient situation.

The domain of administering and monitoring therapeutic interven-tions and regimens includes nursing strategies such as maintaining intra-venous therapy, administering medications safely, combating the hazards of mobility, and wound management as applicable for the patient situation. Nursing interventions also include those things that happen outside of the view of the patient and family, such as getting timely responses from physicians, coping with staff shortages, and prioritizing the needs across multiple patients.

Evaluation

Evaluation of care is based on the patient's outcome and interpretation of the outcome within his or her unique situation. In addition, evaluation from the nurse's perspective may include issues related to the domains of monitoring and ensuring quality healthcare practices and organizational and work-role competencies.

SCENARIO ILLUSTRATING NURSING CARE FRAMED BY *Benner's* PHILOSOPHY

THE FOLLOWING SCENARIO ILLUSTRATES NURSING care of the patient relative to one identified nursing problem framed by Benner's philosophy of clinical wisdom. This scenario is not intended to cover all aspects of care, but rather is intended to stimulate thinking about how specific care might be approached using this philosophy as a framework for practice.

Ms. W. is a young, Caucasian, single mother of three, who presents to the emergency room with multiple bruises in varying stages and a fractured arm. Radiologic exam reveals several additional healed fractures. Ms. W. is not accompanied to the hospital by anyone, but states that her boyfriend lives with her in her apartment.

During the assessment phase of the nursing process, the nurse meets with the patient to discover the patient's concerns and develop a shared understanding of how to proceed. The helping domain will include assessment learning about the patient's unique situation and will include establishment of the healing relationship with Ms. W. By learning about Ms. W.'s situation, beliefs, values, needs, and goals, the nurse develops an understanding of the meaning of this illness experience for her. Assessment will also include needs in the teaching–coaching domain. In this scenario, those needs focus on timing—that is, when the patient is ready to experience a behavior change and coaching so as to make culturally avoided aspects of her illness, such as the ongoing physical abuse, approachable and understandable. In the diagnostic and monitoring domain, the nurse will anticipate future needs of the Ms. W. and assess her potential for wellness as well as ongoing response to suggested interventions and referrals. The nurse and Ms. W. will plan for care based on the results of the assessment.

Care for Ms. W. relative to the helping role will include those competencies listed earlier in the chapter, such as presencing, providing comfort, and maximizing the patient's participation and control in her own recovery through appropriate referrals. Nursing care interventions related to the teaching role will deal with explaining rationales for procedures, teaching related to both procedures and—more importantly—abuse patterns and resources available, and assisting Ms. W. to integrate the implications of illness (abuse and injury) and recovery issues and change into her life situation. As a part of the diagnostic function domain, the nursing interventions for Ms. W. will include documentation of her condition, her interview, and her responses; interventions and referrals; and anticipation of patient care needs. The domain of administering and monitoring therapeutic interventions and regimens for Ms. W. will include nursing strategies such as administering medications safely, combating the hazards of mobility, and wound management. In addition to addressing competencies within the domains, the nurse will remain cognizant of the need to practice with salience and ethical comportment.

Evaluation of the care of Ms. W. is based on both her physical outcome and her interpretation of the outcome within her unique situation. In addition, evaluation from the nurse's perspective may include issues related to the domains of monitoring and ensuring quality healthcare practices and organizational and work-role competencies.

Throughout this process, the theory may be applied simultaneously to other issues as they are identified by Ms. W. and the nurse. If other issues arise during the nursing encounter that fall outside the interaction focus of the theory, nursing interventions will be planned to address those issues using strategies that are congruent with current best clinical practices.

CLASSROOM ACTIVITY 6-1

Form small groups. Each group should add to the plan of care for Ms. W. in the preceding scenario based on other potential or actual nursing diagnoses typical for a patient with same medical diagnosis or symptoms and demographics. Each group should develop a plan for one additional nursing problem using Benner's philosophy as the basis for practice. Each group should then share its plan with the class.

CLASSROOM ACTIVITY 6-2

Form small groups. Using a case study provided by the instructor, develop a plan of care using Benner's philosophy of nursing as the basis for practice. Each group should then share its plan of care with the class.

CLASSROOM ACTIVITY 6-3

Form small groups. Using a case study provided by the instructor, develop a plan of care using one of the theories as the basis for practice; each group should select a different nursing theory. Each group should then share its plan of care with the class and discuss the similarities and differences in care.

REFERENCES

Benner, P. (1984/2001). *From novice to expert: Excellence and power in clinical nursing practice.* Upper Saddle River, NJ: Prentice-Hall.

Benner, P., Hooper-Kyriakidis, P., & Stannard, D. (1999). *Clinical wisdom and interventions in critical care: A thinking-in-action approach.* Philadelphia: Saunders.

Benner, P., Sutphen, M., Leonard, V., Day, L., Shulman, L. S. (2010). *Educating nurses: A call for radical transformation.* San Francisco: Jossey-Bass.

Benner, P., Tanner, C. A., & Chesla, C. A. (1992). From beginner to expert: Gaining a differentiated clinical world in critical care nursing. *ANS Advances in Nursing Science, 14*(3), 13–28.

Benner, P., Tanner, C. A., & Chesla, C. A. (1996). *Expertise in nursing practice: Caring, clinical judgment, and ethics.* New York: Springer.

Benner, P., Tanner, C. A., & Chesla, C. A. (2009). *Expertise in nursing practice: Caring, clinical judgment, and ethics* (2nd ed.). New York: Springer.

Benner, P., & Wrubel, J. (1989). *The primacy of caring: Stress and coping in health and illness.* Menlo Park, CA: Addison-Wesley.

Brykczynski, K. A. (1998). Clinical nursing exemplars describing expert staff nursing practices. *Journal of Nursing Management, 6,* 351–359

Brykczynski, K. A. (2010a). Patricia Benner: Caring, clinical wisdom, and ethics in nursing practice. In M. R. Alligood & A. M. Tomey (Eds.), *Nursing theorists and their work* (7th ed., pp. 137–164). Maryland Heights, MO: Mosby.

Brykczynski, K. A. (2010b). Benner's philosophy in nursing practice. In M. R. Alligood (Ed.), *Nursing theory: Utilization and application* (4th ed., pp. 137–159). Maryland Heights, MO: Mosby.

Day, L., & Benner, P. (2002). Ethics, ethical comportment, and etiquette. *American Journal of Critical Care, 11*(1), 76–79.

Henderson, V. (1989). Foreword. In P. Benner & J. Wrubel (Eds.), *The primacy of caring: Stress and coping in health and illness* (pp. ix–x). Menlo Park, CA: Addison-Wesley.

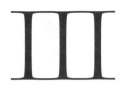

CONCEPTUAL
MODELS

BEHAVIORAL SYSTEM MODEL:
Dorothy Johnson

7

BACKGROUND

DOROTHY E. JOHNSON WAS BORN in 1919 in Savannah, Georgia. She graduated from nursing school in 1938, received her BSN from Vanderbilt University in 1942, and received her MPH from Harvard University in 1948.

Johnson served as faculty at both Vanderbilt University School of Nursing and the University of California in Los Angeles. Over the course of her career, she published more than 30 articles, 4 books, and many reports, and was presented with numerous honors.

According to Johnson (1990), her behavior system model was in the process of development for nearly the entire course of her professional life. The model had roots in the work of behavioral scientists in psychology, sociology, and ethnology, with heavy reliance on systems theory (Loveland-Cherry & Wilkerson, 1989). Johnson's theory was also influenced by Nightingale's belief that nursing's goal is to help individuals prevent or recover from disease or injury, with the focus being placed on the patient rather than on the specific disease (Johnson, 1990). Her initial work began with an effort to develop course content in the basic curriculum by focusing on common human needs, using care and comfort as organizing principles, and stressing tension reduction. Through reasoning, Johnson then began to theorize that nursing's specific contribution to patient welfare was the fostering of efficient and effective behavioral functioning. That perspective led her to accept the theoretical view of the person as a behavioral system, similar to the way that physicians accept the person as a biological system (Fawcett, 2005; Johnson, 1990).

OVERVIEW OF *Johnson's* BEHAVIORAL SYSTEM MODEL

THE GOALS OF NURSING IN Johnson's behavioral system model are to maintain or restore behavioral system balance. Her model for nursing presents the client as a living open system, which is in turn a collection of behavioral subsystems that interrelate to form a behavioral system. Because the subsystems are linked and open, a disturbance in one subsystem will likely have an effect on the other subsystems (Johnson, 1980). Johnson proposed that seven subsystems of behavior exist: achievement, affiliative, aggressive, dependence, sexual, eliminative, and ingestive.

Subsystems include structural components that consist of four elements: (1) drive or a goal, (2) a set, (3) a choice, and (4) an action or behavior. The *drive or goal* of the subsystem reflects the motivation or reasons for the behaviors of the subsystem. Motivational drives direct the activities or behaviors of the subsystems; they may vary from strong to weak and are constantly changing because of maturation, experience, and learning. The *set* comprises the ordinary or normal behaviors that the patient prefers to use to meet the goal of a subsystem. The *choice* represents the options that are available to the patient to meet his or her subsystem goals. This structural component is affected by variables such as gender, age, culture, socioeconomic status, and health status. The final subsystem structural component, an *action or behavior*, emanates as a consequence of the previous three structural components. The question of concern in relation to the structural component of behavior is whether the behavior is efficient and effective in relation to subsystem goal attainment. This is the only structural component that can be directly observed (Johnson, 1980).

Johnson proposed that seven subsystems of behavior exist: achievement, affiliative, aggressive, dependence, sexual, eliminative, and ingestive.

Each subsystem has a function. The **achievement subsystem** functions to control or master an aspect of self or environment to achieve a standard. This subsystem encompasses intellectual, physical, creative, mechanical, and social skills. The **affiliative or attachment subsystem** forms the basis for social organization. Its consequences are social inclusion, intimacy, and the formation and maintenance of strong social bonds. The **aggressive or protective subsystem** functions to protect and preserve the system. The **dependency subsystem** promotes helping or nurturing behaviors. Their consequences include approval, recognition, and physical assistance. The **sexual subsystem** has the function of procreation and gratification and includes development of gender-role identity and gender-role behaviors. The **eliminative subsystem** addresses "when, how, and under what conditions we eliminate," whereas the **ingestive subsystem** "has to do with when, how, what, how much, and under what conditions we eat" (Johnson, 1980, p. 213).

Johnson asserted that each of the subsystems, as well as the system as a whole, has certain functional requirements that must be met through the effort of the individual or through outside assistance for continued growth, development, and viability. These functional requirements include (1) protection from noxious influences with which the system cannot cope, (2) nurturance through input of supplies from the environment (e.g., food, friendship, caring), and (3) stimulation by experiences, events, and behavior that would enhance growth and prevent stagnation (Johnson, 1980, p. 212).

The nursing process for the behavioral system model is known as **Johnson's nursing diagnostic and treatment process**. The components of this process include determination of the existence of a problem, diagnostic classification of problems, management of nursing problems, and evaluation of behavioral system balance and stability.

When using Johnson's model in practice, the focus of the assessment process is obtaining information to evaluate current behavior in terms of past patterns, determining the effects of the current illness on behavioral patterns, and establishing the maximum level of health. The assessment specifically seeks to gather information related to the structure and function of the eight behavioral subsystems as well as the environmental factors that affect the behavioral subsystems (Holaday, 2006). During the assessment phase, the nurse obtains data about the nature of the behavioral functioning related to goal obtainment. These data related to client behavior are couched in terms of whether that behavior is purposeful, orderly, and predictable. The nurse also interviews the client and family to assess the condition of the subsystem structural components and assesses the client's behavior for behavioral system balance and stability. From the data collected, the nurse makes inferences related to the organization, interaction, and integration of the subsystems (Fawcett, 2005).

Problems may be classified as either internal subsystem problems or intersystem problems. Internal subsystem problems may include situations when functional requirements are not met, there is inconsistency or disharmony among components of subsystem, or behavior is not appropriate for the culture. Intersystem problems may include situations in which the behavioral system is dominated by one or two subsystems or in which a conflict exists between two or more subsystems (Fawcett, 2005).

In Johnson's model, the goals of the management of nursing problems are to restore, maintain, or attain balance and stability in the client's behavioral system and to help the client achieve an optimal level of balance and functioning. The goals of management are accomplished through the temporary imposition of external regulatory or control mechanisms, the repair of damaged subsystem structural components, or the fulfillment of subsystem functional requirements (Johnson, 1980, p. 214). The nurse may temporarily impose external regulatory or control mechanisms by setting limits for behavior, inhibiting ineffective behavioral responses, assisting the patient to develop new responses, and reinforcing appropriate behaviors. Repair of damaged structural components includes interventions that influence the patient's drive or motivation or redirect the patient's goals. Interventions also include altering set behaviors through instruction or counseling and adding choices through teaching new skills. The nurse can also intervene to fulfill functional requirements by protecting the patient from overwhelming negative influences that exceed the patient's coping ability, by nurturing the patient through input of adequate essential supplies, and by providing stimulation to enhance growth and prevent stagnation (Fawcett, 2005; Johnson, 1980).

Evaluation is based on the attainment of the goal of balance in the identified subsystems. Evaluation of behavioral system balance and stability is accomplished as the nurse compares the client's behavior after treatment to indices of behavioral system balance and stability (Fawcett, 2005; Johnson, 1980).

> In Johnson's model, the goals of the management of nursing problems are to restore, maintain, or attain balance and stability in the client's behavioral system and to help the client achieve an optimal level of balance and functioning.

IN ADDITION TO THE CONCEPTS already presented, the four metaparadigm concepts of nursing are identified in Johnson's behavioral system model. These concepts are summarized in Table 7-1.

MAJOR CONCEPTS OF NURSING ACCORDING TO *Johnson*

Person

Within the behavioral system model, the person is viewed as a biological being—as a behavioral system with seven subsystems of behavior. According to this model, the role of medicine is to focus on the biological system, and the role of nursing is to focus on the behavioral system.

TABLE 7-1 Metaparadigm Concepts as Defined in Johnson's Theory	
Person (human being)	A biopsychosocial being who is a behavioral system with seven subsystems of behavior
Environment	Includes both the internal and external environments
Health	Efficient and effective functioning of system; behavioral system balance and stability
Nursing	An external regulatory force that acts to preserve the organization and integrity of the patient's behavior at an optimal level under those conditions in which the behavior constitutes a threat to physical or social health or in which illness is found (Johnson, 1980, p. 214)

Environment

In the behavioral system model, the environment includes both the internal and the external environments that are not a part of the individual's behavioral system but that influence the system. Strong environmental forces can disturb the balance of the behavioral system and threaten its stability (Loveland-Cherry & Wilkerson, 1989).

Health

Johnson (1980) refers to both physical and social health in defining the health metaparadigm. According to Johnson, health is determined by the interaction of psychological, social, biological, and physiological factors. Efficient and effective functioning of the system that results in behavioral system balance and stability is equivalent to a state of health. Illness, in contrast, is defined as behavioral system imbalance and instability.

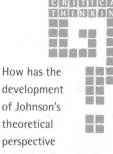

CRITICAL THINKING

How has the development of Johnson's theoretical perspective helped to frame nursing knowledge and influence nursing practice?

Nursing

According to Johnson's behavioral system model, nursing is an external regulatory force that acts to preserve the organization and integrity of the patient's behavior at an optimal level under those conditions in which the behavior constitutes a threat to physical or social health or in which illness is found. This force operates through the imposition of external regulatory or control mechanisms, through attempts to change structural units in desirable directions, or through the fulfillment of the functional requirements of the subsystems. Thus the purpose for nursing practice using Johnson's behavioral system is to facilitate restoration, maintenance, or attainment of behavioral system balance and stability (Johnson, 1980, p. 214). These goals are accomplished through the use of Johnson's nursing diagnostic and treatment process.

THE ANALYSIS PRESENTED HERE CONSISTS of an examination of assumptions and propositions as well as a brief critique of the behavioral system model as proposed by Dorothy Johnson.

> ## ANALYSIS OF *Johnson's* BEHAVIORAL SYSTEM MODEL

Assumptions of the Behavioral System Model

Johnson based her theory on a number of explicit and implicit assumptions. The major assumptions of the theory are as follows:

❖ Behavior is the sum total of physical, biologic, and social factors.

❖ A person is a system of behavior characterized by repetitive, predictable, and goal-directed behaviors that always strive toward balance.

❖ There are different levels of balance and stabilization, and levels are different during different time periods.

❖ Persons expend large amounts of energy attempting to maintain or reestablish behavioral system balance in response to imbalance caused by persistent excessive forces (Holaday, 2010; Meleis, 2007, p. 281).

Propositions of the Behavioral System Model

Primary relationships are seen in the behavioral system model between the person and the environment; between the person, health, and the environment; and between the person, nursing, and health. Primary relationships of the behavioral systems model include the following:

❖ The behavioral system manages its relationship with the environment, which is self-maintaining as long as conditions remain orderly.

❖ Balance is essential for effective and efficient functions of the person; a lack of balance in the structural or functional requirements of the subsystems leads to poor health.

❖ Nursing is an external regulatory force that acts to restore balance to the behavioral system (Holaday, 2010; Johnson, 1980).

Brief Critique of the Behavioral System Model

The behavioral system model was developed by Johnson using inductive reasoning, based on her observations made during many years of nursing practice, as well as on nursing literature and research. The model is fairly simple as far as the number of concepts goes, and the concepts of nursing and behavioral system are described in detail. The model has nearly unlimited applicability with ill persons; however, it has not yet been used as extensively with well persons (Holaday, 2010). Johnson addressed the criticism that the model did not allow for a focus on prevention by stating that "preventive nursing is not possible until problems in the behavioral system are explicated. To the extent that any problem that might arise can be anticipated . . . preventive action is in order" (1990, p. 31).

The concepts within the behavioral system model are clearly and consistently defined (Loveland-Cherry & Wilkerson, 1989), and the comprehensiveness of the model has proven to be adequate for providing direction for nursing research, education, administration, and practice (Fawcett, 2005). Some adaptations of the model have appeared in the literature since the model has been used by others, including the addition of an eighth subsystem dealing with restorative behavior and some alternative interpretations of the functions of subsystems (Fawcett, 2005). In response to these additions and alterations, Johnson has stated, "These changes are such that they alter the fundamental nature of the behavioral system as originally proposed, and I do not agree with them" (1990, p. 27).

Johnson's behavioral system model makes an important contribution to nursing knowledge by directing attention to the person's behavior rather than to the disease state. Johnson used that distinction to clarify the different foci of the disciplines of nursing and medicine (Fawcett, 2005). When beginning her work, she identified that at the time there was no delineated theoretical framework for the discipline of nursing. Thus she began her work in earnest related to the conceptualization of nursing and the other components of the behavioral system model. According to Johnson, only when definitions and specific goals were articulated would nursing be able to begin to speak of a science of nursing (Johnson, 1959).

Johnson's BEHAVIORAL SYSTEM MODEL AS A FRAMEWORK FOR NURSING PRACTICE

THE PURPOSE FOR NURSING PRACTICE using Johnson's behavioral system is to facilitate restoration, maintenance, or attainment of behavioral system balance and stability (Fawcett, 2005). These goals are accomplished through the use of Johnson's nursing diagnostic and treatment process.

THE NURSING PROCESS AND Johnson's BEHAVIORAL SYSTEM MODEL

JOHNSON'S NURSING DIAGNOSTIC AND TREATMENT process includes four components: determination of the existence of a problem, diagnostic classification of problems, management of nursing problems, and evaluation of behavioral system balance and stability.

Assessment and Planning

During the assessment phase of the nursing process, the nurse obtains data about the nature of the behavioral functioning related to goal obtainment. The nurse also obtains data related to client behavior indicating whether that behavior is purposeful, orderly, and predictable. In addition, the nurse interviews the client and family to assess the condition of the subsystem structural components and assesses the client's behavior for behavioral system balance and stability. From the data collected, the nurse makes inferences related to the organization, interaction, and integration of the subsystems.

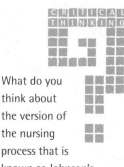

What do you think about the version of the nursing process that is known as Johnson's nursing diagnostic and treatment process? Do you think that it allows the nurse to meet the standards of care practice requirements for assessment, planning, implementation, and evaluation?

Problems may include both internal subsystem problems and inter-system problems. Internal subsystem problems may encompass situations when functional requirements are not met, there is inconsistency or dis-harmony among components of subsystem, or behavior is not appropriate for the culture. Intersystem problems may include situations when the behavioral system is dominated by one or two subsystems or a conflict exists between two or more subsystems (Fawcett, 2005).

Implementation

The goals for the management of nursing problems are to restore, main-tain, or attain the client's behavioral system balance and stability and to help the client achieve an optimal level of balance and functioning (Fawcett, 2005).

Evaluation

Evaluation of behavioral system balance and stability is accomplished as the nurse compares the client's behavior after treatment to indices of behavioral system balance and stability (Fawcett, 2005).

SCENARIO ILLUSTRATING NURSING CARE AND *Johnson's* BEHAVIORAL SYSTEM MODEL

THE FOLLOWING SCENARIO ILLUSTRATES NURS-ING care of the patient relative to one identified nursing problem framed by Johnson's behavior system model. This scenario is not intended to cover all aspects of care, but rather is intended to stimulate thinking about how specific care might be approached using this theory as a framework for practice.

Mr. M. is a 52-year-old married, Caucasian male who is approximately 100 pounds overweight. As a result of his weight gain, Mr. M. has developed hypertension and adult-onset diabetes. He is currently being fol-lowed in an outpatient healthcare setting.

Using Johnson's behavioral system model and the corresponding nursing diagnostic and treatment process, the nurse will begin the assessment process by obtaining information to evaluate current behavior in terms of past patterns, and determining the effects of the current illness on Mr. M.'s behavioral patterns. The assessment specifically seeks to gather information related to the structure and function of the eight behavioral subsystems as well as the environmental factors that affect the behavioral subsystems. Assessment of the subsystems will include four structural components: (1) drive or a goal, (2) set, (3) choice, and (4) action or behavior. In this case, it will focus on when, how, what, how much, and under which conditions Mr. M. eats. After further assessment, it is determined that Mr. M. eats more and more often when he experiences stress.

Once the existence of a problem has been confirmed, the nurse will diagnostically classify the problem. From the data collected, the nurse makes inferences related to the organization, interaction, and integration of Mr. M.'s subsystems and, in collaboration with the patient, plans and sets goals. In this scenario, the patient's blood pressure and diabetes are currently under control, so Mr. M. and the nurse choose to focus on the ingestive subsystem, which is negatively affecting other subsystems; at the same time, current best practices will be observed in providing care related to all identified problems.

The goals of the management of nursing problems are to restore, maintain, or attain the balance and stability of the client's behavioral system and to help the client achieve an optimal level of balance and functioning. To achieve this goal, the nurse may temporarily impose external regulatory or control mechanisms by setting limits for ingestive behavior, inhibiting ineffective behavioral responses in which the patient eats to deal with stressors, assisting the patient to develop new responses to stressors, and reinforcing appropriate behaviors.

Evaluation is accomplished as the nurse compares the client's ingestive behavior as well as the effects of the ingestive subsystem on other subsystems after treatment. The goal of the management for Mr. M. is to restore his behavioral system balance and stability and to help him achieve an optimal level of balance and functioning—in this case, optimal weight for height and age, blood pressure within normal range, and maintenance of blood sugar within normal range.

CLASSROOM ACTIVITY 7-1

Form small groups. Each group should add to the plan of care for Mr. M. in the preceding scenario based on other potential or actual nursing problems typical for a patient with same medical diagnosis or symptoms and demographics, specifically considering other subsystems. Each group should develop a plan for one additional nursing problem using Johnson's theory as the basis for practice. Each group should then share its plan with the class.

CLASSROOM ACTIVITY 7-2

Form small groups. Using a case study provided by the instructor, develop a plan of care using Johnson's nursing theory as the basis for practice. Each group should then share its plan of care with the class.

CLASSROOM ACTIVITY 7-3

Form small groups. Using a case study provided by the instructor, develop a plan of care using one of the theories as the basis for practice; each group should select a different nursing theory. Each group should then share its plan of care with the class and discuss the similarities and differences in care.

REFERENCES

Fawcett, J. (2005). *Contemporary nursing knowledge: Analysis and evaluation of nursing models and theories* (2nd ed.). Philadelphia: F. A. Davis.

Holaday, B. (2006). Johnson's behavioral system model in nursing practice. In M. R. Alligood & A. M. Tomey (Eds.), *Nursing theory: Utilization and application* (3rd ed., pp. 157–180). St. Louis, MO: Mosby.

Holaday, B. (2010). Behavioral system model. In A. M Tomey & M. R. Alligood (Eds.), *Nursing theories and their work* (7th ed., pp. 366–390). Maryland Heights, MO: Mosby.

Johnson, D. E. (1959). The nature of a science of nursing. *Nursing Outlook, 7,* 291–294.

Johnson, D. (1980). The behavioral systems model for nursing. In J. Riehl & C. Roy (Eds.), *Conceptual models for nursing practice* (2nd ed., pp. 207–216). New York: Appleton-Century-Crofts.

Johnson, D. E. (1990). The behavior systems model for nursing. In M. E. Parker (Ed.), *Nursing theories in practice* (pp. 23–32). New York: National League for Nursing.

Loveland-Cherry, C. J., & Wilkerson, S. A. (1989). Dorothy Johnson's behavioral system model. In J. J. Fitzpatrick & A. L. Whall (Eds.), *Conceptual models of nursing* (2nd ed., pp. 147–163). Englewood Cliffs, NJ: Prentice-Hall.

Meleis, A. I. (2007). *Theoretical nursing: Development and progress* (4th ed.). Philadelphia: Lippincott Williams & Wilkins.

INTERACTING SYSTEMS FRAMEWORK AND THEORY OF GOAL ATTAINMENT:
Imogene King

8

LEARNING OBJECTIVES

After completing this chapter the student should be able to

1. Describe the interacting systems that are identified by King

2. Explain the major concepts important to nursing as defined by King

3. Plan nursing care for a patient scenario utilizing King's theory of goal attainment within the context of King's interacting systems framework

KEY TERMS

Interaction–transaction process
Interpersonal systems

Personal systems
Social systems

BACKGROUND

IMOGENE M. KING WAS BORN in 1923 in Iowa. She earned a diploma in nursing in 1945 and a bachelor of science in nursing education in 1948. King worked as a medical–surgical nursing instructor and assistant director of St. John's Hospital School of Nursing from 1947 to 1958. In 1957, she received a master of science in nursing degree. In 1961, she received a doctor of education degree from Teachers College, Columbia University. In 1971, while she was Director at the School of Nursing at Ohio State University, King's first book was published. During the years that followed, King served in various administrative, research, and advisory positions. In addition to writing numerous book chapters and articles, King published a second book in 1981, with a third book to follow in subsequent years. Imogene King retired in 1990 but remained active as a guest lecturer and in community service until her death in 2007 (Sieloff & Messmer, 2010).

OVERVIEW OF *Imogene King's* INTERACTING SYSTEMS FRAMEWORK AND THEORY OF GOAL ATTAINMENT

KING REVEALS IN THE PREFACE of her first book that the purpose of the book is "to propose a conceptual frame of reference for nursing" (1971, p. ix). Moreover, she asserts, "The framework suggests that the essential characteristics of nursing are those properties that have persisted in spite of environmental changes" (p. ix). She continues by explaining that because of "a personal concern about the changes influencing nursing" (p. x), she was prompted to explore several questions, including these:

What is the scope of practice of nursing, and in what kind of settings do nurses perform their functions? Are the current goals of nursing similar to those of the past half century? What are the dimensions of practice that have given the field of nursing a unifying focus over time? (p. x)

Reflection upon these questions led King to select four universal ideas that included social systems, health, perception, and interpersonal relations and to explore the relevance of these ideas to nursing. These ideas provided the general frame of reference for identifying concepts that then suggested more specific directives for nursing practice (King, 1971, p. x).

What resulted was the development of a conceptual framework and the theory of goal attainment. King's conceptual framework is more abstract than her theory and presents a broader view of an area of interest; although conceptual linkages occur in both the framework and the theory, the linkages are more clearly delineated in the theory (Evans, 1991; Meleis, 2007).

Because all systems include the essential elements of structure, function, resources, goal(s), and decision making, King attempted to provide a structure for nursing as a discipline and profession by using a systems framework as a basis for the development of her conceptual framework. In the conceptual framework, the structure of a system is viewed as an open system with semipermeable boundaries between individuals, groups, and society, all of which interact with the environment. The functions of these three systems are identified in the reciprocal relations of individuals as they interact in groups. Resources are essential to perform functions within a structure and attain goals. The allocation of human and material resources involves choice or decision making within the system. Decisions at one level of function influence the behavior at all levels and are reflected in outcomes. The goal is to keep the system in harmony or health (King, 1990, pp. 75–76; 1995, p. 25).

King, in what became known as the interacting systems framework, determined that health concerns related to nursing could be grouped into categories known as dynamic interacting systems. King conceptualized three levels of dynamic interacting systems: **personal systems** (individuals), **interpersonal systems** (groups), and **social systems** (society). Individuals exist within personal systems, and concepts relevant to this system include body image, growth and development, perception, self, space, and time. Interpersonal systems are formed when two or more individuals interact. The concepts important to understanding this system include communication, interaction, role, stress, and transaction. Examples of social systems may include religious systems, educational systems, and healthcare systems. Concepts important to understanding

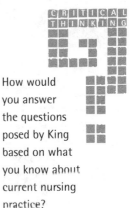

CRITICAL THINKING

How would you answer the questions posed by King based on what you know about current nursing practice?

King conceptualized three levels of dynamic interacting systems: personal systems (individuals), interpersonal systems (groups), and social systems (society).

the social system include authority, decision making, organization, power, and status (Evans, 1991; King, 1981; Sieloff, 2006). These three "systems with identified concepts provide a way of organizing one's knowledge, skills, and values" (King, 1989, p. 151).

King's theory of goal attainment was derived from her interacting systems framework (Sieloff, 2006) and addresses nursing as a process of human interaction (Norris & Frey, 2006). The theory focuses on the interpersonal system interactions in the nurse–client relationship. During the nursing process, the nurse and the client each perceive each other, make judgments, and take action that results in reaction. Interaction results, and if perceptual congruence exists, transactions occur (Sieloff, 2006). Outcomes are defined in terms of goals to be attained. If the goals are related to patient behaviors, then they become criteria by which the effectiveness of nursing care can be measured (King, 1989, p.156).

> King's theory of goal attainment was derived from her interacting systems framework and addresses nursing as a process of human interaction.

MAJOR CONCEPTS OF NURSING ACCORDING TO *King*

IN ADDITION TO THE CONCEPTS already presented, the four metaparadigm concepts of nursing are identified in King's theory. These concepts are summarized in Table 8-1.

Person

The individual is conceptualized as a personal system. The personal system focuses on individual human beings. Characteristics of human beings identified by King include being a complex, open living system that copes with wide range of events, persons, and things over time. Human beings react as a whole and, therefore, must be viewed as an entire living system. The concepts of body image, growth and development, perception, self, space, and time are relevant to the personal system (Evans, 1991).

Environment

King (1990) defines the environment as the social system surrounding the concept in question. It can be both external and internal. The external environment is the context "within which human beings grow, develop,

TABLE 8-1 Metaparadigm Concepts as Defined in King's Model	
Person (human being)	A personal system that interacts with interpersonal and social systems.
Environment	Can be both external and internal. The external environment is the context "within which human beings grow, develop, and perform daily activities" (King, 1981, p. 18); the internal environment of human beings transforms energy to enable them to adjust to continuous external environmental changes (King, 1981, p. 5).
Health	"Dynamic life experiences of a human being, which implies continuous adjustment to stressors in the internal and external environment through optimum use of one's resources to achieve maximum potential for daily living" (King, 1981, p. 5).
Nursing	A process of human interaction with the goal of helping patients achieve to their goals.

and perform daily activities" (King, 1981, p. 18); the internal environment of human beings transforms energy to enable them to adjust to continuous external environmental changes (King, 1981, p. 5). In this holistic view of environment, external and internal aspects of the environment are interrelated (Evans, 1991).

Health

Although the health of individuals and groups is the goal for nursing, health and illness are not seen as a part of a linear continuum by King. She chose not to address the concept of wellness due to the abstract nature of the concept and because it would lend support to the continuum perspective (Evans, 1991; King, 1990). However, the notion of some differences in health states is described as the "level of health." According to King, this level of health affects the individual's ability to perform activities of daily living; in turn, the ability to perform activities of daily living depends on the harmony and balance in the individual's environment (King, 1981, p. 4).

According to King, health is reflected in "dynamic life experiences of a human being, which implies continuous adjustment to stressors in the internal and external environment through optimum use of one's resources to achieve maximum potential for daily living" (King, 1981, p.

5). Health is a "functional state in the life cycle" (p. 5) and illness has to do with "some interference in the cycle" (p. 5).

Nursing

Based on a descriptive study, King formulated the following definition of nursing: "Nursing is a process of human interactions between nurse and client whereby each person perceives the other and the situation, and through communication they set goals, explore means, and agree on means to achieve goals" (King, 1981; 1990, p. 80). Other features of nursing practice include the following:

❖ The nurse and the patient do not know each other.

❖ The nurse is licensed to practice professional nursing.

❖ The patient is in need of the services provided by the nurse.

❖ The nurse and the patient are in a reciprocal relationship in that the nurse has special knowledge and skills to communicate appropriate information so as to help the patient set goals, and the patient has information about self and perceptions of problem that, when communicated to the nurse, will help in mutual goal setting.

❖ The nurse and the patient are in mutual presence, purposefully interacting to achieve goals.

❖ Interactions occur in a two-person group.

❖ Interactions are limited to those between the licensed professional nurse and the patient in need of nursing care.

❖ Interactions take place in natural environments (King, 1981, p. 150).

ANALYSIS OF *King's* THEORY OF GOAL ATTAINMENT

THE ANALYSIS PRESENTED HERE CONSISTS of an examination of assumptions and propositions as well as a brief critique of the theory of goal attainment.

Assumptions of the Theory of Goal Attainment

The theory of goal attainment is based on the following specific assumptions about human beings:

- ❖ Individuals are social beings.

- ❖ Individuals are sentient beings.

- ❖ Individuals are rational beings.

- ❖ Individuals are reacting beings.

- ❖ Individuals are perceiving beings.

- ❖ Individuals are controlling beings.

- ❖ Individuals are purposeful beings.

- ❖ Individuals are action-oriented beings.

- ❖ Individuals are time-oriented beings (King, 1981, p. 143).

The theory is based on the following specific assumptions about nurse–client interactions:

- ❖ Perceptions of nurse and of client influence the interaction process.

- ❖ Goals, needs, and values of nurse and client influence the interaction process.

- ❖ Individuals have a right to knowledge about themselves.

- ❖ Individuals have a right to participate in decisions that influence their life, their health, and community services.

- ❖ Health professionals have a responsibility to share information that helps individuals make informed decisions about their health care.

- ❖ Individuals have a right to accept or reject health care.

- ❖ The goals of health professionals and the goals of recipients of health care may be incongruent (King, 1981, p. 143–144).

Propositions of the Theory of Goal Attainment

Propositional statements are identified by King for the theory of goal attainment and include the following:

❖ If perceptual accuracy is present in nurse–client interactions, transactions will occur.

❖ If the nurse and the client make transactions, goals will be attained.

❖ If goals are attained, satisfactions will occur.

❖ If goals are attained, effective nursing care will occur.

❖ If transactions are made in the nurse–client interactions, growth and development will be enhanced.

❖ If role expectations and role performance as perceived by the nurse and the client are congruent, transactions will occur.

❖ If role conflict is experienced by the nurse, the client, or both, stress in nurse–client interactions will occur.

❖ If nurses with special knowledge and skills communicate appropriate information to clients, mutual goal setting and goal attainment will occur (King, 1981, p. 149).

Brief Critique of the Theory of Goal Attainment

The definitions in King's theory are clear and conceptually derived from the research literature in existence at the time of their publication. The theory of goal attainment has 10 major concepts, making the theory fairly complex although easily understandable. Empirical data were used in the development and refinement of the King's theory, and research continues as part of the testing of conceptual relationships within the theory. In the past, some criticism was leveled at this theory based on the claim that the theory of goal attainment has limited application in areas of nursing in which patients are unable to interact competently with the nurse. King has responded to this criticism by pointing out that 70 percent of communication is nonverbal. This argument must have satisfied at least some of the critics, given that King's conceptual model and theory of goal attainment continue to be used to provide quality, theory-based patient care in practice settings in numerous countries around the world (Sieloff & Messmer, 2010).

KING POSITS THAT NURSING IS a process of interactions that lead to transactions. Transactions lead to goal attainment, and goal attainment is a measure of effective nursing care. Nurse–patient interactions can be classified into one of eight categories:

- ❖ Action
- ❖ Reaction
- ❖ Disturbance
- ❖ Mutual goal setting
- ❖ Exploration of means to achieve the goal
- ❖ Agreement on means to achieve the goal
- ❖ Transaction
- ❖ Attainment of goal (King, 1981; 1990, p. 78, 80)

To implement the theory of goal attainment in practice, the goal-oriented nursing record was proposed (King, 1981, 1990). It consists of a nursing database that assesses patient abilities to perform activities of daily living, perceptions of health concern, and knowledge related to patient's learning needs. From these data, nursing diagnoses are constructed and goals are mutually set with patients. During these interactions, nurses provide information to assist patients in making informed decisions. When goals have been identified, nursing orders have been written based on the goals, and the progress notes indicate that the goals have been attained, effective nursing care has been documented (King, 1990, p. 82–83).

THE MODEL OF TRANSACTIONS, ALSO known as the **interaction–transaction process**, provides a theoretical basis for the nursing process as a method. Application of the model of transactions

King's
INTERACTING SYSTEMS FRAMEWORK AND THEORY OF GOAL ATTAINMENT AS A FRAMEWORK FOR NURSING PRACTICE

THE NURSING PROCESS AND *King's* **INTERACTING SYSTEMS FRAMEWORK AND THEORY OF GOAL ATTAINMENT: THE INTERACTION– TRANSACTION PROCESS**

in practice may be approached using the nursing process where assessment focuses on the perceptions of the nurse and the client, communication of the nurse and the client, and interaction of the nurse and the client. Planning involves a decision about goals and agreement as to how to attain those goals. Implementation focuses on transactions made, and evaluation focuses on goals attained using King's theory (King, 1992).

Assessment (Perception, Communication, Interaction)

During the phase corresponding to the assessment phase of the nursing process, the patient and the nurse perceive each other and the situation. Interaction is an ongoing process characterized by communication. Communication during this phase of the process includes the nurse gathering additional information, validating perceptions, delineating and validating patient concerns, and establishing mutual trust (Frey, 2010; King, 1999). Nursing functions during this phase include viewing, recognizing, observing, and measuring.

Planning (Decision Making, Exploration, Agreement)

Nursing functions during the planning phase include the synthesis, interpretation, and analysis of data within the context of the nursing process, followed by making decisions about mutually set goals. Next, decisions are made related to actions to meet the agreed-upon goals (Frey, 2010; King, 1999). These decisions are made by asking questions such as the following:

- ❖ Which goals will serve the patient's best interest?
- ❖ What are the patient's goals?
- ❖ Are the patient's goals and the nurse's goals for the patient congruent?
- ❖ If the goals are not congruent, what further communication and interaction are needed to achieve congruence?

❖ What are the priority goals?

❖ What does the patient perceive is the best way to attain goals?

❖ Is the patient willing to work toward attainment of goals?

❖ What does the nurse perceive as the best way to attain the goals?
(Frey, 2010, p. 195)

Implementation (Transaction)

The next step of the process results in the occurrence of transactions. Transactions take place as a result of perceiving the person or situation, making judgments about perceptions, and taking action. Reactions to actions lead to interaction between the nurse and the patient, which in turn leads to transactions that reflect a shared view and commitment. Transactions are made and inferred from interactions, although they are not amenable to direct observation (Frey, 2010; King, 1999). During this phase of the process, the nurse will ask questions such as these:

❖ Am I doing what we have agreed upon?

❖ How and when do I carry out the actions?

❖ Why am I carrying out the action?

❖ Is it reasonable to think that carrying out this action will allow attainment of goals? (Frey, 2010, p. 195–196)

CRITICAL THINKING

What do you think about the model of transactions as a theoretical basis for the nursing process? Do you think that it allows the nurse to meet the standards of care practice requirements for assessment, planning, implementation, and evaluation?

Evaluation (Goal Attainment)

The primary aim of the evaluation phase is to assess the attainment of goals and, if goals are not attained, to determine why they are not attained. Unmet goals can result from the identification of incorrect or incomplete data; incorrect interpretation of data as a result of perceptual error, lack of knowledge, or goal conflict; or barriers related to the nurse, patient, or system (Frey, 2010; King, 1999).

SCENARIO ILLUSTRATING NURSING CARE FRAMED BY *King's* SYSTEMS FRAMEWORK AND THEORY OF GOAL ATTAINMENT UTILIZING THE NURSING PROCESS

THE FOLLOWING SCENARIO ILLUSTRATES NURSING care of the patient relative to one identified nursing problem framed by King's theory of goal attainment. This scenario is not intended to cover all aspects of care, but rather is intended to stimulate thinking about how specific care might be approached using this theory as a framework for practice.

Mr. B. is a 78-year-old African American, married male who was referred to the home health nurse after his discharge from the local hospital. He has been prescribed a low-sodium diet due to fluid volume overload secondary to congestive heart failure.

During the initial visit, the nursing assessment focuses on the perceptions of the nurse and the client, communication of the nurse and the client, and interaction of the nurse and the client. The nurse begins by asking Mr. B. questions about his perception of the situation and his conclusions related to the situation. The nurse also asks the same questions of herself. Communication includes the nurse gathering additional information, validating her perceptions of Mr. B., validating the concerns of Mr. B., and establishing mutual trust. Nursing functions during assessment include viewing, recognizing, observing, and measuring; they reveal that Mr. B. consumes a diet high in sodium.

Planning for the care of Mr. B. will involve decisions about goals and agreement as to how to attain goals. These decisions are made by the nurse asking questions such as the following (adapted from Frey, 2010, p. 195): (1) Which goals will serve Mr. B's best interest? (2) What are Mr. B.'s goals? (3) Are Mr. B.'s goals and the nurse's goals for Mr. B. congruent? (4) If the goals are not congruent, what further communication and interaction are needed to achieve congruence? (5) What are the priority goals? (6) What does Mr. B. perceive to be the best way to attain goals? (7) Is Mr. B. willing to work toward attainment of goals? (8) What does the nurse perceive as the best way to attain the goals?

There is agreement that Mr. B. needs to adhere to the prescribed low-sodium diet. To achieve that goal as well as his ultimate goal of not being hospitalized again for fluid retention, Mr. B. will require some additional information related to his dietary restrictions.

The next step of the process results in the occurrence of transactions. During this phase of the process, the nurse and Mr. B. participate in teaching sessions related to his low-sodium diet. The nurse will need to ask questions to evaluate whether she is doing what she and Mr. B. agreed upon as well as questions related to the feasibility of meeting the goals based on the transaction.

The primary aim of the evaluation phase is to assess if the goals set by the nurse and Mr. B. have been attained and, if goals were not attained, then to determine why they were not attained. Throughout this model of transactions process, the nurse continues to assess and intervene to apply the model simultaneously to problems other than the low-sodium diet as indicated by the condition of Mr. B. and current best clinical practices.

CLASSROOM ACTIVITY 8-1

Form small groups. Each group should add to the plan of care for Mr. B. in the preceding scenario based on other potential or actual nursing problems typical for a patient with same medical diagnosis or symptoms and demographics. Each group should develop a plan for one additional nursing problem using King's theory as the basis for practice. Each group should then share its plan with the class.

CLASSROOM ACTIVITY 8-2

Form small groups. Using a case study provided by the instructor, develop a plan of care using King's nursing theory as the basis for practice. Each group should then share its plan of care with the class.

CLASSROOM ACTIVITY 8-3

Form small groups. Using a case study provided by the instructor, develop a plan of care using one of the theories as the basis for practice; each group should select a different nursing theory. Each group should then share its plan of care with the class and discuss the similarities and differences in care.

REFERENCES

Evans, C. S. (1991). *Imogene King: A conceptual framework for nursing.* Newbury Park, CA: Sage.

Frey, M. A. (2010). King's conceptual system and theory of goal attainment in nursing practice. In M. A. Alligood (Ed.), *Nursing theory: Utilization and application* (4th ed., pp. 187–210). Maryland Heights, MO: Mosby.

King, I. M. (1971). *Toward a theory for nursing: General concepts of human behavior.* New York: John Wiley and Sons.

King, I. M. (1981). *A theory of nursing: Systems, concepts, process.* New York: John Wiley and Sons.

King, I. M. (1989). King's general systems framework and theory. In J. P. Riehl-Sisca (Ed.), *Conceptual models for nursing practice* (3rd ed., pp. 149–158). Norwalk, CT: Appleton & Lange.

King, I. M. (1990). King's conceptual framework and theory of goal attainment. In M. E. Parker (Ed.), *Nursing theories in practice* (pp. 73–84). New York: National League for Nursing.

King, I. M. (1992). King's theory of goal attainment. *Nursing Science Quarterly, 5*(1), 19–26.

King, I. M. (1995). The theory of goal attainment. In M. A. Frey & C. L. Sieloff (Eds.), *Advancing King's systems framework and theory of nursing* (pp. 23–32). Thousand Oaks, CA: Sage.

King, I. M. (1999). A theory of goal attainment: Philosophical and ethical implications. *Nursing Science Quarterly, 12*(4), 292–296.

Meleis, A. I. (2007). *Theoretical nursing: Development and progress* (4th ed.). Philadelphia: Lippincott Williams & Wilkins.

Norris, D., & Frey, M. A. (2006). King's system framework and theory in nursing practice. In M. R. Alligood & A. M. Tomey (Eds.), *Nursing theory: Utilization and application* (3rd ed., pp. 181–205). St. Louis, MO: Mosby.

Sieloff, C. L. (2006). Imogene King: Interacting systems framework and middle range theory of goal attainment. In A. M. Tomey & M. R. Alligood (Eds.), *Nursing theorists and their work* (6th ed., pp. 297–317). St. Louis, MO: Mosby.

Sieloff, C. L., & Messmer, P. R. (2010). Conceptual system and middle range theory of goal attainment. In A. M Tomey & M. R. Alligood (Eds.), *Nursing theories and their work* (7th ed., pp. 286–308). Maryland Heights, MO: Mosby.

SCIENCE OF UNITARY HUMAN BEINGS:
Martha Rogers

9

LEARNING OBJECTIVES

After completing this chapter the student should be able to

1. Identify and describe the concepts specific to the science of unitary human beings as proposed by Rogers

2. Explain the major concepts important to nursing as defined by Rogers

3. Plan nursing care for a patient scenario utilizing Rogers' science of unitary human beings

KEY TERMS

Helicy
Integrality

Resonancy

BACKGROUND

MARTHA ELIZABETH ROGERS WAS BORN on May 12, 1914, in Dallas, Texas, but was raised in Tennessee. She studied science at the University of Tennessee from 1931 until 1933 and received her diploma in nursing from Knoxville General Hospital School of Nursing in 1936. Shortly thereafter, she received a bachelor of science degree from George Peabody College in Nashville, Tennessee. In addition, Rogers earned a master of arts degree in public health nursing from Teachers College in 1945, a master of public health degree in 1952, and a doctor of science degree from Johns Hopkins University in 1954.

Rogers' early nursing career focused on rural public health nursing and visiting nursing. From 1954 until 1979, she was a professor of nursing at New York University, where from 1954 until 1975 she also served as the department chair of the Division of Nursing. From 1979 until her death in 1994, she held the title of Professor Emeritus.

During her professional career, Rogers wrote three books and more than 200 articles. She lectured in nearly every state in the United States as well as in many other countries around the world. She received numerous honorary doctorates and awards to acknowledge her many contributions to nursing.

Rogers gave credit to scientists from multiple disciplines for influencing her development of the science of unitary human beings. Rogerian science emerged from an interrelationship of sciences such as anthropology, sociology, psychology, religion, philosophy, astronomy, history, biology, physics, mathematics, and literature as well as from Nightingale's proposals "placing human beings within the framework of the natural world" (Gunther, 2010a, p. 243).

OVERVIEW OF
Martha Rogers'
SCIENCE OF
UNITARY HUMAN
BEINGS

ACCORDING TO ROGERS (1994), NURSING is a learned profession, both a science and an art. The art of nursing is the creative use of the science of nursing for human betterment.

Rogers' theory asserts that human beings are dynamic energy fields, which are integrated with environmental energy fields. She asserts that a person and his or her environment form a single unit. As such, the human does not adapt to the environment and the environment does not cause anything to happen to the individual; rather, the person and the environment change together. Once change occurs, neither the person nor the environment can return to the former state (Johnson & Webber, 2010). Both human energy fields and environmental fields are open systems, pandimensional in nature and in a constant state of change. Pattern is the identifying characteristic of energy fields.

Rogers identified the principles of helicy, resonancy, and integrality as part of her work in describing the nature of change within human and environmental energy fields. Collectively, these principles are known as the principle of homeodynamics. The **helicy** principle describes the unpredictable but continuous, nonlinear evolution of energy fields, as evidenced by a spiral development that is a continuous, nonrepeating, and innovative patterning that reflects the nature of change. **Resonancy** is depicted as a wave frequency and an energy field pattern evolution from lower- to higher-frequency wave patterns; it is reflective of the continuous variability of the human energy field as it changes. The principle of **integrality** emphasizes the continuous mutual process of person and environment (Rogers, 1970; 1992).

Rogers used two widely recognized toys to help illustrate her theory and the constant interaction of the human–environment process. The Slinky illustrates the openness, rhythm, motion, balance, and expanding nature of the human life process, which is continuously evolving (Rogers, 1970). The kaleidoscope illustrates the changing patterns that appear to be infinitely different (Johnson & Webber, 2010, p. 142).

IN ADDITION TO THE CONCEPTS already presented, the four metaparadigm concepts of nursing are identified in Rogers' theory of unitary human beings. These concepts are summarized in Table 9-1.

The art of nursing is the creative use of the science of nursing for human betterment.

CRITICAL THINKING

How has the development of Rogers' theoretical perspective affected the development of nursing knowledge and the practice of nursing?

MAJOR CONCEPTS OF NURSING ACCORDING TO *Rogers*

TABLE 9-1 Metaparadigm Concepts as Defined in Roger's Theory	
Person (human being)	An irreducible, irreversible, pandimensional, negentropic energy field identified by pattern; the unitary human being develops through three principles: helicy, resonancy, and integrality (Rogers, 1992)
Environment	An irreducible, pandimensional, negentropic energy field, identified by pattern, manifesting characteristics different from those of the parts, and encompassing all that is other than any given human field (Rogers, 1992)
Health	Health and illness are a part of a continuum (Rogers, 1970)
Nursing	Seeks to promote symphonic interaction between human and environmental fields, to strengthen the integrity of the human field, and to direct and redirect patterning of the human and environmental fields for realization of maximum health potential (Rogers, 1970)

Person

The person is defined as an irreducible, irreversible, pandimensional, negentropic energy field, identified by pattern and manifesting characteristics that are specific to the whole and that cannot be predicted from knowledge of the parts (Rogers, 1992, p. 27). The unitary human being develops through three principles: helicy, resonancy, and integrality (Rogers, 1992).

Environment

The environment is defined as an irreducible, pandimensional, negentropic energy field, identified by pattern and manifesting characteristics different from those of the parts and encompassing all that is other than any given human field (Rogers, 1992, p. 27). The human field and the environmental field coexist without limits and boundaries, with the environment being viewed as a whole with the human energy field embedded within it.

Health

In Rogers' (1970) theory, health and illness are a part of a continuum, albeit one that is not explicitly defined. Rogers views the concepts of health and illness as manifestations of pattern. She uses the term "passive health" to refer to wellness or the absence of disease and major illness (Rogers, 1970).

CRITICAL THINKING

What do you think about the abstract conceptualization of person and environment as proposed in Rogers' theoretical framework? Do these conceptualizations adequately explain the phenomena of interest to nursing?

Nursing

Rogers views nursing as both an art and a science. Nursing seeks to promote symphonic interaction between human and environmental fields, to strengthen the integrity of the human field, and to direct and redirect patterning of the human and environmental fields for realization of maximum health potential (Rogers, 1970). Thus the focus of nursing is on the unitary human being and his or her environment.

THE ANALYSIS PRESENTED HERE CONSISTS of an examination of assumptions and propositions as well as a brief critique of the science of unitary human beings as proposed by Martha Rogers.

> ## ANALYSIS OF *Rogers'* SCIENCE OF UNITARY HUMAN BEINGS

Assumptions of Rogers' Science of Unitary Human Beings

Rogers (1970) identified five assumptions that support and connect the concepts within her conceptual model:

❖ "Man is a unified whole possessing his own integrity and manifesting characteristics more than and different from the sum of his parts" (p. 47).

❖ "Man and environment are continuously exchanging matter and energy with one another" (p. 54).

❖ "The life process evolves irreversibly and unidirectionally along the space–time continuum" (p. 59).

❖ "Pattern and organization identify man and reflect his innovative wholeness" (p. 65).

❖ "Man is characterized by the capacity for abstraction and imagery, language and thought, sensation, and emotion" (p. 73).

The first four assumptions relate to all living systems including the person. The fifth assumption relates only to the human being.

Propositions of Rogers' Science of Unitary Human Beings

The relational propositions of the science of unitary human beings link the four metaparadigm concepts of nursing as summarized here:

1. For nurses, the focus consists of long-established concern with people and the world they live in. It is the natural forerunner of an organized, abstract system encompassing people and their environments (Rogers, 1992, p. 28).

2. The nurse is an environmental component for the individual receiving services (Rogers, 1992, p. 61).

3. The primary focus of nursing is to promote health (Rogers, 1992, p. 61).

4. The purpose of nurses is to promote well-being for all persons, wherever they are (Rogers, 1992, p. 28).

5. The purpose of nursing is to promote human betterment wherever people are, on planet earth or in outer space (Rogers, 1992, p. 33).

The concepts of health, environment, and person are linked in the first two propositions. The third proposition links nursing and health. Propositions 4 and 5 link person, nursing, and health, and the last proposition provides linkages between all four metaparadigm concepts (Fawcett, 2005, p. 326).

Brief Critique of Rogers' Science of Unitary Human Beings

The science of unitary human beings was developed using deductive logic and demonstrates both logical congruence and internal consistency. The model is abstract and complex; however, ongoing work has simplified, operationalized, and clarified many of the concepts and relationships, resulting in the development of testable theories derived from the model. While the model initially had many critics, the Rogerian model has gained in popularity as scientific knowledge has evolved. The focus on the concepts within the model is on understanding human evolution, and the emphasis is on integrality of the human–environmental relationship. Nevertheless, researchers have demonstrated that Rogers' model has applications in all areas of nursing, including practice, education, and research (Gunther, 2010a). In addition to the Rogerian model's other contributions, three theories of nursing have been derived from the science of unitary human beings: the theory of accelerating evolution, the theory of rhythmical correlates of change, and the theory of paranormal phenomena (Fawcett, 2005, p. 19).

Rogers' model is an abstract system of ideas but is applicable to practice, with nursing care focused on pattern appraisal and patterning activities.

ROGERS' MODEL IS AN ABSTRACT system of ideas but is applicable to practice, with nursing care focused on pattern appraisal and patterning activities. Pattern appraisal involves a comprehensive assessment of environmental field patterns and human field patterns of communication, exchange, rhythms, dissonance, and harmony through the use of cognitive input, sensory input, intuition, and language. Patterning activities may include interventions such as meditation, imagery, journaling, and modifying surroundings. Evaluation is ongoing and requires a repetition of the appraisal process (Gunther, 2006).

Rogers' **SCIENCE OF UNITARY HUMAN BEINGS AS A FRAMEWORK FOR NURSING PRACTICE**

IN THIS SECTION, ROGERS' SCIENCE of unitary human beings is discussed in the context of the steps of the nursing process.

THE NURSING PROCESS AND *Rogers'* **SCIENCE OF UNITARY HUMAN BEINGS**

Assessment

The assessment process begins with the appraisal, which seeks to identify patterns. Pattern appraisal requires an assessment that incorporates cognitive input, sensory input, intuition, and language. During an interview process, the patient is encouraged to reflect on patterns that include nutrition, exercise, sleep and wake cycle, work, leisure, and relationships (Gunther, 2010b).

Planning

Once the patient and the nurse reach consensus regarding the pattern appraisal, the planning can begin related to the process of patterning.

Implementation

Nursing action focuses on mutual patterning of the human–environmental field. The goal of the nurse is to promote symphonic rhythms of this field. Patterning activities can be developed to address dissonance that may be described by the patient in terms such as pain, discomfort, or anxiety (Gunther, 2010b).

Patterning activities may include the nurse assisting the patient with meditation, imagery, visualization, or therapeutic touch when there is a primary focus on human field patterning. The practice known as "centering" is vital to many patterning activities. When centering, the patient focuses on his or her core or energy field. The purpose of patterning is to heal the physical body or to modify the perception of dissonance (Gunther, 2010b).

The environment is the other component of the human–environmental field and, as such, may promote either health or dissonance. The key point to remember in considering environmental field patterning is the importance of interrelationship. The nurse works with the patient in the context of the family and community, which together create a situation of energy patterns flowing through energy patterns. Thus the family must be involved in the patterning process. According to this model, when there is harmony of the fields, the potential for change increases. Within the Rogerian model, the anticipated change is reflected in harmonious patterns or a decrease in dissonance for the patient (Gunther, 2010b).

Evaluation

Evaluation using Rogers' model is ongoing and consists of a repetition of the appraisal process. Emphasis is placed on identifying perceptions of dissonance related to the initial pattern appraisal. This process continues as long as the nurse–patient relationship continues (Gunther, 2010b).

THE FOLLOWING SCENARIO ILLUSTRATES NURS-ING care of the patient relative to one identified nursing problem framed by Rogers' science of unitary human beings. This scenario is not intended to cover all aspects of care, but rather is intended to stimulate thinking about how specific care might be approached using this theory as a framework for practice.

SCENARIO ILLUSTRATING NURSING CARE FRAMED BY *Rogers'* SCIENCE OF UNITARY HUMAN BEINGS UTILIZING THE NURSING PROCESS

Mrs. M. is a 53-year-old Caucasian who is sedentary. She has experienced some weight gain over the past year and has noticed a decrease in her endurance when she is climbing stairs in her home and office building. Mrs. M. is visiting the nurse in the outpatient health-care setting.

The assessment process for Mrs. M. will begin with the appraisal and identification of patterns. This process will incorporate an interview between Mrs. M. and the nurse. Mrs. M. will be encouraged to reflect on patterns that include nutrition, exercise, sleep and wake cycle, work, leisure, and relationships. Given her current chief complaint, however, the major focus at this time will be on exercise patterns. Pattern appraisal for Mrs. M. will also involve a comprehensive assessment of environmental field patterns and human field patterns of communication, exchange, rhythms, dissonance, and harmony.

Once Mrs. M. and the nurse reach consensus regarding the pattern appraisal, the planning can begin related to the process of patterning. Planned human field patterning activities may include the nurse assisting Mrs. M. with interventions such as meditation, imagery, journaling, or modifying surroundings. To be successful in human field patterning, the nurse will assist Mrs. M. to center, or focus on her core energy field. The nurse and Mrs. M. will also plan for the family of Mrs. M. to attend the next clinic visit: When there is harmony of energy fields flowing through energy fields at the family and community levels, there is an increased potential for change.

Actual nursing for Mrs. M. will focus on pattern appraisal and patterning activities that will increase her amounts of exercise and physical endurance. The level of exercise chosen will be based on current best practice and the physical assessment of Mrs. M. Evaluation is ongoing and requires a repetition of the appraisal. Throughout the ongoing appraisal process, the nurse will continue to assess and intervene so as to apply the model simultaneously to other identified problems as indicated by the condition of Mrs. M. and current best clinical practices.

CLASSROOM ACTIVITY 9-1

Form small groups. Each group should add to the plan of care for Mrs. M. in the preceding scenario based on other potential or actual nursing problems typical for a patient with same medical diagnosis or symptoms and demographics. Each group should develop a plan for one additional nursing problem using Rogers' theory as the basis for practice. Each group should then share its plan with the class.

CLASSROOM ACTIVITY 9-2

Form small groups. Using a case study provided by the instructor, develop a plan of care using Rogers' nursing theory as the basis for practice. Each group should then share its plan of care with the class.

CLASSROOM ACTIVITY 9-3

Form small groups. Using a case study provided by the instructor, develop a plan of care using one of the theories as the basis for practice; each group should select a different nursing theory. Each group should then share its plan of care with the class and discuss the similarities and differences in care.

REFERENCES

Fawcett, J. (2005). *Contemporary nursing knowledge: Analysis and evaluation of nursing models and theories* (2nd ed.). Philadelphia: F.A. Davis.

Gunther, M. (2006). Rogers' science of unitary human beings in nursing practice. In M. R. Alligood & A. M. Tomey (Eds.), *Nursing theory: Utilization and application* (3rd ed., pp. 283–306). St. Louis, MO: Mosby.

Gunther, M. (2010a). Unitary human beings. In M. R. Alligood & A. M. Tomey (Eds.), *Nursing theorists and their work* (7th ed.). Maryland Heights, MO: Mosby.

Gunther, M. (2010b). Rogers' science of unitary human beings in nursing practice. In R. A. Alligood (Ed.). *Nursing theory: Utilization and application* (4th ed.). Maryland Heights, MO: Mosby.

Johnson, B. M., & Webber, P. B. (2010). A*n introduction to theory and reasoning in nursing* (3rd ed.). Philadelphia: Lippincott, Williams, & Wilkins.

Rogers, M. E. (1970). *An introduction to the theoretical basis of nursing.* Philadelphia: F. A. Davis.

Rogers, M. E. (1992). Nursing science and the space age. *Nursing Science Quarterly, 5,* 27–34.

Rogers, M. E. (1994). The science of unitary human beings: Current perspectives. *Nursing Science Quarterly, 7,* 33–35.

10

ROY ADAPTATION MODEL:
Sister Callista Roy

LEARNING OBJECTIVES

After completing this chapter the student should be able to

1. Describe the concepts of the Roy adaptation model as proposed by Roy

2. Explain the major concepts important to nursing as defined by Roy

3. Plan nursing care for a patient scenario utilizing the Roy adaptation model

KEY TERMS

Adaptation

Adaptive modes

Cognator subsystem

Regulator subsystem

BACKGROUND

SISTER CALLISTA ROY WAS BORN in 1939 in Los Angeles, California. She received a baccalaureate degree in nursing in 1963 from Mount Saint Mary's College. In addition to earning a master's degree in nursing in 1966 from the University of California–Los Angeles, Roy earned a master's degree in sociology in 1973, followed by a doctorate in sociology in 1977, both from the University of California (Phillips, 2010, p. 335).

Roy developed the basic concepts of her model while she was a graduate student at the University of California–Los Angeles after begin challenged by Dorothy Johnson in a seminar to develop a conceptual model for nursing. The Roy adaptation model was first published in 1970. Since that time, Roy has published many books and articles, and has presented numerous lectures focusing on the model and its use in nursing practice. She has also continued to refine and redefine the model (Roy, 2009; Roy & Andrews, 1991; 1999) and has been awarded many honors for her contributions to nursing theory, practice, research, and education (Phillips, 2010).

Roy credits Harry Helson's adaptation theory for playing a key role in her early thinking and development of her own model. She also credits Rapoport's definition of systems as well as concepts from Lazarus and Selye (Roy & Roberts, 1981). In addition, Roy acknowledges the contributions made by other faculty and students to the development of the model. The Roy adaptation model is currently one of the most widely used frameworks in nursing practice, being applied by hundreds of thousands of nurses in countries all over the world.

OVERVIEW OF THE *Roy* ADAPTATION MODEL

THE ROY ADAPTATION MODEL PRESENTS the person as a holistic adaptive system in constant interaction with the internal and the external environment. The main task of the human system is to maintain integrity in the face of environmental stimuli (Phillips, 2010). The goal of nursing is to foster successful adaptation.

According to Roy and Andrews (1999), **adaptation** refers to "the process and outcome whereby thinking and feeling persons as individuals or in groups, use conscious awareness and choice to create human and environmental integration" (p. 54). Adaptation leads to optimal health and well-being, to quality of life, and to death with dignity (Andrews & Roy, 1991). The adaptation level represents the condition of the life processes. Three levels are described by Roy: integrated, compensatory, and compromised life processes. An integrated life process may change to a compensatory process, which attempts to reestablish adaptation. If the compensatory processes are not adequate, compromised processes result (Roy, 2009, p. 33).

Coping processes in the Roy adaptation model include both innate coping mechanisms and acquired coping mechanisms. Innate coping processes are genetically determined or common to the species; they are generally viewed as automatic processes. In contrast, acquired coping processes are learned or developed through customary responses (Roy, 2009, p. 41).

The processes for coping in the Roy adaptation model are further categorized as "the regulator and cognator subsystems as they apply to individuals, and the stabilizer and innovator subsystems as applied to groups" (p. 33). A basic type of adaptive process, the **regulator subsystem** responds through neural, chemical, and endocrine coping channels. Stimuli from the internal and external environment act as inputs through the senses to the nervous system, thereby affecting the fluid, electrolyte, and acid–base balance, as well as the endocrine system. This information is all channeled automatically, with the body producing an automatic, unconscious response to it (p. 41).

The second adaptive process, the **cognator subsystem**, responds through four cognitive–emotional channels: perceptual and information processing, learning, judgment, and emotion. Perceptual and information processing includes activities of selective attention, coding, and memory. Learning involves imitation, reinforcement, and insight. Judgment includes problem solving and decision making. Defenses are used to seek relief from anxiety and make affective appraisal and attachments through the emotions (p. 41).

The cognator–regulator and stabilizer–innovator subsystems function to maintain integrated life processes. These life processes—whether

> The adaptation level represents the condition of the life processes. Three levels are described by Roy: integrated, compensatory, and compromised life processes.

integrated, compensatory, or compromised—are manifested in behaviors of the individual or group. Behavior is viewed as an output of the human system and takes the form of either adaptive responses or ineffective responses. These responses serve as feedback to the system, with the human system using this information to decide whether to increase or decrease its efforts to cope with the stimuli (Roy, 2009, p. 34).

Although one can identify specific processes inherent in the regulator–cognator subsystems, it is not possible to directly observe the functioning of these systems. The behaviors can be observed in four categories, or **adaptive modes**: physiologic–physical mode, self-concept–group identify mode, role function mode, and interdependence mode. It is through these four modes that responses to and interaction with the environment can be carried out and adaptation can be observed (p. 43).

Behavior in the *physiologic–physical mode* is the manifestation of the physiologic activities of all cells, tissues, organs, and systems making up the body. Five basic needs exist: oxygenation, nutrition, elimination, activity and rest, and protection. In addition, four processes are involved in physiologic adaptation: the senses; fluid, electrolyte, and acid–base balance; neurologic function; and endocrine function. The underlying need for the physiologic mode is physiologic integrity (p. 43). When viewing the first mode in relationship to a group of individuals, it is appropriate to use the terminology "physical mode" and to look at the group manifestation of adaptation in terms of basic operating resources, because the basic need associated with the physical mode for a group is resource adequacy or wholeness achieved by adapting to changes in physical resource needs (Roy, 2009, p. 43–44).

The *self-concept–group identity mode* includes the components of the physical self, including body sensation and body image, and the personal self, including self-consistency, self-ideal, and moral–ethical–spiritual self. The basic need underlying the self-concept mode for the individual is psychic and spiritual integrity—that is, the need to know who one is so that one can be or exist with a sense of unity (p. 44). "Group identity" is the term used to refer to the second mode with groups. This mode comprises interpersonal relationships, group self-image, social milieu, culture, and shared responsibility of the group. Identity integrity is the need underlying this group adaptive mode (p. 44).

The *role function mode* focuses on the roles of the person in society and the roles within a group. The basic need underlying the role function mode is social integrity—that is, the need to know who one is in relation to others so that one will know how to act (p. 44).

Finally, the *interdependence mode* is a category of behavior related to interdependent relationships. This mode focuses on interactions related to the giving and receiving of love, respect, and value. The basic need of this mode is relational integrity, or the feeling of security in nurturing relationships. Thus it follows that two specific relationships are the focus within this mode for the individual: significant others and support systems. For the group, the interdependence mode relates to the social context in which the group operates; important factors in this case include infrastructure and member capability (Roy, 2009, p. 45).

In the Roy adaptation model, three classes of stimuli form the environment: the focal stimulus, contextual stimuli, and residual stimuli.

❖ "The focal stimulus is the internal or external stimulus most immediately in the awareness of the individual or group— the object or event most present in the consciousness" (p. 35).

❖ "Contextual stimuli are all other stimuli present in the situation that contribute to the effect of the focal stimulus. That is, contextual stimuli are all the environmental factors that present to the human adaptive system from within or outside but which are not the center of attention or energy" (p. 35). Even though the contextual stimuli are not the center of attention, these factors do influence how people deal with the focal stimulus.

❖ Residual stimuli are environmental factors within or outside human systems, the effects of which are unclear in the situation. The effects of these stimuli may be unclear if there is no awareness on the part of the patient that a stimulus is an influence, or it may not be clear to the observer that these stimuli are having an influence on the human system (p. 36).

MAJOR CONCEPTS OF NURSING ACCORDING TO *Roy*

In addition to the concepts already presented, the four metaparadigm concepts of nursing are identified in the Roy adaptation model. These concepts are summarized in Table 10-1.

Person

According to the Roy adaptation model, humans are holistic, adaptive systems. "The human system is described as a whole with parts that function as unity for some purpose. Human systems include people as individuals, or in groups, including families, organizations, communities, and society as a whole" (Roy & Andrews, 1999, p. 31). The person is the main focus of nursing and is the recipient of nursing care. The person is specifically defined as "an adaptive system with cognator and regulator subsystems acting to maintain adaptation in the four adaptive modes" (Roy, 2009, p. 12).

Environment

Environment is the second major concept of the model. It is understood as the world within and around humans as adaptive systems (Roy, 2009, p. 46). The environment refers to "all conditions, circumstances, and

▨ TABLE 10-1 Metaparadigm Concepts as Defined in the Roy Adaptation Model	
Person	"An adaptive system with cognator and regulator subsystems acting to maintain adaptation in the four adaptive modes" (Roy, 2009, p. 12)
Environment	"All conditions, circumstances, and influences surrounding and affecting the development and behavior of persons and groups, with particular consideration of mutuality of person and earth resources" (Roy, 2009, p. 12)
Health	"A state and process of being and becoming integrated and whole that reflects person and environment mutuality" (Roy, 2009, p. 12)
Nursing	The goal of nursing is "to promote adaptation for individuals and groups in the four adaptive modes, thus contributing to health, quality of life, and dying with dignity by assessing behavior and factors that influence adaptive abilities and to enhance environmental factors" (Roy, 2009, p. 12)

influences surrounding and affecting the development and behavior of persons and groups, with particular consideration of mutuality of person and earth resources" (p. 12). It is the changing environment that stimulates the person to make adaptive responses (Andrews & Roy, 1991, p. 18). However, any environmental change—even if positive—demands increasing energy to adapt to the situation. Factors in the environment that affect the person are categorized as focal, contextual, and residual stimuli (Phillips, 2010, p. 343).

Health

Health is "a state and process of being and becoming integrated and whole that reflects person and environment mutuality" (Roy, 2009, p. 12). In her early writings, Roy wrote about health as existing along a continuum; she now views this conceptualization of health as "simplistic and unrealistic since it does not accommodate the coexistence of wellness and illness and excludes individuals with chronic disabilities or terminal illness who, in spite of their condition, are dealing effectively with life's challenges" (p. 46–47). During the 1990s, Roy's writings began to focus on health as a process in which health and illness can coexist (Roy & Andrews, 1999; Phillips, 2010, p. 342). In either conceptualization, health is viewed as a reflection of adaptation (Andrews & Roy, 1991, p. 21).

Nursing

Roy defines nursing as a "health care profession that focuses on human life processes and patterns of people with a commitment to promote health and full life-potential for individuals, families, groups, and the global society" (Roy, 2009, p. 3). She defines nursing as the science and practice. The goal of nursing is "to promote adaptation for individuals and groups in the four adaptive modes, thus contributing to health, quality of life, and dying with dignity by assessing behavior and factors that influence adaptive abilities and to enhance environmental factors" (Roy, 2009, p. 12).

The goal of nursing is "to promote adaptation for individuals and groups in the four adaptive modes, thus contributing to health, quality of life, and dying with dignity by assessing behavior and factors that influence adaptive abilities and to enhance environmental factors."

Analysis of the Roy Adaptation Model

The analysis presented here consists of an examination of assumptions and propositions as well as a brief critique of the adaptation model of nursing.

Assumptions of the Roy Adaptation Model

Assumptions included in Roy's model are classified into three categories: philosophic assumptions, scientific assumptions, and cultural assumptions. Philosophic assumptions of the model include the following:

❖ Persons have a mutual relationship with the world and a God-figure.

❖ Human meaning is rooted in an omega point convergence of the universe.

❖ God is intimately revealed in the diversity of creation and is the common destiny of creation.

❖ Persons use human creative abilities of awareness, enlightenment, and faith.

❖ Persons are accountable for entering the process of deriving, sustaining, and transforming the universe (Roy, 2009, p. 31).

Scientific assumptions of the model include the following:

❖ Systems of matter and energy progress to higher levels of complex self-organization.

❖ Consciousness and meaning are constitutive of person and environment integration.

❖ Awareness of self and environment is rooted in thinking and feeling.

❖ Human decisions are accountable for integration of creative processes.

❖ Thinking and feeling mediate human action.

❖ System relationships include acceptance, protection, and fostering interdependence.

❖ Persons and earth have common patterns and integral relations.

❖ Person and environment transformations are created in human consciousness.

❖ Integration of human environment meanings results in adaptation (Roy, 2009, p. 31).

Cultural assumptions include the following:

❖ Experiences within a specific culture will influence how each element of the Roy adaptation model is expressed.

❖ Within a culture, there may be a concept that is central to the culture and that will influence some or all of the elements of the Roy adaptation model to a greater or lesser extent.

❖ Cultural expressions of the elements of the Roy adaptation model may lead to changes in practice activities such as nursing assessment.

❖ As Roy adaptation model elements evolve within a cultural perspective, implications for education and research may differ from the experience in the original culture (Roy, 2009, p. 31).

Propositions of the Roy Adaptation Model

The following are the relational propositions of the Roy adaptation model (Fawcett, 2005, p. 382–383):

❖ Stimuli from the internal and external environments (through the senses) serve as inputs to the nervous system and affect the fluid, electrolyte, and acid–base balance, as well as the endocrine system. This information is channeled automatically in the appropriate manner, and an automatic, unconscious response is produced (Roy & Andrews, 1999, p. 46).

❖ Internal and external stimuli, including psychological, social, physical, and physiological factors, serve as inputs to the cognator subsystem (Roy & Andrews, 1999, p. 47).

❖ Stimuli and adaptation level serve as input to human adaptive systems; processing of this input through control processes results in behavioral responses (Roy & Andrews, 1999, p. 43).

❖ Human systems, as individuals, families, groups, organizations, or communities, must sense changes in the environment and make adaptations in the way they function to accommodate new environmental requirements (Roy & Andrews, 1999, p. 44).

❖ Adaptation level affects the human system's ability to respond positively in a situation (Roy & Andrews, 1999, p. 36).

❖ The changing environment stimulates the person to make adaptive responses. As the environment changes, the person has the opportunity to continue to grow, to develop, and to enhance the meaning of life for everyone (Andrews & Roy, 1991, p. 18).

❖ The characteristics of the internal and external stimuli influence the adequacy of cognitive and emotional processes (Roy & Andrews, 1999, p. 547).

❖ The characteristics of the internal and external stimuli influence (behavioral) responses (Roy & Andrews, 1999, p. 547).

❖ Human beings are described as adaptive systems that are constantly growing and developing within changing environments. Health for human adaptive systems can be described as a reflection of this interaction or adaptation (Roy & Andrews, 1999, p. 53–54).

❖ The goal of nursing is the promotion of adaptation in each of the four adaptive modes, thereby contributing to health, quality of life, or dying with dignity (Roy & Andrews, 1999, p. 55).

❖ The general goal of nursing intervention is to maintain and enhance adaptive behavior and to change ineffective behavior to adaptive (Roy & Andrews, 1999, p. 81).

❖ It is the nurse's role to promote adaptation in situations of health and illness and to enhance the interaction of human systems with the environment, thereby promoting health (Roy & Andrews, 1999, p. 55).

Brief Critique of the Roy Adaptation Model

The concepts of the Roy adaptation model are clearly and consistently defined. The model is internally consistent, even though it is a complex model with several major concepts, subconcepts, and many relational statements. It has the level of complexity required to make it broad in scope and generalizable for both practice and research; however, once learned, the model is logical and easy to understand (Phillips, 2010).

THE ROY ADAPTATION MODEL IS commonly used in nursing practice. To use the model in practice, the nurse follows Roy's six-step nursing process:

1. Assess the behaviors manifested from the four adaptive modes (physiological–physical mode, self-concept–group identity mode, role function mode, and interdependence mode).

2. Assess and categorize the stimuli for those behaviors.

3. Make a nursing diagnosis based on the person's adaptive state.

4. Set goals to promote adaptation.

5. Implement interventions aimed at managing stimuli to promote adaptation.

6. Evaluate achievement of adaptive goals (Phillips, 2010).

Andrews and Roy (1986) pointed out that by manipulating the stimuli rather than the patient, the nurse enhances "the interaction of the person with their environment, thereby promoting health" (p. 51).

> ## THE *Roy* ADAPTATION MODEL AS A FRAMEWORK FOR NURSING PRACTICE

ROY SPECIFICALLY ADDRESSES INCORPORATION OF a six-step nursing process within the context of her model, stressing that although steps are discussed separately for clarity, the process is ongoing and simultaneous (Roy, 2009, p. 57). Roy also states in relationship to each of the steps of the nursing process that "nurses rely on highly developed technical, interpersonal, and intuitive skills as they assess and initiate interventions involving approaches such as physical care, anticipatory guidance, health teaching, and counseling" (p. 59).

> ## THE NURSING PROCESS AND THE *Roy* ADAPTATION MODEL

Assessment

The first step of the process is the assessment of behavior—after all, behavior is the indicator of how a human adaptive system manages to cope with, or adapt to, changes in health status. Behaviors may be either observable or non-observable (Roy, 2009, p. 58). In the nursing situation, the primary concern is behavior that requires further adaptive responses as a result of environmental changes straining the coping processes of the adaptive system. The nurse must know how to assess for these behaviors, compare them to specific criteria to evaluate their contribution to the maintenance of integrity, and identify the strengths of the coping processes and the demands faced (p. 59).

During the assessment phase of the nursing process, the nurse systematically considers behaviors manifested from the four adaptive modes and assesses the stimuli for those behaviors, categorizing them as focal, contextual, or residual stimuli (Phillips, 2010, p. 435). The nurse uses observational skills, intuition, accurate measures (e.g., blood pressure reading, eye chart, or assessment scale), and interviewing skills to systematically collect data related to behaviors (Roy, 2009, p. 59–60).

The nurse must then make a tentative judgment of the behavior. In making this initial judgment as to whether a behavior is adaptive or ineffective, the nurse must continually involve the patient. Ultimately, the patient's perceptions associated with the effectiveness of behaviors are essential in determining if the behavior is adaptive or ineffective (p. 61).

In addition to the assessment of behaviors, the nurse must identify the internal and external stimuli that are influencing behaviors. The skills used for assessing stimuli are the same ones that the nurse used in assessing behaviors—namely, astute observation, sensitive intuition, accurate measurement, and perceptive interview. To set priorities, the nurse, in collaboration with the patient, identifies the focal, contextual, and residual stimuli that are influencing behavior (p. 62). In addition, "the nurse identifies the particular stimulus of the adaptation level, that is, integrated, compensatory, and compromised life processes that contribute to adaptive or ineffective behavior" (p. 62).

Analysis of the data results in a statement or nursing diagnosis reflective of the patient's adaptive state. In setting up a nursing diagnosis within the framework of her adaptation model, Roy suggests that nurses develop statements that match behaviors and the most relevant stimuli. This type of wording of the diagnosis facilitates the step of goal setting (p. 66–67).

Planning

During the next phase of the nursing process, the nurse and the patient set goals to promote adaptation. Goal setting within the framework of Roy's model involves the statement of behavioral outcomes of nursing care that will promote adaptation. "The goal statement should designate not only the behavior to be observed but the way the behavior will change (as observed, measured, or subjectively reported) and the time from in which the goal is to be attained" (Roy, 2009, p. 77).

Implementation

During the implementation phase of the process, the nurse determines how best to assist the patient in attaining his or her goals and chooses interventions to promote the desired adaptation through either changing stimuli or strengthening adaptive processes (Roy, 2009, p. 78). The identification of possible approaches to nursing intervention includes the selection of which stimuli to change. To make this decision, the nurse lists the stimuli affecting specific behaviors and identifies the relevant coping processes. Then the consequences of changing the stimulus or affecting a coping process are identified together with the probability (low, moderate, or high) of their occurrence. In collaboration with the patient, the nurse judges the outcome of the consequence as either desirable or undesirable (p. 79). Once the appropriate nursing intervention has been selected, the nurse works with the patient to initiate steps that will alter the stimulus and enhance coping (p. 80).

Evaluation

Evaluation focuses on judging the effectiveness of the nursing intervention in relation to the behavior of the individual or group. To determine if the adaptive goals have been met, the nurse uses the same skills as were employed in the assessment phase of the process—observation, intuition, measurement, and interviewing (Roy, 2009, p. 81).

CRITICAL THINKING

What do you think about the six-step version of the nursing process advocated for use with the Roy adaptation model? Do you believe that it allows the nurse to meet the standards of care practice requirements for assessment, planning, implementation, and evaluation?

SCENARIO ILLUSTRATING NURSING CARE FRAMED BY THE *Roy* ADAPTATION MODEL UTILIZING THE NURSING PROCESS

THE FOLLOWING SCENARIO ILLUSTRATES NURSING care of the patient relative to one identified nursing problem framed by Roy's adaptation model. This scenario is not intended to cover all aspects of care, but rather is intended to stimulate thinking about how specific care might be approached using this theory as a framework for practice.

Mrs. M. is a 37-year-old single mother with two school-age children. Mrs. M. suffered multiple facial injuries as a result of a motor vehicle accident several months ago. The injuries have healed without complication, but she has moderate residual scarring.

Assessment of Mrs. M. begins with the behaviors manifested from the four adaptive modes. The nurse uses observational skills, intuition, measurements, and interviewing skills to collect data. The nurse involves Mrs. M. in the assessment to verify the nurse's own perceptions. The nurse verifies that Mrs. M. has generally adapted well following the motor vehicle accident. The exception is the self-concept mode: Some of her behaviors are ineffective in relation to adaptation, as evidenced by Mrs. M.'s avoidance of social gatherings, wearing dark glasses and big hats, and wearing heavy makeup to cover her scars.

Next, the nurse and Mrs. M. set goals to promote adaptation. Goal setting for Mrs. M. within the framework involves statements of measurable behavioral outcomes of nursing care that will promote adaptation related to body image within the self-concept adaptive mode. The nurse, in collaboration with Mrs. M., chooses interventions based on current best practices to promote adaptation by either changing stimuli or strengthening Mrs. M.'s adaptive processes. Evaluation focuses on judging the effectiveness of the nursing interventions in relation to Mrs. M.'s behaviors. In addition, if any other nursing problems are uncovered during the assessment, the nurse addresses those problems simultaneously using the process described and incorporating best practices to provide appropriate nursing care.

CLASSROOM ACTIVITY 10-1

Form small groups. Each group should add to the plan of care for Mrs. M. in the preceding scenario based on other potential or actual nursing problems typical for a patient with same medical diagnosis or symptoms and demographics. Each group should develop a plan for one additional nursing problem using Roy's theory as the basis for practice, while considering at least one of the four adaptive modes. Each group should then share its plan with the class.

CLASSROOM ACTIVITY 10-2

Form small groups. Using a case study provided by the instructor, develop a plan of care using Roy's nursing theory as the basis for practice. Each group should then share its plan of care with the class.

CLASSROOM ACTIVITY 10-3

Form small groups. Using a case study provided by the instructor, develop a plan of care using one of the theories as the basis for practice; each group should select a different nursing theory. Each group should then share its plan of care with the class and discuss the similarities and differences in care.

REFERENCES

Andrews, H. A., & Roy, Sr. C. (1986). *Essentials of the Roy adaptation model.* Norwalk, CT: Appleton-Century-Crofts.

Andrews, H. A., & Roy, Sr. C. (1991). Essentials of the Roy adaptation model. In Sr. C. Roy & H. A. Andrews (Eds.), *The Roy adaptation model: The definitive statement* (pp. 2–25). Norwalk, CT: Appleton & Lange.

Fawcett, J. (2005). *Contemporary nursing knowledge development: Analysis and evaluation of nursing models and theories* (2nd ed.). Philadelphia: F. A. Davis.

Phillips, K. D. (2010). Sister Callista Roy: Adaptation model. In A. M. Tomey & M. R. Alligood (Eds.), *Nursing theorists and their work* (7th ed., pp. 335–365). Maryland Heights, MO: Mosby.

Roy, Sr. C. (1970). Adaptation: A conceptual framework for nursing. *Nursing Outlook, 18,* 42–45.

Roy, Sr. C. (2009). *The Roy adaptation model* (3rd ed.). Upper Saddle River, NJ: Pearson.

Roy, Sr. C., & Andrews, H. A. (1991). *The Roy adaptation model: The definitive statement.* Norwalk, CT: Appleton & Lange.

Roy, Sr. C., & Andrews, H. A. (1999). *The Roy adaptation model* (2nd ed.). Stamford, CT: Appleton & Lange.

Roy, Sr. C., & Roberts, S. (1981). *Theory construction in nursing: An adaptation model.* Englewood Cliffs, NJ: Prentice-Hall.

THE NEUMAN SYSTEMS MODEL:
Betty Neuman

LEARNING OBJECTIVES

After completing this chapter the student should be able to

1. Describe and explain the major concepts of the Neuman systems model as proposed by Neuman

2. Explain the major concepts important to nursing as defined by Neuman

3. Plan nursing care for a patient scenario utilizing the Neuman systems model

KEY TERMS

Created environment

Extrapersonal stressors

Flexible line of defense

Interpersonal stressors

Intrapersonal stressors

Lines of resistance

Neuman systems model nursing
   process format

Normal line of defense

Prevention-as-intervention

Primary prevention-as-intervention

Reconstitution

Secondary prevention-as-intervention

Tertiary prevention-as-intervention

BACKGROUND

BETTY NEUMAN WAS BORN IN 1924 in Ohio. After graduating from Peoples Hospital School of Nursing in Ohio in 1947, she moved to California, where she earned a baccalaureate degree in public health and psychology in 1957 and a master's degree in mental health, public health consultation, in 1966 from the University of California–Los Angeles. Neuman completed a doctoral degree in clinical psychology at Pacific Western University in 1985 (Freese & Lawson, 2010, p. 309).

Neuman initially developed her systems model as a teaching tool to assist students in expanding their understanding of the impact of patient variables beyond the context of the medical model. She first published the model in the early 1970s (Neuman, 1974; Neuman & Young, 1972) and then, after continued development, published the model in book form in 1982 (Neuman, 1982). She then continued to refine the model, with her subsequent books reflecting those refinements (Neuman, 1989; 1995; 2002). In addition to writing books, Neuman has been involved in numerous other publications, presentations, and consultations regarding the application and use of the model. She is currently retired and living in Ohio (Freese & Lawson, 2010).

The Neuman systems model is based on general systems theory. However, in her development of the model, Neuman synthesized knowledge from several disciplines, in addition to incorporating her own philosophical beliefs and clinical nursing expertise. For example, the model draws from gestalt theory descriptions of homeostasis, Marxist philosophy as it relates to the property of parts being determined by the larger whole of the system, de Chardin's philosophy of the wholeness of life, Selye's definition of stress, and Caplan's definition of levels of prevention (Freese & Lawson, 2010, p. 310).

OVERVIEW OF THE *Neuman* SYSTEMS MODEL

ACCORDING TO NEUMAN (2002, P. 3), "The Neuman Systems Model is a unique, systems-based perspective that provides a unifying focus for approaching a wide range of nursing concerns." Part of the uniqueness derives from the model's focus on wellness of the client system in relation to the environmental stressors and the client system's reaction to stress (Neuman, 2002). In the Neuman systems model, the client system in interaction with the environment is the domain of nursing concern, although the client system can be defined as a single client, a group, a number of groups, or a social issue (Neuman, 2002, p.3).

The Neuman systems model is a wellness model based on general systems theory in which the client system is exposed to environmental stressors from within and without the system. In the model, the focus is on the client system in relationship to environmental stressors. The client system is protected by a circular series of buffers known as lines of defense that minimize the effects of stressors. Progressing inward, three lines of defense are encountered: the flexible line of defense, the normal line of defense, and lines of resistance. The greater the quality of the client system's health, the greater the levels of protection provided by the various lines of defense (Geib, 2006). Additional description of the concepts of the model is provided in the next section. An overview and diagram of the model are provided on the Neuman systems model website (http:// neumansystemsmodel.org/NSMdocs/nsm_powerpoint_overview.htm).

> In the Neuman systems model, the client system in interaction with the environment is the domain of nursing concern, although the client system can be defined as a single client, a group, a number of groups, or a social issue.

IN ADDITION TO THE CONCEPTS already presented, the four metaparadigm concepts of nursing are identified and explicated in the Neuman systems model. These concepts are summarized in Table 11-1.

Person

The person is viewed as a client or client system. Neuman selected the term "client" for use in her model out of respect for client–caregiver collaborative relationships and because of the wellness perspective assumed by the model. Within the model, the client or client system may be an individual, a family, a group, a community, or a social issue. The model components are as applicable to a broad

> **MAJOR CONCEPTS OF NURSING ACCORDING TO THE *Neuman* SYSTEMS MODEL**

TABLE 11-1 Metaparadigm Concepts as Defined in Neuman's Model

Person (client system)	A composite of physiological, psychological, sociocultural, developmental, and spiritual variables in interaction with the internal and external environment. Represented by a central structure, lines of defense, and lines of resistance (Neuman, 2002).
Environment	All internal and external factors or influences surrounding the client system. Three relevant environments indentified are the internal environment, the external environment, and the created environment (Neuman, 2002, p. 18).
Health	Health is equated with optimal system stability; it is viewed on a continuum of wellness to illness (Neuman, 2002, p. 23).
Nursing	Prevention as intervention; concerned with all potential stressors.

system, such as the global community, as they are to a one-client system (Neuman, 2002, p. 15).

The client system is a composite of five interacting variables, which are present in varying degrees of development:

❖ The physiological variable: bodily structure and internal function

❖ The psychological variable: mental processes and interactive environmental effects

❖ The sociocultural variable: combined effects of social cultural conditions and influences

❖ The developmental variable: age-related development processes and activities

❖ The spiritual variable (spiritual beliefs and influences) (p. 16–17)

Because the spiritual variable is open to more interpretation, Neuman (p. 16) describes it in considerable detail as it is understood within the context of her systems model.

Neuman uses the analogy of the "seed" to describe the spiritual variable. It is assumed that each person is born with a spiritual energy force or "seed" within the spiritual variable. The "seed or human spirit with its enormous energy potential lies on a continuum of dormant, unacceptable, or undeveloped to recognition, development, and positive system

CRITICAL THINKING

Can you think of any additional client system variables to add to Neuman's list of five client system variables that make up the person?

influence" (Neuman, 2002, p. 16). The "natural seed must have environmental catalysts such as timing, warmth, moisture, and nutrients to burst forth with the energy that transforms it into a living form . . . The human spirit combines with the power of the Holy Spirit as a gift from God when the innate human force, or 'seed' becomes catalyzed by some life event" (p. 16). It is assumed that spiritual development in varying degrees empowers the client system toward well-being by positively directing spiritual energy for use first by the mind and then by the body. As a consequence, thought patterns are positively affected and the body becomes increasingly nourished and sustained through the positive use of spiritual energy empowerment (p. 16).

The client system is represented structurally in the model as a series of concentric rings or circles surrounding a basic structure. These flexible concentric circles represent normal lines of defense and lines of resistance that function to preserve client system integrity by acting as protective mechanisms for the basic structure. The basic structure or central core consists of basic survival factors common to the species, innate or genetic features, and strengths and weaknesses of the system. The **flexible line of defense** forms the outer boundary of the defined client system; it protects the normal line of defense. The **normal line of defense** represents what the client has become or the usual wellness state. Adjustment of the five client system variables to environmental stressors determines its level of stability. The series of concentric broken circles surrounding the basic structure are known as **lines of resistance**. They become activated following invasion of the normal line of defense by environmental stressors.

An interactive relationship exists among all lines of defense and resistance: Each line contains the five system variables and functions to protect the system components. Input, outputs, and feedback across these lines provide corrective action to change, enhance, and stabilize the system (p. 17–18).

Environment

The environment is defined by Neuman as "all internal and external factors or influences surrounding the identified client or client system" (2002, p. 18). The Neuman systems model identifies three relevant environments:

the internal environment, the external environment, and the created environment.

The internal environment "consists of all forces or interactive influences internal to or contained solely within the boundaries of the defined client/client system" (p. 18). It correlates with the intrapersonal factors or stressors found in the Neuman systems model.

The external environment "consists of all forces or interactive influences external to or existing solely outside of the defined client/client system" (p. 18). It correlates with both the interpersonal and extrapersonal factors and stressors (p. 18).

The third environment of the Neuman systems model is the **created environment**, which "represents an open system exchanging energy with both the internal and external environment" (Neuman, 1989; 1990a; 2002). The created environment, which is developed unconsciously by the client, is a symbolic expression of system wholeness that "acts as an immediate or long-range safe reservoir for existence or the maintenance of system integrity" (Neuman, 2002, p. 19). It may be expressed consciously or unconsciously and functions to insulate the client from environmental stressors by providing a mechanism for protective coping since coping is directly related to perception (p. 19–20).

In the Neuman systems model, environmental stressors are classified as intrapersonal, interpersonal, or extrapersonal depending on their relationship to the client system:

❖ **Intrapersonal stressors** are internal environmental forces that occur within the boundary of the client system. They may include, for example, conditioned responses or autoimmune responses (Neuman, 2002, p. 22).

❖ **Interpersonal stressors** are "external environmental interaction forces that occur outside the boundaries of the client system at the proximal range" (p. 22). They may include, for example, communication patterns or role expectations.

❖ **Extrapersonal stressors** are "external environmental interaction forces that occur outside the boundaries of the client system at the distal range" (p. 22). They may include, for example, social policies or financial concerns.

Health

In the Neuman systems model, health is conceptualized as existing on a continuum, where wellness and illness represent the opposite ends of the continuum. Actually, Neuman visualizes this continuum as a vertical half-circle rather than a horizontal line. Health for the client is equated with optimal system stability. It is envisioned as a manifestation of living energy available to preserve and enhance system integrity and as being at various changing levels—rising or falling throughout the life span in response to basic structure factors and client response to environmental stressors (Neuman, 2002, p. 23).

Nursing

The major concern of nursing is keeping the client system stable through accurately assessing the current effects and possible effects of environmental stressors and through assisting the client during the adjustments required to achieve an optimal level of wellness. The nurse uses three levels of prevention-as-intervention—primary, secondary, and tertiary—to keep the system stable. In keeping the system stable, the nurse creates linkages among the metaparadigm concepts of nursing (Neuman, 2002, p. 25).

The nurse uses three levels of prevention-as-intervention—primary, secondary, and tertiary—to keep the system stable.

ANALYSIS OF THE *Neuman* SYSTEMS MODEL

THE ANALYSIS PRESENTED HERE CONSISTS of an examination of assumptions and propositions as well as a brief critique of the Neuman systems model.

Assumptions of the Neuman Systems Model

Basic assumptions of the Neuman systems model include the following statements as identified by Fawcett (2005, p. 168–169):

❖ Provided support factors are in place, the client system constantly monitors self by making adjustments as needed to retain, attain, and maintain stability for an optimal health state (Neuman, 1990a, p. 129).

❖ The client is an open system that interacts with the environment so as to promote harmony and balance between the internal and external environment. The client is a composite of physiologic, psychologic, sociocultural, developmental, and spiritual variables that are viewed as parts of the whole. Ideally, the client system adjusts successfully to internal and external environmental stressors, thereby maintaining the normal wellness level or system stability (Neuman, 1990b, p. 259).

❖ Each client system is unique; each system is a composite of common known factors or innate characteristics within a normal, given range of response, contained within a basic structure (Neuman, 2002, p. 14).

❖ Each person is born with a spiritual energy force or "seed" within the spiritual variable, as identified in the basic structure of the client system (Neuman, 2002, p. 16).

❖ Spiritual development in varying degrees empowers the client system toward well-being by positively directing spiritual energy for use first by the mind and then by the body (Neuman, 2002, p. 16).

❖ The environment contains both internal and external stressors and resistance factors. Stressors are considered neutral; the client encounter determines whether the outcome is beneficial or noxious (Neuman, 1990b, p. 259).

❖ The client engages in a constant, dynamic energy exchange with the environment (Neuman, 2002, p. 14).

Health represents a usual dynamic stability state of the normal line of defense. A reaction to stressors occurs when the normal line of defense is penetrated, leading to illness symptoms. The client's position on the wellness–illness continuum is related to the amount of available energy stored and/or used by the system in retaining, attaining, and maintaining system stability (Neuman, 1990b, p. 259).

Nursing is concerned with reduction of potential or actual stressor reactions through use of primary, secondary, or tertiary prevention, as an intervention to retain, attain, and maintain an optimal wellness level. The goal of nursing is optimal client system stability or wellness. Perceptual distortions between the client and the nurse, as well as goal plans, are mutually negotiated and resolved (Neuman, 1990b, p. 259).

Propositions of the Neuman Systems Model

Relational propositions for the Neuman systems model as presented by Fawcett (2005, p. 177, 180) are listed here:

- The client is a system capable of input and output related to intrapersonal, interpersonal, and extrapersonal environmental influences, interacting with the environment by adjusting to it or adjusting the environment to itself (Neuman, 2002, p. 23–24).

- Input, output, and feedback between the client and the environment are circular in nature. The client and the environment have a reciprocal relationship, the outcome of which is corrective or regulative for the system (p. 23).

- Many known, unknown, and universal environmental stressors exist. Each stressor differs in its potential for disturbing a client's usual level of stability or normal line of defense (14).

- When the cushioning effect of the flexible line of defense is no longer capable of protecting the client system against an environmental stressor, the stressor breaks through the normal line of defense. At this point, the interrelationships of the physiological, psychological, sociocultural, developmental, and spiritual variables determine the nature and degree of the system's reaction to the stressor (p. 14).

- Lines of resistance in the client system are activated to combat potential or actual stressor reactions (Neuman, 1990b, p. 259).

- The client is an interacting open system in total interface with internal and external environmental forces or stressors. The client is in constant change, with reciprocal environmental interaction at all times moving either toward a dynamic state of stability or wellness or toward one of illness in varying degrees (Neuman, 2002, p. 12).

❖ The process of interaction and adjustment results in varying degrees of harmony, stability, or balance between the client and the environment (p. 23).

❖ The major concern for nursing is keeping the client system stable by accurately assessing the current effects and possible effects of environmental stressors and assisting the client in making the adjustments required for an optimal level of wellness (p. 25).

❖ In keeping the system stable, the nurse creates linkage among the client, environment, health, and nursing (p. 25).

Brief Critique of the Neuman Systems Model

The Neuman systems model is a comprehensive conceptual model that clearly operationalizes the concepts that are relevant to nursing. These concepts, while abstract, are familiar to nurses and are congruent with the traditional understanding of the nursing metaparadigm. The model is complex, yet organized in a logical manner. Thus it is easy for nurses to understand for use in practice and research. The scope of the model is broad, allowing for its use for individuals, families, groups, or communities. Neuman's model also incorporates the concepts of levels of prevention that are familiar not only to nurses but also to members of other healthcare disciplines. The Neuman systems model has been used extensively in a wide variety of nursing situations (Freese & Lawson, 2010, p. 321).

THE *Neuman* SYSTEMS MODEL AS A FRAMEWORK FOR NURSING PRACTICE

USING THE NEUMAN SYSTEMS MODEL as a framework for providing nursing care involves intervention at three levels of prevention: primary prevention intervention, secondary prevention intervention, and tertiary prevention intervention. The **prevention-as-intervention** format or mode identifies the entry-point condition of the client system into the healthcare system. It also indicates the general type of intervention or action required. Note, however, that the prevention-as-intervention mode allows for simultaneous multilevel intervention as required by the client system (Neuman, 2002, p. 25).

Primary prevention–as–intervention is used for primary prevention as wellness retention—that is, to protect the client system's normal line of defense or usual wellness state by strengthening the flexible line of defense. The goal is to promote wellness by stress prevention and reduction of risk factors (p. 25).

If the primary prevention-as-intervention was unsuccessful or not provided, then **secondary prevention–as–intervention** would be provided. This modality is used for secondary prevention as wellness attainment—that is, to protect the basic structure by strengthening the internal lines of resistance. The goal is to provide appropriate treatment of symptoms so as to achieve optimal client system stability or wellness and energy conservation (p. 26). If following treatment, secondary intervention-as-prevention "fails to reconstitute the client system, death occurs as a result of the failure of the basic structure to support the intervention" (p. 28). **Reconstitution** is the determined energy increase related to the degree of reaction and is identified as beginning at any point following treatment. Complete reconstitution may progress well beyond the previous normal line of defense, it may stabilize the system at a lower level, or it may return to the level prior to illness (p. 28).

The **tertiary prevention–as–intervention** modality is used for tertiary prevention as wellness maintenance—that is, to protect the client system's reconstitution or return to wellness following treatment (p. 28). Tertiary prevention can begin at any point in client reconstitution after treatment once some degree of client system stability has occurred. The goal is to maintain optimal wellness by supporting existing strengths and conserving client system energy (p. 28).

THE NURSING PROCESS AND THE *Neuman* SYSTEMS MODEL

T HE **NEUMAN SYSTEMS MODEL NURSING process format** has been specifically designed for use with the Neuman systems model. This nursing process has been developed so that it applies to three categories: nursing diagnosis, nursing goals, and

What do you think about the Neuman systems model nursing process format as designed for the Neuman systems model? Do you believe that the three categories—nursing diagnosis, nursing goals, and nursing outcomes—allow the nurse to meet the standards of care practice requirements for assessment, planning, implementation, and evaluation?

nursing outcomes. When using the Neuman systems model, the nurse is concerned with acquiring comprehensive client system data. The process allows for full explanation of the client system condition and provides a rationale for nursing actions. The unique features of the Neuman systems model nursing process are the determination of perceptions of the client system and the caregiver and the mutual determination of client intervention goals. Outcomes are based on prevention-as-intervention modalities (Neuman, 2002, p. 30).

Nursing Diagnosis Category (Assessment)

The nurse–patient relationship begins with the initial contact and is perceived as a partnership. Systemic data collection occurs through the physical assessment and interview process in an ongoing partnership, including validation of the data collected with the client and resolution of any perceptual discrepancies. Assessment includes physiological, psychological, developmental, sociocultural, and spiritual variables; basic structure, function, strengths, and resources of the client system; potential and actual environmental stressors; and characteristics of the client's flexible and normal lines of defense, lines of resistance, degree of reaction, and reconstitution (Geib, 2010, p. 244).

Based on the assessment, variances from wellness are identified and diagnoses are identified and prioritized. The guidelines for use of the Neuman systems model in practice stipulate that the diagnostic taxonomy employed reflects the following categories: client system (individual, family, group, or community), response level (primary, secondary, or tertiary), subsystem response (five variables), stressor source (intrasystem, intersystem, or extrasystem), and stressor type (five variables) (Freese, Neuman, & Fawcett, 2002, p. 38; Geib, 2010, p. 245–246).

Nursing Goals (Planning and Implementation)

Goals and interventions are developed in partnership with the client. Specific outcome goals, along with primary prevention-as-intervention, secondary prevention-as-intervention, and tertiary prevention-as-intervention modalities, are developed to promote optimal client system stability (Geib, 2010, p. 244).

Nursing Outcomes (Implementation and Evaluation)

During this phase of the process, the nurse implements the planned primary prevention-as-intervention, secondary prevention-as-intervention, and tertiary prevention-as-intervention modalities. The nurse evaluates and modifies these interventions as necessary, working in partnership with the client, based on the client system stability (Geib, 2010, p. 245).

THE FOLLOWING SCENARIO ILLUSTRATES NURSING care of the patient relative to one identified nursing problem framed by the Neuman systems model. This scenario is not intended to cover all aspects of care, but rather is intended to stimulate thinking about how specific care might be approached using this theory as a framework for practice.

SCENARIO ILLUSTRATING NURSING CARE FRAMED BY THE *Neuman* SYSTEMS MODEL UTILIZING THE *Neuman* SYSTEMS MODEL NURSING PROCESS FORMAT

Ms. B. is a 32-year-old, obese single mother of three who presents to the clinic. Systemic data collection occurs through physical assessment and interview with Ms. B. The assessment includes physiological, psychological, developmental, sociocultural, and spiritual variables; basic structure, function, strengths, and resources available to Ms. B.; potential and actual environmental stressors; and characteristics of Ms. B.'s flexible and normal lines of defense, lines of resistance, degree of reaction, and reconstitution. Based on the assessment, it is determined that Ms. B. is experiencing an actual nutritional imbalance—more than body requirements—related to family and environmental stressors.

The nurse, in partnership with Ms. B., develops goals and interventions. Specific outcome goals for Ms. B. include secondary prevention-as-intervention modalities to assist Ms. B. in addressing her current family and environmental stressors as well as interventions aimed at expanding her flexible line of defense so as to promote system stability. In addition, if any other nursing problems are uncovered in additional variables; basic structure, function, strengths, and resources; stressors; or lines of defense during the assessment, the nurse addresses those problems simultaneously using the process described and incorporating best practices to provide appropriate nursing care.

CLASSROOM ACTIVITY 11-1

Form small groups. Each group should add to the plan of care for Ms. B. in the preceding scenario based on other potential or actual nursing problems typical for a patient with same medical diagnosis or symptoms and demographics. Each group should develop a plan for one additional nursing problem using Neuman's theory as the basis for practice. Each group should then share its plan with the class.

CLASSROOM ACTIVITY 11-2

Form small groups. Using a case study provided by the instructor, develop a plan of care using the Neuman systems model as the basis for practice. Each group should then share its plan of care with the class.

CLASSROOM ACTIVITY 11-3

Form small groups. Using a case study provided by the instructor, develop a plan of care using one of the theories as the basis for practice; each group should select a different nursing theory. Each group should then share its plan of care with the class and discuss the similarities and differences in care.

REFERENCES

Fawcett, J. (2005). *Contemporary nursing knowledge: Analysis and evaluation of nursing models and theories* (2nd ed.). Philadelphia: F. A. Davis.

Freese, B. T., & Lawson, T. G. (2010). Betty Neuman: Systems model. In M. R. Alligood & A. M. Tomey (Eds.), *Nursing theorists and their work* (7th ed., pp. 309–334). Maryland Heights, MO: Mosby.

Freese, B. T., Neuman, B., & Fawcett, J. (2002). Guidelines for Neuman systems model-based clinical practice. In B. Neuman & J. Fawcett (Eds.), *The Neuman systems model* (4th ed., pp. 37–42). Upper Saddle River, NJ: Prentice Hall.

Geib, K. M. (2006). Neuman's systems model in nursing practice. In M. R. Alligood & A. M. Tomey (Eds.), *Nursing theory: Utilization and application* (3rd ed., pp. 229–254). St. Louis, MO: Mosby.

Geib, K. M. (2010). Neuman's systems model in nursing practice. In M. R. Alligood (Ed.), *Nursing theory: Utilization and application* (4th ed., pp. 235–260). Maryland Heights, MO: Mosby.

Neuman, B. (1974). The Betty Neuman health care systems model: A total person approach to patient problems. In J. P. Riehl & C. Roy (Eds.), *Conceptual models for nursing practice* (2nd ed., pp. 119–134). New York: Appleton-Century-Crofts.

Neuman, B. (1982). *The Neuman systems model: Application to nursing education and practice.* Norwalk, CT: Appleton-Century-Crofts.

Neuman, B. (1989). *The Neuman systems model* (2nd ed.). Norwalk, CT: Appleton & Lange.

Neuman, B. (1990a). Health on a continuum based on the Neuman systems model. *Nursing Science Quarterly, 3,* 129–135.

Neuman, B. (1990b). The Neuman systems model: A theory for practice. In M. E. Parker (Ed.), *Nursing theories in practice* (pp. 241–261). New York: National League for Nursing.

Neuman, B. (1995). The Neuman systems model (3rd ed.). Norwalk, CT: Appleton & Lange.

Neuman, B. (2002). The Neuman systems model. In B. Neuman & J. Fawcett (Eds.), *The Neuman systems model* (4th ed., pp. 3–34). Upper Saddle River, NJ: Prentice Hall.

Neuman, B., & Young, R. J. (1972). A model for teaching total person approach to patient problems. *Nursing Research, 21,* 264–269.

THE CONSERVATION MODEL:
Myra Estrin Levine

LEARNING OBJECTIVES

After completing this chapter the student should be able to

1. Identify and describe the major concepts of the conservation model as proposed by Levine

2. Explain the major concepts important to nursing as defined by Levine

3. Plan nursing care for a patient scenario utilizing Levine's conservation model

KEY TERMS

Conservation

Conservation of energy

Conservation of personal integrity

Conservation of social integrity

Conservation of structural integrity

BACKGROUND

MYRA ESTRIN LEVINE WAS BORN in Chicago in 1920. She earned a diploma in nursing from Cook County School of Nursing in 1944, followed by a bachelor of science degree in nursing from the University of Chicago. In 1962, she received a master's of science degree in nursing from Wayne State University and then enrolled in postgraduate work at the University of Chicago.

Levine held many positions during her career. She was at various times a private duty nurse, supervisor, administrator, civilian nurse in the U.S. Army, and professor. She taught in four different schools of nursing—the Cook County Hospital School of Nursing, Loyola University, Rush University, and the University of Illinois—in the United States, and she served as a visiting professor at two schools of nursing in Israel—Tel Aviv University and Ben-Gurion University of the Negev (Johnson & Webber, 2010).

Levine did not set out to develop a theory of nursing, but rather sought to create a structure for teaching curriculum in nursing that would incorporate all major nursing concepts and focus on maintaining the patient's ability to adapt (Levine, 1973). Authors and other theorists who contributed to Levine's thinking included von Bertalanffy (open system), Erikson (developmental theories), Selye (stress and adaptation), and Nightingale (ideas about observations) (Johnson & Webber, 2010; Schaefer, 2010a).

Levine was a dynamic speaker and a prolific writer. Her contributions to the profession of nursing were recognized through numerous honors, including her being a charter fellow in the American Academy of Nursing and an honorary doctorate from Loyola University. Levine died in 1996 at the age of 75 (Schaefer, 2010a).

OVERVIEW OF THE CONSERVATION MODEL

A BRIEF DISCUSSION OF THE VALUE system upon which Levine's conservation model is built will enhance understanding of the concepts of this model. Levine believed that the foundational belief of the sanctity of life provided the structure for all moral systems and that all of the efforts of the healing sciences were founded upon the holiness and wholeness of the human being (Levine, 1989a, p. 125). She also deliberately used the word "patient" in all of her publications rather than the word "client" to describe the recipient of care. She explained that the Latin root word for "client" means "follower"; given that this usage is reminiscent of a paternalistic relationship, she suggested, it ought to be forbidden in nursing on moral grounds. In contrast, the word "patient" comes from the Latin word for "suffering" (Levine, 1989a, p. 126). According to Levine (1990, p. 199), it is the condition of suffering that allows the patient to set independence aside and accept the services of another person.

Levine introduced the conservation principles in *Nursing Forum* (1967). Two years later, she published her textbook *Introduction to Clinical Nursing* (1969a), which was an application of the framework. She used the term **conservation** to label the framework because it was derived from the Latin word meaning "to keep together" (Pieper, 1989, p. 137).

The goals of the conservation model are achieved through interventions geared toward the four conservation principles:

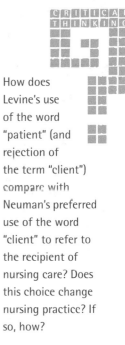

CRITICAL THINKING

How does Levine's use of the word "patient" (and rejection of the term "client") compare with Neuman's preferred use of the word "client" to refer to the recipient of nursing care? Does this choice change nursing practice? If so, how?

❖ The principle of **conservation of energy** addresses the requirement of individuals in relation to a balance of energy and a constant renewal of energy to maintain life processes and activities.

❖ The principle of **conservation of structural integrity** addresses healing as a process of restoring structural and functional integrity through conservation and defense of wholeness, in which those individuals with permanent effects of illness or loss of structure are guided to a new level of adaptation (Levine, 1991, 1996).

❖ The principle of **conservation of personal integrity** recognizes the sanctity of life that is manifest in all persons and "includes recognition of the holiness of each person" (Levine, 1996, p. 40). This principle encompasses the ideas that self-worth and identity are important and, therefore, that nurses should show patients respect (Schaefer, 2010a, p. 229).

❖ The principle of **conservation of social integrity** reminds the nurse that life gains meaning through social communities and that the meaning of health is socially determined (Schaefer, 2010a, p. 229).

The four foundational principles of the conservation model are the conservation of energy, the conservation of structural integrity, the conservation of personal integrity, and the conservation of social integrity.

Three major concepts form the basis of the conservation model and its assumptions: conservation, wholeness, and adaptation. *Conservation*, according to Levine, "describes the way complex systems are able to continue to function even when severely challenged" (1990, p. 192). It is through the process of conservation that persons are able to face challenges, adapt, and maintain their uniqueness. The primary focus of conservation is keeping together the wholeness of the person.

The second major concept in the conservation model is *wholeness* (or *holism*). Levine based her definition of wholeness on Erickson's description of wholeness of an open system because she believed that this definition provided the option of exploring the parts of the whole to understand the whole. Integrity refers to the oneness of the person (Schaefer, 2010a, p. 227).

The third major concept in the conservation model is *adaptation*. According to Levine, "adaptation is the process of change whereby the individual retains his integrity within the realities of his internal and external environment" (1973, p. 11). Conservation is the outcome of adaptation. Levine identified three characteristics of adaptation: historicity, specificity, and redundancy (1991). Levine believed that every person has "fixed patterns of responses uniquely designed to ensure success in essential life activities, and demonstrating that adaptation is both historical and specific" (1991, p. 5). Redundancy represents the fail-safe options available to persons to ensure adaptation. Loss of redundant choices through trauma, age, disease, or environmental changes may make it difficult for the person to maintain life (Schaefer, 2010a, p. 227).

MAJOR CONCEPTS OF NURSING ACCORDING TO THE CONSERVATION MODEL

The capacity of the person to adapt to the environmental condition is called the organismic response. There are four levels of organismic response integration: fight or flight, inflammatory response, response to stress, and perceptual awareness (Schaefer, 2010a, p. 228). Nursing care focuses on the management of these responses (Levine, 1969a).

IN ADDITION TO THE CONCEPTS already presented, the four metaparadigm concepts of nursing are identified in Levine's conservation model. These concepts are summarized in Table 12-1.

TABLE 12-1 Metaparadigm Concepts as Defined in Levine's Model	
Person	A "system of systems, [that] in its wholeness expresses the organization of all the contributing parts" (Levine, 1991, pp. 8–9); may be an individual, an individual in a group, or an individual in a community (Levine, 1973)
Environment	The context in which individuals live their lives; each individual has both internal and external environments
Health	Health and disease are patterns of adaptive changes; the concept of health implies wholeness and integrity, whereas disease represents the person's effort to protect self-integrity
Nursing	"Nursing is human interaction" (Levine, 1973, p. 1) and the goal of nursing is to promote adaptation and maintain wholeness (Levine, 1971a, p. 258)

Person

Levine views the person as a "system of systems, [that] in its wholeness expresses the organization of all the contributing parts" (1991, p. 8–9). Levine stresses the holistic nature of persons. She equates wholeness with integrity and integrity with concepts of freedom of choice, sense of identity, and self-worth (Levine, 1991).

Levine also views life as "a process of change" (1989b, p. 326). Persons, as systems of systems, experience life as change through constant adaptation with the goal of conservation. The person can be defined as an individual; an individual in a group, such as a family; or an individual in a community (Levine, 1973) who is in constant interaction with the environment.

Environment

The environment is the context in which individuals live their lives and each individual has both internal and external environments. The internal environment includes physiological and pathophysiological factors within the patient that are challenged by changes in the external environment. The external environment consists of factors that impose on and challenge the person.

Levine acknowledges three levels of environment: perceptual, operational, and conceptual (Levine, 1973). The perceptual environment includes aspects of the world that persons interpret through the senses. The operational environment includes elements of the environment that physically affect persons but may not be perceived. The conceptual environment includes cultural patterns that affect behavior (Schaefer, 2010b, p. 214–215).

Health

Levine views health and disease as patterns of adaptive changes (Levine, 1971a), where the ultimate goal is well-being. The concept of health implies wholeness and integrity, whereas disease presents the person's "effort to protect self-integrity" (Levine, 1971a, p. 257). According to Levine (1973), disease is unregulated and undisciplined change rather than sequential and orderly change, and it must be stopped to prevent death.

In addition, health is socially defined according to the person being able to function in a reasonably normal manner. The definition of health is expected to change over time for individuals (Levine, 1969b).

Nursing

"The nurse enters into a partnership of human experience where sharing moments in time—some trivial, some dramatic—leaves its mark forever on each patient."

According to Levine, "Nursing is human interaction" (1973, p. 1). Elaborating upon the essence of nursing, Levine states that "The nurse enters into a partnership of human experience where sharing moments in time—some trivial, some dramatic—leaves its mark forever on each patient" (1977, p. 845). The goal of nursing is to promote adaptation and maintain wholeness (Levine, 1971a, p. 258). This goal is accomplished through the conservation of energy and structural, personal, and social integrity (Levine, 1991).

ANALYSIS OF THE CONSERVATION MODEL

THE ANALYSIS PRESENTED HERE CONSISTS of an examination of assumptions and propositions as well as a brief critique of the conservation theory as proposed by Levine.

Assumptions of the Conservation Model

Although Levine did not specifically state assumptions, the following statements have been identified as assumptions (Fawcett, 2005; Schaefer, 1996, 2010a):

❖ The person can be understood only in the context of his or her environment (Levine, 1973), including the context of place or time (Levine, 1990, p. 197).

❖ Persons are sentient, thinking, future-oriented and past-aware individuals (Levine, 1989b, p. 326).

❖ "Every self-sustaining system monitors its own behavior by conserving the use of resources required to define its unique identity" (Levine, 1991, p. 1).

❖ Human beings respond in a singular, yet integrated, fashion (Levine, 1971b).

Propositions of the Conservation Model

The relational propositions of Levine's conservation model as identified by Fawcett (2005, p. 144–145) are listed here:

❖ The conservation model emphasizes that the environment is not a passive stage setting, but rather that the person is an active participant in exploring, seeking, and testing the world he or she inhabits (Levine, 1992, p. 41).

❖ The individual is always within an environmental milieu, and the consequences of his or her awareness of the environment persistently influence the person's behavior at any given moment (Levine, 1973, p. 444).

❖ The person's presence in the environment also influences it and, therefore, the kind of information available from it (Levine, 1973, p. 446).

❖ The individual protects and defends himself or herself within the environment by gaining all the information he or she can about it (Levine, 1973, p. 451).

❖ The interaction at the interface between the individual and the environment is an orderly, sometimes predictable, but always limited process. The consequence of the interaction is invariably the product of the characteristics of the individual and the external factors; the process of the interaction is adaptation (Levine, 1989b, p. 326).

❖ The ability of every individual not only to survive but also to flourish is a consequence of the competence of the person's interactions with the environments in which he or she functions (Levine, 1991, p. 4–5).

❖ The person cannot be described apart from the specific environment in which he or she is found. The precise environment necessarily completes the wholeness of the individual (Levine, 1989b, p. 325).

❖ The goal of conservation is health (Levine, 1990, p. 193).

❖ Conservation of the integrity of the person is essential to assuring health and providing the strength needed to confront disability. Indeed, the importance of conservation in the treatment of illness is precisely focused on the reclamation of wholeness or health (Levine, 1991, p. 3).

❖ The environment is not always "user-friendly." Successful engagement with the environment depends on the individual's repertoire—that store of adaptations which is either built into the genes or achieved through life experiences. While redundant or backup systems may offer options when the initial response is insufficient, health and safety are products of a competent conservation (Levine, 1990, p. 193).

❖ The nurse cannot enter another person's environment without becoming an essential factor in it (Levine, 1992, p. 41).

❖ The nurse participates actively in every patient's environment, and much of what the nurse does supports the patient's adaptations as he or she struggles in the predicament of illness (Levine, 1973, p. 13).

❖ Even in the presence of disease, the organism responds wholly to the environmental interaction in which it is involved. A considerable element of nursing care is devoted to restoring the symmetry of response—symmetry that is essential to the well-being of the organism (Levine, 1969b, p. 98).

Brief Critique of the Conservation Model

The conservation model was initially derived from deductive logic by integrating theories and concepts from the humanities, sciences of nursing, physiology, psychology, and sociology (Schaefer, 2010a, p. 231). Inductive reasoning was used to further develop the model as Levine lived the model in practice (Schaefer, 2010a, p. 233). The resulting model is clear, simple, and easily generalizable. Although it includes numerous terms, all are defined clearly and in a manner that lends to the internal consistency to the model. Levine's model has been used in both research and practice. According to Mefford (2004), the conservation model provides a basis for many other theories for practice, including the theory of conservation, the theory of therapeutic intention, the theory of redundancy, and the theory of health promotion for preterm infants.

THE CONSERVATION MODEL AS A FRAMEWORK FOR NURSING PRACTICE

NURSING CARE USING LEVINE'S CONSERVATION model focuses on the management of the four organismic responses (Levine, 1969a) while addressing the conservation principles. Levine emphasizes the importance of observation in nursing practice where observation is continuous, repetitive, and changing (Levine, 1973, p. 24) as part of the effort to assess wholeness, adaptation, and conservation.

THE NURSING PROCESS AND THE CONSERVATION MODEL

LEVINE USES THE TERM "NURSING process" in her model but does not intend it as it exists in the current nursing jargon. Indeed, she recommends that the nurse use the steps of the scientific method for establishing guidelines of patient care. However, for the sake of discussion, consistency, and comparison, Levine's conservation model will be described here in the context of the steps of the nursing process.

Assessment

The assessment process of nursing is emphasized in the conservation model, with nursing interventions being planned only after the nurse has

What do you think about Levine's view that the nurse should use steps of the scientific method for establishing guidelines of patient care rather than the standard nursing process? Do you think that this approach allows the nurse to meet the standards of care practice requirements for assessment, planning, implementation, and evaluation?

made an accurate assessment of the patient's needs. Collection of data through interviewing and observation is emphasized in the assessment phase. The nurse observes the patient with specific consideration of conservation principles and organismic responses to illness.

Observation is also a tool for directing care, so it must be shared among professionals. Levine (1966) recommended the use of trophicognosis—a scientific method for gathering data into a usable form, reaching nursing care judgments, and communicating information—as an alternative to nursing diagnosis.

Planning

The nurse seeks validation with the patient related to the identified problem. The nurse hypothesizes about the problem and the solution to develop the plan of care (Schaeder, 2010b, p. 219).

Implementation

Interventions are essentially a testing of the hypotheses formulated in the previous phase of the process. Interventions are designed based on addressing the conservation principles (Schaefer, 2010b, p. 219). Even though nursing interventions may focus at a particular time on one of the conservation principles, nurses must continue to recognize the ongoing influence of the other three principles (Levine, 1990). Rationales for nursing interventions are also highly emphasized by Levine.

Evaluation

Evaluation is based on observations of the organismic responses to the interventions and judgments as to whether the hypotheses are supported. If the hypotheses are not supported, then the plan is revised and new hypotheses are proposed (Schaefer, 2010b, p. 220).

THE FOLLOWING SCENARIO ILLUSTRATES NURS-
ING care of the patient relative to one identified
nursing problem framed by Levine's conservation model. This scenario is not intended to cover all
aspects of care, but rather to stimulate thinking about
how specific care might be approached using this theory as a framework for practice.

> **SCENARIO ILLUSTRATING NURSING CARE FRAMED BY THE CONSERVATION MODEL UTILIZING THE NURSING PROCESS**

Mrs. C. is an 85-year-old recent widow who has been
discharged from the acute care setting after an exacerbation of congestive heart failure. The nurse who
visits Mrs. C. will collect data through interview and
observation related to the conservation principles—
including conservation of energy, conservation of structural integrity, conservation of personal integrity, and conservation of social integrity—in an
effort to promote adaptation and maintain wholeness. The assessment
reveals that Mrs. C. is specifically struggling with wholeness to in relation
to conservation of structural integrity as she adapts to a new lifestyle,
specifically in relation to the dietary sodium restriction.

Trophicognosis for Mrs. C. might be fluid volume excess. The nurse
validates the problem with Mrs. C. and hypothesizes a solution. Because
interventions will be designed to address the specific conservation principle, the intervention for Mrs. C. will focus on guiding Mrs. C. to a new
level of adaptation in relation to her dietary restrictions. Evaluation is
based on observations of Mrs. C.'s capacity to adapt and the nurse's judgment as to whether the hypotheses are supported. The nurse will also
apply the model simultaneously to other conservation principles and
other identified problems as indicated by the condition of Mrs. C. and
current best practices.

CLASSROOM ACTIVITY 12-1

Form small groups. Each group should add to the plan of care for Mrs. C. in the preceding scenario based on other potential or actual nursing problems typical for a patient with the same medical diagnosis or symptoms and demographics. Each group should develop a plan for one additional nursing problem using Levine's conservation theory as the basis for practice. Each group should then share its plan with the class.

CLASSROOM ACTIVITY 12-2

Form small groups. Using a case study provided by the instructor, develop a plan of care using Levine's nursing theory as the basis for practice. Each group should then share its plan of care with the class.

CLASSROOM ACTIVITY 12-3

Form small groups. Using a case study provided by the instructor, develop a plan of care using one of the theories as the basis for practice; each group should select a different nursing theory. Each group should then share its plan of care with the class and discuss the similarities and differences in care.

REFERENCES

Fawcett, J. (2005). *Contemporary nursing knowledge: Analysis and evaluation of nursing models and theories* (2nd ed.). Philadelphia: F. A. Davis.

Johnson, B. M., & Webber, P. B. (2010*). An introduction to theory and reasoning in nursing* (3rd ed.). Philadelphia: Lippincott Williams & Wilkins.

Levine, M. E. (1966). Trophicognosis: An alternative to nursing diagnosis. *American Nurses Association Regional Clinical Conferences, 2*, 55–70.

Levine, M. E. (1967). The four conservation principles of nursing. *Nursing Forum, 6*, 45–59.

Levine, M. E. (1969a). *Introduction to clinical nursing.* Philadelphia: F. A. Davis.

Levine, M. E. (1969b). The pursuit of wholeness. *American Journal of Nursing, 69*, 93–98.

Levine, M. E. (1971a). Holistic nursing. *Nursing Clinics of North America, 6*, 253–263.

Levine, M. E. (1971b). *Renewal for nursing.* Philadelphia: F. A. Davis.

Levine, M. E. (1973). *Introduction to clinical nursing* (2nd ed.). Philadelphia: F. A. Davis.

Levine, M. E. (1977). Nursing ethics and the ethical nurse. *American Journal of Nursing, 77*(5), 845–849.

Levine, M. E. (1989a). Beyond dilemma. *Seminars in Oncology Nursing, 4*, 124–128.

Levine, M. E. (1989b). The conservation principles of nursing: Twenty years later. In J. P. Riehl (Ed.), *Conceptual models for nursing practice* (3rd ed., pp. 325–337). Norwalk, CT: Appleton & Lange.

Levine, M. E. (1990). Conservation and integrity. In M. E. Parker (Ed.), *Nursing theories in practice* (pp. 189–201). New York: National League for Nursing.

Levine, M. E. (1991). The conservation principles: A model for health. In K. Schaefer & J. Pond (Eds.), *Levine's conservation model: A framework for nursing practice* (pp. 1–11). Philadelphia: F. A. Davis.

Levine, M. E. (1992). Nightingale redux. In F. N. Nightingale, *Notes on nursing: What it is, what it is not* (commemorative edition, pp. 39–43). Philadelphia: Lippincott.

Levine, M. E. (1996). The conservation principles: A retrospective. *Nursing Science Quarterly, 9*(1), 38–41.

Mefford, L. C. (2004). A theory of health promotion for preterm infants based on Levine's conservation model of nursing. *Nursing Science Quarterly, 17*(3), 260–266.

Pieper, B. A. (1989). Levine's nursing model: The conservation principles. In J. J. Fitzpatrick & A. L. Whall (Eds.), *Conceptual models of nursing: Analysis and application* (2nd ed., pp. 137–146). Norwalk, CT: Appleton & Lange.

Schaefer, K. M. (1996). Levine's conservation model: Caring for women with chronic illness. In P. H. Walker & B. Neuman (Eds.), *Blueprint for use of nursing models: Education, research, practice and administration* (pp. 187–227). New York: National League for Nursing.

Schaefer, K. M. (2010a). Myra Estrin Levine: The conservation model. In M. R. Alligood & A. M. Tomey (Eds.), *Nursing theorists and their works* (7th ed., pp. 225–241). Maryland Heights, MO: Mosby.

Schaefer, K. M. (2010b). Levine's conservation model in nursing practice. In M. R. Alligood (Ed.), *Nursing theory: Utilization and application* (4th ed., pp. 211–233). Maryland Heights, MO: Mosby.

SELF-CARE DEFICIT THEORY OF NURSING:
Dorothea Orem

LEARNING OBJECTIVES

After completing this chapter the student should be able to

1. Identify and explain the three theories associated with the self-care deficit theory of nursing

2. Explain the major concepts important to nursing as defined by Orem

3. Plan nursing care for a patient scenario utilizing Orem's self-care deficit nursing theory

KEY TERMS

Developmental self-care requisites
Self-care agency

Therapeutic self-care demand
Universal self-care requisites

BACKGROUND

DOROTHEA ELIZABETH OREM WAS BORN in Baltimore, Maryland, in 1914. Orem earned a diploma of nursing in the 1930s, a bachelor of science degree in nursing education in 1939, and a master of science degree in nursing education in 1946. Both of the latter degrees came from the Catholic University of America.

Orem's career included a variety of nursing experiences in pediatrics, adult medical and surgical units, emergency rooms, operating rooms, and private duty; she also practiced in roles that included consultant, director, professor, theorist, and author. The self-care deficit theory of nursing for which Orem is well known was formulated incrementally during her early career and subsequently refined throughout her career and retirement. For example, Orem's definition of nursing was formulated in 1956; in 1959, she introduced the basic ideas of the self-care framework. Orem's first book, *Nursing: Concepts of Practice,* was published in 1971. However, it was not until 1985 that Orem introduced the three theories associated with the self-care framework. Orem retired in 1986 and lived in Savannah, Georgia, until her death in 2007 at the age of 92 years (Berbiglia & Banfield, 2010).

OVERVIEW OF *Orem's* SELF-CARE DEFICIT THEORY OF NURSING

THE SELF-CARE DEFICIT NURSING THEORY has been one of the most commonly used nursing theories in the practice setting. Orem's initial purpose in the development of what expanded into the theory was to define nursing's concern and nursing's goal as a part of curriculum development. Her definition of nursing's concern included "man's need for self-care action and the provision and management of it on a continuous basis in order to sustain life and health, recover from disease or injury, and cope with their effects" (Orem, 1959, p. 3). Her definition of nursing's goal comprised, more simply, "overcoming human limitations" (Orem, 1959, p. 4).

Orem described her model as a general theory that is made up of three related theories. The general theory of self-care deficit nursing posits that when the patient or family members are unable to provide care to the patient, a self-care demand exists that can be met by the nurse. The three interrelated theories include the theory of self-care, the theory of self-care deficit, and the theory of nursing systems. According to Orem, "the three-part theory focuses not on individuals, but on persons in relations. Each of the three theories has as its focus a specific dimension of the person: the theory of self-care focuses on the self, the I; the theory of self-care deficit focuses on you and me; and the theory of nursing system focuses on we, persons in community" (1990, p. 49). These three theories in relationship constitute Orem's general theory of nursing known as the self-care deficit theory of nursing (Berbiglia, 2010; Orem, 1990; Taylor, 2006).

Theory of Self-Care

The theory of self-care describes why and how people care for themselves and suggests that nursing is required in case of inability to perform self-care as a result of limitations. This theory includes the concepts of self-care agency, therapeutic self-care demand, and basic conditioning factors.

Self-care agency is an acquired ability of mature and maturing persons to know and meet their requirements for deliberate and purposive action to regulate their own human functioning and development (Orem, 2001, p. 492). The concept of self-care agency has three dimensions: development, operability, and adequacy. Development and operability are identified in terms of the kinds of self-care operations individuals can consistently and effectively perform. Adequacy is measured in terms of the number and kinds of operations in which persons can engage and the operations required to meet a self-care demand (Fawcett, 2005, p. 237; Orem, 2001, p. 256).

According to Orem (2001, p. 491), **therapeutic self-care demand** consists of the summation of care measures necessary to meet all of an individual's known self-care requisites.

Basic conditioning factors refer to those factors that affect the value of the therapeutic self-care demand or self-care agency of an individual. Ten factors are identified: age, gender, developmental state, health state, pattern of living, healthcare system factors, family system factors, sociocultural factors, availability of resources, and external environmental factors (Orem, 2001).

Three theories in relationship constitute Orem's self-care deficit theory of nursing, each of which has as its focus a specific dimension of the person: "The theory of self-care focuses on the self, the I; the theory of self-care deficit focuses on you and me; and the theory of nursing system focuses on we, persons in community."

Orem identifies three types of self-care requisites that are integrated into the theory of self-care and provide the basis for self-care. **Universal self-care** requisites are those found in all human beings and are associated with life processes. These requisites include the following needs:

- ❖ Maintenance of sufficient intake of air
- ❖ Maintenance of sufficient intake of water
- ❖ Maintenance of sufficient intake of food
- ❖ Provision of care associated with elimination processes and excrements
- ❖ Maintenance of a balance of activity and rest
- ❖ Maintenance of a balance between solitude and social interaction
- ❖ Prevention of hazards to human life, human functioning, and human well-being
- ❖ Promotion of human functioning and development within social groups in accordance with human potential, known limitations, and the human desire to be normal (Orem, 1985, p. 90–91)

Developmental self-care requisites are related to different stages in the human life cycle and might include events such attending college, marriage, and retirement. Broadly speaking, the development self-care requisites include the following needs:

- ❖ Bringing about and maintenance of living conditions that support life processes and promote the processes of development—that is, human progress toward higher levels of organization of human structures and toward maturation
- ❖ Provision of care either to prevent the occurrence of deleterious effects of conditions that can affect human development or to mitigate or overcome these effects from various conditions (Orem, 1985, p. 96)

Health–deviation self-care requisites are related to deviations in structure or function of a human being. There are six categories of health-deviation requisites:

- ❖ Seeking and securing appropriate medical assistance

❖ Being aware of and attending to the effects and results of illness states

❖ Effectively carrying out medically prescribed treatments

❖ Being aware of and attending to side effects of treatment

❖ Modifying self-concept in accepting oneself in a particular state of health

❖ Learning to live with the effects of illness and medical treatment (Orem, 1985, p. 99–100)

Theory of Self-Care Deficit

The theory of self-care deficit explains that maturing or mature adults deliberately learn and perform actions to direct their survival, quality of life, and well-being; put more simply, it explains why people can be helped through nursing. According to Orem, nurses use five methods to help meet the self-care needs of patients:

❖ Acting for or doing for another

❖ Guiding and directing

❖ Providing physical or psychological support

❖ Providing and maintaining an environment that supports personal development

❖ Teaching (Johnson & Webber, 2010; Orem, 1995; 2001)

Theory of Nursing Systems

The theory of nursing systems describes and explains relationships that must exist and be maintained for the product (nursing) to occur (Berbiglia, 2010; Taylor, 2006). Three systems can be used to meet the self-requisites of the patient: the wholly compensatory system, the partially compensatory system, and the supportive-educative system.

❖ In the *wholly compensatory system*, the patient is unable to perform any self-care activities and relies on the nurse to perform care.

❖ In the *partially compensatory system*, both the patient and the nurse participate in self-care activities, with the responsibility for care shifting from the nurse to the patient as the self-care demand changes.

❖ In the *supportive-educative system,* the patient has the ability for self-care but requires assistance from the nurse in decision making, knowledge, or skill acquisition. The nurse's role is to promote the patient as a self-care agent.

The system selected depends on the nurse's assessment of the patient's ability to perform self-care activities and self-care demands (Johnson & Webber, 2010; Orem, 1995; 2001).

MAJOR CONCEPTS OF NURSING ACCORDING TO *Orem*

IN ADDITION TO THE CONCEPTS already presented, the four metaparadigm concepts of nursing are identified in Orem's theory. These concepts are summarized in Table 13-1. As described by Orem, the concepts of person, environment, health, and nursing are interrelated.

Person

In Orem's self-care deficit nursing theory, the person is viewed biologically, symbolically, and socially but as an integrated whole (Johnson, 1989). A person is defined as the patient in the care of a

TABLE 13-1 Metaparadigm Concepts as Defined by Orem's Theory	
Person (patient)	A person under the care of a nurse; a total being with universal, developmental, and health deviation needs, who is capable of self-care
Environment	Physical, chemical, biologic, and social contexts within which human beings exist. Environmental components include environmental factors, environmental elements, environmental conditions, and the developmental environment (Orem, 1985).
Health	"A state characterized by soundness or wholeness of developed human structures and of bodily and mental functioning" (Orem, 1995, p. 101)
Nursing	Therapeutic self-care designed to supplement self-care requisites. Nursing actions fall into one of three categories: wholly compensatory, partly compensatory, or supportive-educative system (Orem, 1985).

nurse—that is, as a total being with universal, developmental, and health deviation needs, who is capable of self-care.

Environment

While the environment includes the physical, chemical, biologic, and social contexts within which human beings exist, the environmental components include environmental factors, environmental elements, environmental conditions, and the developmental environment (Orem, 1985). As such, the environment is defined as a subcomponent of the person. The person and the environment make up an integrated system, given that environmental factors influence the health needs of patients and, therefore, may be modified by the nurse to affect the patient. For example, to address developmental self-care requisite needs, the provision of an environment conducive to appropriate development might be offered as a method of assisting the patient relative to that category of therapeutic self-care demands (Johnson, 1989).

Health

Orem defines health as "a state characterized by soundness or wholeness of developed human structures and of bodily and mental functioning" (1995, p. 101). Orem's definition of health includes the capacity to live within the physical, biological, and social environments and to achieve a level of innate potential. Nevertheless, because this view of health is somewhat dependent upon the environment, it can be expected that variations in the definition of health will emerge (Johnson, 1989).

Nursing

Nursing agency in Orem's theory refers to the developed capabilities of persons educated as nurses that allow them to act, to know, and to help patients to meet their therapeutic self-care demands and to regulate the development or exercise of the patient's self-care agency. Nursing actions fall into one of three categories: wholly compensatory, partly compensatory, or supportive-educative system (Orem, 1995). The goal or broad purpose of nursing agency, according to Orem (2001, p. 289), is to compensate

Nursing actions fall into one of three categories: wholly compensatory, partly compensatory, or supportive-educative system.

for or overcome known or emerging health-derived or health-associated limitations. This goal is accomplished through either helping the patient accomplish therapeutic self-care, helping the patient move toward responsible self-care, or helping the patient's caregiver become competent in proving and managing the patient's care using nursing supervision and consultation (Orem, 1985).

ANALYSIS OF *Orem's* SELF-CARE DEFICIT NURSING THEORY

THE ANALYSIS PRESENTED HERE CONSISTS of an examination of assumptions and propositions as well as a brief critique of the self-care deficit nursing theory.

Assumptions of Orem's Self-Care Deficit Nursing Theory

Orem's self-care deficit nursing theory is based on both explicit and implicit assumptions. Explicit assumptions are as follows:

- ❖ Nursing is a deliberate, purposeful helping service performed by nurses.

- ❖ Persons are capable and willing to perform self-care for self and for dependent family members.

- ❖ Self-care is part of life that is necessary for health, human development, and well-being.

- ❖ Education and culture influence individuals.

- ❖ Self-care is learned through human interaction and communication.

- ❖ Self-care includes deliberate and systematic actions to meet a known need for care.

- ❖ Human agency is exercised in discovering, developing, and transmitting to others ways and means to identify needs for and make inputs to self and others.

- ❖ Each person possesses powers and capabilities, personal dispositions, talents, interests, and values (Meleis, 2007).

Implicit assumptions of Orem's theory include the following:

❖ People should be self-reliant and responsible for their own care needs as well as others in the family who are not able to care for themselves.

❖ People are individuals (entities) who are distinct from others and from their environment (Meleis, 2007).

Propositions of Orem's Self-Care Deficit Nursing Theory

The self-care deficit theory of nursing includes several general propositions, which are outlined here (Meleis, 2007):

❖ Human beings have capabilities to provide their own self-care or care for dependents to meet universal, developmental, and health-deviation self-care requisites. These capabilities are learned and recalled.

❖ Self-care abilities are influenced by age, developmental state, experiences, and sociocultural background.

❖ Self-care deficits should balance self-care demands and self-care capabilities.

❖ Self-care or dependent care is mediated by age, developmental stage, life experiences, sociocultural orientation, health, and resources.

❖ Therapeutic self-care includes actions of nurses, patients, and others who regulate self-care capabilities and meet self-care needs.

❖ Nurses assess the abilities of patients to meet their self-care needs and their potential of not performing their self-care.

❖ Nurses engage in selecting valid and reliable processes, technologies, or actions for meeting self-care needs.

In addition to these general propositions, each of the three individual theories also has its own set of propositions.

Brief Critique of Orem's Self-Care Deficit Nursing Theory

The terms used in Orem's theory are defined precisely and used consistently across the model as well as within the three theories that make up the model. A limited number of terms are used in the theory, giving it simplicity; at the same time, the concepts are developed with sufficient depth to give the theory the level of complexity necessary to describe and understand nursing as a human practice discipline (Berbiglia & Banfield, 2010).

The theory possesses the characteristics of both generality and empirical precision. Orem addresses the issue of generality by stating that "the self-care deficit theory of nursing is not an explanation of the individuality of a particular concrete nursing practice situation, but rather the expression of a singular combination of conceptualized properties" (1995, p. 166–167), thus making the theory useful in a wide variety of nursing practice situations. Even so, data collected in nursing practice situations can be categorized according to the concepts in the theory.

One of the invaluable contributions of the self-care deficit nursing theory is that it clearly differentiates the focus of nursing from that of other disciplines and provides a unique focus for nursing. In addition, Orem's work provides a structure for the organization of existing nursing knowledge and the generation of new knowledge (Berbiglia & Banfield, 2010).

Orem's SELF-CARE DEFICIT NURSING THEORY AS A FRAMEWORK FOR NURSING PRACTICE

DELIVERING NURSING CARE UTILIZING OREM'S self-care deficit nursing theory may occur at one of the three levels of prevention: primary, secondary, and tertiary. According to Orem, nursing care aimed at universal self-care or developmental self-care, when therapeutic, represents the primary level of prevention. By comparison, nursing care focusing on health-deviation self-care, when therapeutic, represents the secondary or tertiary level of prevention (Orem, 2001, p. 202).

OREM CONSIDERED THE CRITICAL THINK-ING process commonly known as the nursing process to be a component of what she termed the professional–technical system dimension of the concept of nursing agency. Orem (2001) designed a version of the nursing process that is known as the "practice methodology" for the self-care framework. This practice methodology is defined in terms of four operations: diagnostic operations, prescriptive operations, regulatory operations, and control operations.

> **THE NURSING PROCESS AND** *Orem's* **SELF-CARE DEFICIT NURSING THEORY**

Diagnostic Operations

Diagnostic operations—the first phase of the process—begin with the establishment of the nurse–patient relationship and progress to contracting with the patient to identify current and potential therapeutic self-care demands. Assessment of conditioning factors, self-care agency, and a review of universal, developmental, and health deviation self-care requisites and self-care actions also occur in the diagnostic operations phase. An analysis of the assessment data results in a diagnosis related to self-care demands and self-care deficits that reflects the adequacy of self-care agency (Berbiglia, 2010).

Prescriptive Operations

The prescriptive operations phase includes determining the ideal therapeutic self-care demand for the patient. This occurs as the nurse reviews possible helping methods and identifies the most appropriate methods based on the existing conditioning factors. In addition, the prescriptive operations phase is the time when the nurse and the patient plan actions to meet the therapeutic self-care demands and adjust those actions as self-care requisites change. Prioritization of therapeutic self-care demands must occur in this phase prior to determining the nursing and patient actions. Priority must be given to those therapeutic self-care demands that are most essential to physiological processes. As such, top priority is reserved for self-care demands that are essential to life processes. The goal of the second priority level is to prevent personal harm, injury, or

CRITICAL THINKING

How has the development of Orem's theoretical perspective helped to frame nursing knowledge and alter the practice of the nurse?

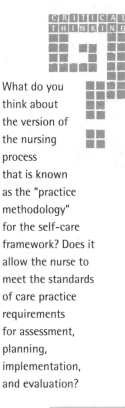

What do you think about the version of the nursing process that is known as the "practice methodology" for the self-care framework? Does it allow the nurse to meet the standards of care practice requirements for assessment, planning, implementation, and evaluation?

health deterioration. Third-priority actions are those that will maintain or promote health, and fourth-priority actions contribute to well-being (Berbiglia, 2010).

Regulatory Operations

The interventions that emerge from the prescriptive phase are used in the regulatory operations phase to design, plan, and produce the regulatory nursing system. During this phase, emphasis is placed on the development of self-care agency (Berbiglia, 2010, p. 269).

Control Operations

Evaluation occurs during the control operations phase of the process. It is during this phase that the effectiveness of interventions and patient outcomes are evaluated. A review of regulatory operations should occur to evaluate for correctness and appropriateness. In addition, patient outcomes should be evaluated in relation to functioning, developmental change, and adaptation to changes in level of self-care ability (Berbiglia, 2010).

SCENARIO ILLUSTRATING NURSING CARE USING *Orem's* SELF-CARE DEFICIT NURSING THEORY UTILIZING THE NURSING PROCESS

THE FOLLOWING SCENARIO ILLUSTRATES NURSING care of the patient relative to one identified nursing problem framed by Orem's self-care deficit nursing theory. This scenario is not intended to cover all aspects of care, but rather to stimulate thinking about how specific care might be approached using this theory as a framework for practice.

Mrs. F. is an 87-year-old patient who has been admitted to the acute care setting with left-side weakness. Diagnostic operations will include the development of a therapeutic relationship between the nurse and Mrs. F. as well as an assessment of conditioning factors, an assessment of self-care agency, and a review of universal, developmental, and health deviation self-care requisites and self-care actions. Through this process, the nurse determines that Mrs. F. requires assistance to safely ambulate and requires moderate assistance with performance of activities of daily living.

During the prescriptive operations phase, the nurse reviews possible helping methods and identifies the most appropriate methods based on Mrs. F.'s existing conditioning factors, including her age, gender, resources, family system, developmental stage, and health state. Priority must be given to those therapeutic self-care demands that are most essential to maintaining physiological processes and to preventing harm.

During the regulatory operations phase, emphasis is placed on the development of self-care agency. This means that the nurse will assist Mrs. F. in the provision of self-care requisites as necessary until Mrs. F. can safely assume responsibility for her own self-care. The nurse will move from provision of care to assisting with care and then to supporting and guiding the Mrs. F. so that she is able to safely care for herself.

During the control operations phase, the nurse makes judgments about the quality of self-care, the development of self-care agency, and the nursing assistance still required by Mrs. F. Based on these judgments the nurse recommends adjustments in nursing care. It is important to note that the nurse also applies the model simultaneously to other self-care deficits and other identified problems as indicated by the condition of Mrs. F. and current best nursing practices.

CLASSROOM ACTIVITY 13-1

Form small groups. Each group should add to the plan of care for Mrs. F. in the preceding scenario based on other potential or actual nursing problems typical for a patient with the same symptoms and demographics. Each group should develop a plan for one additional nursing problem using Orem's theory as the basis for practice. Each group should then share its plan with the class.

CLASSROOM ACTIVITY 13-2

Form small groups. Using a case study provided by the instructor, develop a plan of care using Orem's nursing theory as the basis for practice. Each group should then share its plan of care with the class.

CLASSROOM ACTIVITY 13-3

Form small groups. Using a case study provided by the instructor, develop a plan of care using one of the theories as the basis for practice; each group should select a different nursing theory. Each group should then share its plan of care with the class and discuss the similarities and differences in care.

REFERENCES

Berbiglia, V. A. (2010). Orem's self-care deficit theory in nursing practice. In M. R. Alligood (Ed.). *Nursing theory: Utilization and application* (4th ed., pp. 261–286). Maryland Heights, MO: Mosby.

Berbiglia, V. A., & Banfield, B. (2010). Self-care deficit theory of nursing. In M. R. Alligood & A. M. Tomey (Eds.), *Nursing theorists and their work* (7th ed., pp. 265–285). Maryland Heights, MO: Mosby.

Fawcett, J. (2005). *Contemporary nursing knowledge: Analysis and evaluation of nursing models and theories* (2nd ed.). Philadelphia: F. A. Davis.

Johnson, B. M., & Webber, P. B. (2010). *An introduction to theory and reasoning in nursing* (3rd ed.). Philadelphia: J. B. Lippincott.

Johnson, R. L. (1989). Orem's self-care model for nursing. In J. J. Fitzpatrick & A. L. Whall (Eds.), *Conceptual models of nursing: Analysis and application* (2nd ed., pp. 165–184). Norwalk, CT: Appleton & Lange.

Meleis, A. I. (2007). *Theoretical nursing: Development and progress* (4th ed.). Philadelphia: J. B. Lippincott.

Orem, D. (1959). *Guides for developing curriculum for the education of practical nurses.* Washington, DC: U.S. Government Printing Office.

Orem, D. (1985). *Nursing: Concepts of practice* (3rd ed.). St. Louis, MO: Mosby.

Orem, D. (1990). A nursing practice theory in three parts, 1956–1989. In M. E. Parker (Ed.), *Nursing theories in practice* (pp. 47–60). New York: National League for Nursing.

Orem, D. (1995). *Nursing: Concepts of practice* (5th ed.). St. Louis, MO: Mosby.

Orem, D. (2001). *Nursing: Concepts of practice* (6th ed.). St. Louis, MO: Mosby.

Taylor, S. G. (2006). Self-care deficit theory of nursing. In A. M. Tomey & M. R. Alligood (Eds.), *Nursing theorists and their work* (6th ed., pp. 267–296). St. Louis, MO: Mosby.

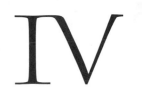

NURSING
THEORIES

THEORY OF INTERPERSONAL RELATIONS:
Hildegard Peplau

LEARNING OBJECTIVES

After completing this chapter the student should be able to

1. Identify and explain the concepts important to the theory of interpersonal relations as proposed by Peplau

2. Explain the major concepts important to nursing as defined by Peplau

3. Plan nursing care for a patient scenario utilizing Peplau's theory of interpersonal relations

KEY TERMS

Orientation phase

Pattern integrations

Resolution (termination) phase

Working phase

BACKGROUND

HILDEGARD PEPLAU WAS BORN IN 1909 in Pennsylvania as the daughter of immigrant parents. She graduated with a diploma from Pottstown Hospital School of Nursing in 1931. In 1943, she received a bachelor of arts degree in interpersonal psychology from Bennington College, Vermont, followed by a master of arts degree in psychiatric nursing from Teachers College, Columbia University in 1947. In 1953, Peplau received an EdD in curriculum development, also from Columbia University (Howk, 2002, p. 379).

Peplau is considered the mother of psychiatric nursing. Although she is best known for the development of the theory of interpersonal relations, she also made significant contributions to the profession of nursing, influencing professional, educational, and practice standards of nursing through emphasizing the importance of professional self-regulation. In addition, Peplau introduced the concept of advanced nursing practice (Howk, 2002, p. 379).

Peplau's work was built upon her personal and practice experiences, including her experiences with professionals from psychiatry, medicine, education, and sociology. She made a strong commitment to incorporate established knowledge into her framework at a time when theory development in the discipline of nursing was very new relative to theory development in related disciplines. Peplau's work was influenced by Freud, Maslow, and Sullivan's interpersonal relationship theories, and by the psychoanalytical model (Haber, 2000; Howk, 2002; Pokorny, 2010). Her understanding of the effects of illness on individuals and families was influenced by her early-life experiences during the great influenza epidemic of 1918 as well as her later clinical observations. Peplau's clinical and teaching experiences were quite varied. She worked as a supervisor for an operating room and infirmary; she practiced in psychiatric facilities; during World War II, she worked in a neuropsychiatric hospital. She taught graduate-level psychiatric nursing at Columbia University and Rutgers University. After her retirement in 1974, she served as a visiting professor at the University of Leuven in Belgium, where she helped to establish the first graduate-level nursing program in Europe (Howk, 2002, p. 380).

In addition, Peplau was an active leader in nursing organizations. She was executive director and president of the American Nurses Association, director of the New Jersey State Nurses' Association, a member of the Expert Advisory Council of the World Health Organization, the National Nurse Consultant to the Surgeon General of the Air Force, and a nursing consultant to the U.S. Public Health Service and National Institute of Mental Health. She also served on editorial boards for psychiatric and mental health professional journals (Howk, 2002, p. 380).

Peplau was honored for her many contributions to the profession of nursing by induction into the American Academy of Nursing's Living Legends Hall of Fame. She was an elected fellow in the American Academy of Nurses and Sigma Theta Tau. Peplau died at the age of 89 in 1999 in her home in California (Howk, 2002, p. 380).

THE THEORY OF INTERPERSONAL RELATIONS is a middle-range theory focusing on the relationship between the nurse and the patient. In her theory, Peplau addresses all of nursing's metaparadigm concepts, but remains primarily concerned with one aspect of nursing: how persons relate to one another. According to Peplau, the nurse–patient relationship is the center of nursing (Young, Taylor, & McLaughlin-Renpenning, 2001).

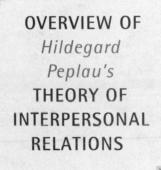

OVERVIEW OF
Hildegard Peplau's
THEORY OF INTERPERSONAL RELATIONS

Peplau (1952) originally described four phases in nurse–patient relationships that overlap and occur over the time of the relationship: orientation, identification, exploitation, and resolution. In 1997, Peplau combined the phase of identification and exploitation, resulting in three phases: orientation, working, and termination. Nevertheless, most other theorists still consider the phases of identification and exploitation to be subphases of the working phase. During the **orientation phase,** a health problem has emerged that results in a "felt need," and professional assistance is sought (p. 18). In the **working phase**, the patient identifies those who can help and the nurse permits exploration of feelings by the patient. During this phase, the nurse can begin to focus the patient on the achievement of new goals. The

According to Peplau, the nurse–patient relationship is the center of nursing.

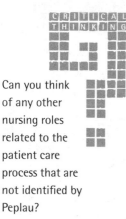

Can you think of any other nursing roles related to the patient care process that are not identified by Peplau?

resolution (termination) phase is the time when the patient gradually adopts new goals and frees himself or herself from identification with the nurse (Peplau, 1952).

As the patient progresses through these phases, he or she assumes roles such as patient and stranger. The patient may also take on the roles or behaviors of an infant, child, adolescent, and adult person depending on his or her personality and level of previous development. However, because the person, as the patient, is probably encountering the stress of illness, he or she may regress to an earlier level of development in relation to his or her role or behavior. The role of the nurse during the various phases of interaction is, in turn, affected by the role of the patient (Blake, 1980).

Peplau (1952) originally described six nursing roles that emerge during the phases of the nurse–patient relationship: the role of the stranger, the role of the resource person, the teaching role, the leadership role, the surrogate role, and the counseling role. Refinement of the theory over Peplau's career resulted in the following list of nursing roles: teacher, resource, counselor, leader, technical expert, and surrogate.

❖ As a teacher, the nurse provides knowledge about a need or problem.

❖ In the role of a resource, the nurse provides information to understand a problem.

❖ In the role of counselor, the nurse helps recognize, face, accept, and resolve problems.

❖ As a leader, the nurse initiates and maintains group goals through interaction.

❖ As a technical expert, the nurse provides physical care using clinical skills.

❖ As a surrogate, the nurse may take the place of another (Johnson & Webber, 2010, p. 125).

Peplau (1952) also described four psychobiological experiences: needs, frustration, conflict, and anxiety. According to Peplau, these experiences "all provide energy that is transformed into some form of action" (p. 71) and provide a basis for goal formation and nursing interventions

(Howk, 2002). Anxiety is an energy that emerges in response to a perceived threat to the biological or psychological security of a person. This threat generally occurs in relationship to communications with others. Peplau viewed anxiety and illness as having a direct relationship. Specifically, in illness, the anxiety needed for growth is bound. A major goal of nursing is to assess the degree of anxiety, the ways in which it is communicated, and its effect on the patient's ability to learn and maintain healthy behavior patterns and to implement strategies to effectively reduce levels of anxiety. Through interpersonal interaction, the nurse facilitates the patient's ability to transform symptom-bound energy into problem-solving energy, with a resultant reduction in anxiety as the patient moves toward health (Reed & Johnston, 1989, p. 59).

People generally develop patterns of behaviors in response to anxiety. In some persons, the problems created by the pattern of response may be the factor that precipitates the patient–nurse relationship. In other persons, the patient–nurse relationship may be initiated because the pattern of response is inadequate to address the anxiety. Because communication is so closely linked with anxiety, Peplau also addresses the concept of communication, noting that communication involves both verbal and nonverbal communication as well as the symbolic meanings behind communications. She further adds that it is the responsibility of the nurse to assess communication factors and to influence the patient's communication in such a way that contributes to health (Reed & Johnston, 1989, p. 53–54).

In addition to anxiety and communication, the concept of **pattern integrations** is a component included in the application of the theory. The concept of pattern integrations refers to the identification of patterns within the interpersonal relationship between two or more persons that link or bind them and enable them to transform energy into patterns of action that bring satisfaction or security in the face of a recurring problem. Four types of integrating patterns are possible:

❖ *Complementary* patterns occur when the behavior of one person fits with and complements the behavior of the other.

❖ *Mutual* patterns occur when the same or similar behaviors are used by both persons.

❖ *Alternating* patterns occur when different behaviors used by two persons alternate between the two persons.

❖ *Antagonistic* patterns may occur if the behaviors of two persons do not fit but the relationship continues (Fawcett, 2005, p. 540).

Peplau, as one of the first theorists since Nightingale to present a theory for nursing, is considered a pioneer in the area of theory development in nursing. It has been suggested that the publication of Peplau's book in 1952 created a paradigm change in the nature of the relationship between the patient and the nurse. Prior to her book, nursing practice involved acting on, to, or for the patient, such that the patient was considered an object of nursing actions. Peplau's work was the force behind the conceptualization of the patient as a *partner* in the nursing process (Howk, 2002, p. 379–380). Peplau's model continues to be used extensively by clinicians, especially those in mental health nursing. Peplau, however, believed that psychodynamic nursing transcended all clinical nursing specialties and that all nursing was based on the interpersonal process and relationship that develops between the nurse and the client (Forchuk, 1995, p. 464).

MAJOR CONCEPTS OF NURSING ACCORDING TO *Peplau*

IN ADDITION TO THE CONCEPTS already presented, the four metaparadigm concepts of nursing are identified in Peplau's theory. These concepts are summarized in Table 14-1.

TABLE 14-1 Metaparadigm Concepts as Defined in Peplau's Theory	
Person	Encompasses the patient (one who has problems for which expert nursing services are needed or sought) and the nurse (a professional with particular expertise) (Peplau, 1992, p. 14)
Environment	Forces outside the organism within the context of culture (Peplau, 1952, p. 163)
Health	"Implies forward movement of personality and other ongoing human processes in the direction of creative, constructive, productive, personal, and community living" (Peplau, 1952, p. 12)
Nursing	The therapeutic, interpersonal process between the nurse and the patient

Person

Peplau views the person in terms of an organism that lives in an unstable equilibrium (Peplau, 1952). The term "person" encompasses both the patient (the individual who has problems for which expert nursing services are needed or sought) and the nurse (a professional with particular expertise) (Peplau, 1992, p. 14).

Environment

Peplau views the environment in terms of "existing forces outside the organism and in the context of culture" (Peplau, 1952, p. 163). As such, the environment encompasses physiological, psychological, and social components that are fluid and that may be either illness maintaining or health promoting (Peplau, 1952, p. 82). She adds that "general conditions that are likely to lead to heath always include the interpersonal process" (Howk, 2002, p. 384; Peplau, 1952, p. 14).

Health

Peplau views health as a word symbol that "implies forward movement of personality and other ongoing human processes in the direction of creative, constructive, productive, personal, and community living" (Peplau, 1952, p. 12). However, in the discussion of illness, it must be noted that Peplau believes that a direct relationship exists between anxiety and illness. In illness, energy from anxiety needed for growth is instead bound in nonhealthy symptoms.

Nursing

Peplau views nursing as a "significant, therapeutic, interpersonal process" (Peplau, 1952, p. 16) between the nurse and the patient that functions cooperatively with other processes to make health possible for individuals. "Nursing is an educative instrument, a maturing force that aims to promote forward movement of personality in the direction of creative, constructive, productive, personal, and community living" (Peplau, 1952, p. 16).

ANALYSIS OF THE THEORY OF INTERPERSONAL RELATIONS

THE ANALYSIS PRESENTED HERE CONSISTS of an examination of assumptions and propositions as well as a brief critique of Peplau's theory of interpersonal relations.

Assumptions of the Theory of Interpersonal Relations

Peplau made the implicit assumption that "the nursing profession has legal responsibility for the effective use of nursing and for its consequences to patients" (1952, p. 6). Peplau (1952, p. xii) also identifies two explicit assumptions that guide her theory:

❖ "The kind of person that the nurse becomes makes a substantial difference in what each patient will learn as he or she receives nursing care."

❖ "Fostering personality development toward maturity is a function of nursing and nursing education. Nursing uses principles and methods that guide the process toward resolution of interpersonal problems."

Propositions of the Theory of Interpersonal Relations

The only relational proposition that can be identified in Peplau's theory is that nursing actions or processes are beneficial to human beings. However, because the nurse–patient relationship is viewed as one concept within the theory, it can be argued that the theory omits relational propositions. Nonrelational propositions include the following (Fawcett, 2005):

❖ The nurse–patient relationship is an interpersonal process made up of four components: the client, the nurse, the professional expertise of the nurse, and the client's problem or need for which expert nursing serves are sought (Peplau, 1992).

❖ The nurse–patient relationship is an interpersonal process that comprises three sometime overlapping or interlocking phases (Peplau, 1952).

CRITICAL THINKING

How has the development of Peplau's theoretical perspective helped to frame nursing knowledge and influence nursing practice?

Brief Critique of Peplau's Theory of Interpersonal Relations

Peplau's theorizing was primarily inductive and based on observations in her clinical work and environment. Her theory also had foundations in existing, established theory. Peplau's theory is clear and easy to understand, and its basic concepts are defined and assumptions are stated. The theory can be generalized and tested and has been utilized in practice, education, and research.

A CENTRAL FEATURE IN THE CLINICAL methodology when using Peplau's theory of interpersonal relations is the nurse's ability "to interpret observations and to guide the patient's work in formulating his or her own interpretations of personal experience" (Peplau, 1992, p. 18). According to Peplau, "Observation, communication, and recording are all interlocking performances in interpersonal relations that make it possible for nurses to study what is happening in their contact with patients" (1952, p. 309). This is a vital component of the assessment, data analysis, and evaluation of nursing care.

WHILE THE NURSING PROCESS IS not explicitly mentioned in Peplau's theory, the various phases known as the nursing process can be identified for the sake of examination, consistency, and comparison.

> *Peplau's*
> **THEORY OF INTERPERSONAL RELATIONS AS A FRAMEWORK FOR NURSING PRACTICE**

> **THE NURSING PROCESS AND** *Peplau's* **THEORY OF INTERPERSONAL RELATIONS**

Assessment

The nurse who is practicing using Peplau's theory of interpersonal relations would work in the orientation phase as a counselor to establish a relationship with the patient and family and to identify actual or potential problems.

Planning

By the end of the orientation phase, the nurse and the patient are no longer strangers and are ready to move into the working phase of the relationship so that planning can begin and problems that have been identified can be resolved.

Implementation

Once the working phase of the relationship is achieved, the nurse–patient partnership is clarified to agree upon the level of dependence/independence expected by the patient. Once a problem has been identified and clarified, the nurse takes on the role of teacher and resource to provide information about the problem and types of assistance available. The nurse is ultimately responsible for setting goals that move the patient toward independence. Throughout this process the nurse supports the patient's abilities (Johnson & Webber, 2010, p. 125).

Evaluation

Evaluation is based upon the patient's achievement of the goals set during an earlier phase of the nurse process. The termination phase occurs when the patient's problem is resolved and the patient is ready for independence from the nurse (Johnson & Webber, 2010, p. 125).

SCENARIO ILLUSTRATING NURSING CARE FRAMED BY *Peplau's* THEORY OF INTERPERSONAL RELATIONS IN NURSING UTILIZING THE NURSING PROCESS

THE FOLLOWING SCENARIO ILLUSTRATES NURSING care of the patient relative to one identified nursing problem framed by Peplau's theory of interpersonal relations in nursing. This scenario is not intended to cover all aspects of care, but rather to stimulate thinking about how specific care might be approached using this theory as a framework for practice.

Mr. B. is a young adult male who presents to the clinic with symptoms of anxiety and fatigue, with a history of chemical dependency and alcohol abuse. The nurse works in the orientation phase as a counselor to establish a relationship with Mr. B. and his family and to identify actual or potential problems. By the end of the orientation phase, the nurse and Mr. B. are no longer strangers and are ready to move into the working phase of the relationship, so that planning can begin and problems that have been identified can be resolved. The problem identified for Mr. B. is ineffective coping related to situational stressors.

Once the working phase of the relationship is achieved, the nurse–patient partnership is clarified to agree upon the level of dependence/independence expected by Mr. B. The nurse takes on the role of teacher and resource to provide information related to effective coping strategies and the assistance available to Mr. B. During this phase, the nurse allows Mr. B. to explore his feelings and guides Mr. B. to set goals that gradually increase his level of independence. The resolution or termination phase occurs over time as Mr. B. adopts new goals and frees himself from identification with the nurse.

Throughout this process, the model may be applied simultaneously to other problems as they are identified by Mr. B. and the nurse during their therapeutic relationship. Goals are identified and strategies that are congruent with current best clinical practices are planned to address those issues.

CLASSROOM ACTIVITY 14-1

Form small groups. Each group should add to the plan of care for Mr. B. in the preceding scenario based on other potential or actual nursing problems typical for a patient with the same medical diagnosis or symptoms and demographics. Each group should develop a plan for one additional nursing problem using Peplau's theory as the basis for practice. Each group should then share its plan with the class.

CLASSROOM ACTIVITY 14-2

Form small groups. Using a case study provided by the instructor, develop a plan of care using Peplau's nursing theory as the basis for practice. Each group should then share its plan of care with the class.

CLASSROOM ACTIVITY 14-3

Form small groups. Using a case study provided by the instructor, develop a plan of care using one of the theories as the basis for practice; each group should select a different nursing theory. Each group should then share its plan of care with the class and discuss the similarities and differences in care.

REFERENCES

Blake, M. (1980). The Peplau developmental model for nursing practice. In J. P. Riehl & C. Roy (Eds.), *Conceptual models for nursing practice* (2nd ed., pp. 53–59). New York: Prentice Hall.

Fawcett, J. (2005). *Contemporary nursing knowledge development: Analysis and evaluation of nursing models and theories* (2nd ed.). Philadelphia: F. A. Davis.

Forchuk, C. (1995). Hildegard E. Peplau: Interpersonal nursing theory. In C. M. McQuiston & A. A. Webb (Eds.), *Foundations of nursing theory: Contributions of 12 key theorists* (pp. 457–514). Thousand Oaks, CA: Sage.

Haber, J. (2000). Hildegard E. Peplau: The psychiatric nursing legacy of a legend. *Journal of the American Psychiatric Nurses Association, 6,* 56–62.

Howk, C. (2002). Hildegard E. Peplau: Psychodynamic nursing. In A. M. Tomey & M. R. Alligood (Eds.), *Nursing theorists and their work* (5th ed., pp. 379–398). St. Louis, MO: Mosby.

Johnson, B. M., & Webber, P. B. (2010). *An introduction to theory and reasoning in nursing* (3rd ed.). Philadelphia: Lippincott Williams & Wilkins.

Peplau, H. (1952). *Interpersonal relations in nursing.* New York: G. P. Putnam's Sons.

Peplau, H. E. (1992). Interpersonal relations: A theoretical framework for application in nursing practice. *Nursing Science Quarterly, 5,* 13–18.

Peplau, H. E. (1997). Peplau's theory of interpersonal relations. *Nursing Science Quarterly, 10*(4), 162–167.

Pokorny, M. E. (2010). Nursing theorists of historical significance. In M. R. Alligood & A. M. Tomey (Eds.), *Nursing theorists and their work* (7th ed., pp. 54–68). Maryland Heights, MO: Mosby.

Reed, P. G., & Johnston, R. L. (1989). Peplau's nursing model: The interpersonal process. In J. J. Fitzpatrick & A. L. Whall (Eds.), *Conceptual models of nursing: Analysis and application* (2nd ed., pp. 49–67). Norwalk, CT: Appleton and Lange.

Young, A., Taylor, S. G., & McLaughlin-Renpenning, K. (2001). *Connections: Nursing research, theory, and practice.* St. Louis, MO: Mosby.

THEORY OF CULTURE CARE DIVERSITY AND UNIVERSALITY:
Madeleine Leininger

15

BACKGROUND

MADELEINE LEININGER WAS BORN IN Nebraska in 1925. She began her nursing career after she graduated with a diploma from St. Anthony's School of Nursing in Denver, Colorado. In 1950, Leininger received a bachelor's degree in biological science with a minor in philosophy and humanistic studies from Benedictine College in Atchison, Kansas. She then worked as a an instructor, staff nurse, and head nurse on a medical–surgical unit and opened a new psychiatric unit as director of nursing services at St. Joseph's Hospital in Omaha, Nebraska. During that time, she also enrolled in advanced study in nursing at Creighton University in Omaha (McFarland, 2010, p. 454).

In 1954, Leininger received a master's degree in psychiatric nursing from Catholic University of America in Washington, D.C. She then joined the faculty at the University of Cincinnati in Ohio, where she began the world's first master's-level clinical specialist program in child psychiatric nursing. She also initiated and directed the first graduate nursing program in psychiatric nursing at the University of Cincinnati and the Therapeutic Psychiatric Nursing Center. During this same period, she wrote one of the first basic psychiatric nursing text books (McFarland, 2010, p. 454–455).

It was during her time in Cincinnati that Leininger noticed a lack of understanding among staff related to cultural factors influencing the behaviors of children. She observed differences in responses to care and treatments among children from diverse cultural backgrounds. A short time later, Margaret Mead came to the University of Cincinnati as a visiting professor in the Department of Psychiatry. Leininger discussed with Mead the potential interrelationships between nursing and anthropology. She ultimately decided to pursue her interests with focused doctoral study on cultural, social, and psychological anthropology at the University of Washington. After receiving her doctoral degree, Leininger taught the first course in transcultural nursing at the University of Colorado in 1966 (McFarland, 2010, p. 455).

Throughout her long career, Leininger has held faculty and administrative appointments at many prestigious universities, written more than 30 books, lectured extensively, founded the National Transcultural Nursing

Society, and founded and served as editor of the *Journal of Transcultural Nursing*. She has received numerous awards and honors for her lifetime of contributions to nursing practice.

A CCORDING TO LEININGER, THE CULTURE care diversity and universality theory has features that distinctly set it apart from other nursing theories. For example, it is the only theory that focuses on holistic and comprehensive culture care. It can be used in any culture because it includes multiple holistic factors that are universally found across cultures. It is the only theory that focuses on discovering factors influencing human care such as worldview, social structure factors, language, generic and professional care, ethnohistory, and environmental context (Leininger, 2002; McFarland, 2010).

> # OVERVIEW OF
> *Madeleine Leininger's*
> # CULTURE CARE DIVERSITY AND UNIVERSALITY THEORY

Leininger succinctly identified the main features of the theory of culture care diversity and universality by stating that **transcultural nursing** is "a substantive area of study and practice focused on comparative cultural care (caring) values, beliefs, and practices of individuals or groups of similar or different cultures with the goal of providing culture-specific and universal nursing care practices in promoting health or well-being or to help people face unfavorable human conditions, illness, or death in culturally meaningful ways" (1995, p. 58). Universality of care reveals the common nature of human beings; diversity of care reveals the variability and unique features of persons. Consistent with the focus of her theory, Leininger defines the concepts of nursing in a manner that causes the nurse to specifically consider culture in the delivery of competent nursing care.

According to Leininger (2001), three modalities guide nursing judgments, decisions, and actions so that the nurse can provide culturally congruent care that is beneficial, satisfying, and meaningful to the persons the nurse serves. These three modes include cultural care preservation and/or maintenance, cultural care accommodation and/or negotiation, and cultural care repatterning or restructuring. The nurse using Leininger's theory plans and makes decisions with clients with respect to these three

> Leininger defines the concepts of nursing in a manner that causes the nurse to specifically consider culture in the delivery of competent nursing care.

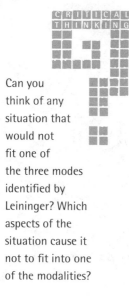

Can you think of any situation that would not fit one of the three modes identified by Leininger? Which aspects of the situation cause it not to fit into one of the modalities?

modes of action. All three care modalities require joint participation by the nurse and patient to achieve nursing care that is culturally congruent (Leininger, 2001).

Leininger provides specific definitions of the three modalities that are central to the nursing theory. **Culture care preservation or maintenance** refers to those assistive, supportive, facilitative, or enabling professional actions and decisions that help people of a specific culture to maintain meaningful care values and lifeways for their well-being, to recover from illness, or to deal with a handicap or dying. **Culture care accommodation or negotiation** refers to those assistive, supportive, facilitative, or enabling professional actions and decisions that help people of a specific culture or subculture adapt to or to negotiate with others for meaningful, beneficial, and congruent health outcomes. **Culture care repatterning or restructuring** refers to the assistive, supportive, facilitative, or enabling professional actions and decisions that help patients reorder, change, or modify their lifeways for new, different, and beneficial health outcomes (Leininger & McFarland, 2006).

Leininger developed the **sunrise model**, which she revised in 2004. She labeled this model as "an enabler," to clarify that while it depicts the essential components of the theory of culture care diversity and universality, it is a visual guide for exploration of cultures. The Sunrise Enabler is available online at the following address: http://wps.prenhall.com/wps/media/objects/2602/2664849/figs_tables/f02_01.pdf.

The Sunrise Enabler symbolizes the rising of the sun (care). The upper half of the circle depicts the components of the social structure and worldview factors that influence care and health through language, ethnohistory, and environmental context. These factors influence the folk, professional, and nursing systems, which are found in the middle part of the model. Nursing acts as a bridge between the folk and professional systems. The Sunrise Enabler depicts human beings as inseparable from their cultural background and social structure, worldview, history, and environmental context. Gender, race, age, and class are also embedded in the social structure factors (Leininger, 1991).

L EININGER DOES NOT ACCEPT THAT the concepts of person, health, environment, and nursing constitute the metaparadigm for nursing (Luna & Cameron, 1989). Nevertheless, Leininger does provide definitions for these concepts within the context of her theory. The metaparadigm nursing concepts are summarized in Table 15-1.

MAJOR CONCEPTS OF NURSING ACCORDING TO *Leininger*

Person

Leininger views human beings as "cultural beings who have survived through time and place because of their ability to care for infants, young and older adults in a variety of environments and ways" (Leininger, 1985, p. 210). Viewing human as cultural beings supports the idea that humans cannot be separated from or understood outside the context of their cultural background. Human beings include individuals, families, cultural groups, communities, and institutions.

Environment

The environmental context is the totality of an event, situation, or experience that gives meaning to human expressions, interpretations, and social interactions in physical, ecological, sociopolitical, and cultural settings

TABLE 15-1 Metaparadigm Concepts as Defined in Leininger's Theory	
Person	Human being, family, group, community, or institution
Environment (environmental context)	Totality of an event, situation, or experience that gives meaning to human expressions, interpretations, and social interactions in physical, ecological, sociopolitical, and/or cultural settings (Leininger, 1991)
Health	A state of well-being that is culturally defined, valued, and practiced (Leininger, 1991, p. 46)
Nursing	Activities directed toward assisting, supporting, or enabling with needs in ways that are congruent with the cultural values, beliefs, and lifeways of the recipient of care (Leininger, 1996)

(Leininger, 1991). Environment is a broad concept that is largely external to humans but exerts daily influence on them (Luna & Cameron, 1989).

Health

According to Leininger, health is more than just the absence of disease or a point on a continuum. The focus of health is on the positive state of well-being; however, it is a state of well-being that is culturally defined, valued, and practiced (Leininger, 1991, p. 46). Health as a concept is also embedded in the social structure (Leininger, 1985, p. 209). As a consequence, the definition of health tends to vary from culture to culture because of differences in values, social structure, and worldview. For these reasons, the nature, meaning, and structure of health must be discovered from the perspective of the patient's unique cultural background (Luna & Cameron, 1989).

Nursing

Nursing is defined by Leininger as "a learned humanistic art and science that focuses upon personalized care behaviors, functions, and processes directed toward promoting and maintaining health behaviors or recovery from illness" (1984, p. 5). Nursing is a transcultural care profession that is unique because human care activities are directed toward assisting, supporting, or enabling persons with needs in ways that are respectful of and congruent with the cultural values, beliefs, and lifeways of the recipients of care (Leininger, 1995).

ANALYSIS OF THE THEORY OF CULTURE CARE DIVERSITY AND UNIVERSALITY

THE ANALYSIS PRESENTED HERE CONSISTS of an examination of assumptions and propositions as well as a brief critique of Leininger's theory of culture care diversity and universality.

Assumptions of the Theory of Culture Care Diversity and Universality

Thirteen major assumptions support Leininger's theory of culture care diversity and universality:

1. Care is the essence of nursing and a distinct, dominant, central, and unifying focus.

2. Culturally based care (caring) is essential for well-being, health, growth, and survival, and to face handicaps or death.

3. Culturally based care is the most comprehensive and holistic means to know, explain, interpret, and predict nursing care phenomena and to guide nursing decisions and actions.

4. Transcultural nursing is a humanistic and scientific care discipline and profession with the central purpose of serving individuals, groups, communities, societies, and institutions.

5. Culturally based caring is essential to curing and healing: There can be no curing without caring, but caring can exist without curing.

6. Concepts, meanings, expressions, patterns, processes, and structural forms of care vary transculturally with diversities (differences) and some universalities (commonalities).

7. Every human culture has generic (lay, folk, or indigenous) care knowledge and practices, and usually professional care knowledge and practices, which vary transculturally and individually.

8. Culture care values, beliefs, and practices are influenced by and tend to be embedded in the worldview, language, philosophy, religion (and spirituality), kinship, social, political, legal, educational, economic, technological, ethnohistorical, and environmental context of cultures.

9. Beneficial, healthy, and satisfying culturally based care influences the health and well-being of individuals, families, groups, and communities within their environmental contexts.

10. Culturally congruent and beneficial nursing care can occur only when care values, expressions, or patterns are known and used explicitly for appropriate, safe, and meaningful care.

11. Culture care differences and similarities exist between professional and client-generic care in human cultures worldwide.

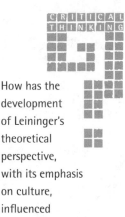

How has the development of Leininger's theoretical perspective, with its emphasis on culture, influenced professional nursing practice?

12. Cultural conflicts, cultural imposition practices, cultural stresses, and cultural pain reflect a lack of the culture care knowledge that is needed to provide culturally congruent, responsible, safe, and sensitive care.

13. The ethnonursing qualitative research method provides an important means to accurately discover and interpret emic and etic embedded, complex, and diverse culture care data (Leininger, 1991, p. 44–45).

Propositions of the Theory of Culture Care Diversity and Universality

In developing her theory, Leininger (2002) formulated four major propositions:

❖ Culture care expressions, meanings, patterns, and practices are diverse, yet have shared commonalities and some universal attributes.

❖ The worldview consists of multiple social structure factors, such as religion, economics, cultural values, ethnohistory, environmental context, language, and generic and professional care, that are critical influencers of cultural care patterns to predict health, well-being, illness, healing, and ways people face disabilities and death.

❖ Generic emic (folk) and professional etic care in different environmental context can greatly influence health and illness outcomes.

❖ Three major action and decision modes provide ways to give culturally congruent, safe, and meaningful health care to cultures: culture care preservation or maintenance, culture care accommodation or negotiation, and culture care repatterning or restructuring. Decision and action modes based on culture care are predicted as key factors to arrive at congruent, safe, and meaningful care.

Brief Critique of Theory of Culture Care Diversity and Universality

Leininger's theory is broad but has specific applicability to individuals and groups when the goal is providing nursing care that is culturally appropriate. Her theory is qualitatively oriented and, therefore, is not generalizable; nevertheless, it is amenable to research within qualitative parameters. The concepts are well organized and defined for study in specific cultures. Rendering culturally specific care has become a key goal in nursing, and the theory of culture care diversity and universality provides a mechanism to accomplish this goal within the discipline of nursing, making it timely in terms of practice, education, and research (McFarland, 2010).

Nursing care driven by Leininger's theory of culture care diversity and universality will begin with being culturally aware and sensitive to each culture, whether it is the culture of an individual patient or the culture of a community or institution. The nurse uses the Sunrise Enabler as a visual guide as he or she systematically explores the components of the culture within the context of the theory so as to achieve the goal of providing competent culturally based care (Morgan, 2010).

The nurse using Leininger's theory plans and makes decisions with clients with respect to the three modes of action. All three care modalities require cooperation of the nurse and the patient, who work together to identify, plan, implement, and evaluate nursing care with respect to the cultural congruence of the care (Leininger, 2001).

> Leininger's
> **THEORY OF CULTURE CARE DIVERSITY AND UNIVERSALITY AS A FRAMEWORK FOR NURSING PRACTICE**

> **THE NURSING PROCESS AND** Leininger's **THEORY OF CULTURE CARE DIVERSITY AND UNIVERSALITY**

Assessment

During the assessment phase, the nurse uses participation, observation, and interviews within the culture to discover the worldview of the member of the culture as well as the patient's cultural and social dimensions, which requires consideration of cultural values, lifeways, influence of language, ethnohistory, and environmental context. Next, the nurse analyzes the information that has been gathered to discover patterns and themes; he or she considers care options based on the assessment data, with the goal of discovering the generic care, nursing care, and professional systems of care recommended (Morgan, 2010, p. 417).

Planning

During the planning phase, the nurse develops a plan of care based on the data gathered and presents the plan to the patient for review and modification. This process should result in culture care preservation or maintenance, accommodation or negotiation, and repatterning or restructuring (Morgan, 2010, p. 417).

All three care modalities require cooperation of the nurse and the patient, who work together to identify, plan, implement, and evaluate nursing care with respect to the cultural congruence of the care.

Implementation

During the implementation or intervention phase, the nurse implements the plan to promote health and well-being.

Evaluation

The nurse observes whether the process has resulted in culturally congruent nursing care.

SCENARIO ILLUSTRATING NURSING CARE FRAMED BY *Leininger's* THEORY OF CULTURE CARE DIVERSITY AND UNIVERSALITY UTILIZING THE NURSING PROCESS

THE FOLLOWING SCENARIO ILLUSTRATES NURSING care of the patient relative to one identified nursing problem framed by Leininger's theory of culture care diversity and universality. This scenario is not intended to cover all aspects of care, but rather to stimulate thinking about how specific care might be approached using this theory as a framework for practice.

Mr. H. is a 52-year-old Native American who is a member of the Choctaw tribe in Mississippi. Mr. H. is overweight and has come to the clinic with his wife, who is also overweight. He complains of symptoms congruent with elevated blood pressure.

The nurse at the clinic is not a member of Mr. H.'s culture but has worked in this clinic—which serves a medical home for the local Choctaw community—for many years. In the past, she has participated in the culture (albeit as an outsider), observed members of the cultural group, and interviewed members of the cultural group. Thus she is familiar with the worldview of the members of the culture, although she acknowledges that the worldviews of different generations within the Choctaw group tend to differ somewhat. In general, she knows the lifeways, cultural values, and environmental context of this particular cultural group. She is also familiar with patterns within the Choctaw group, many of whom suffer from diseases associated with being overweight such as hypertension and diabetes. Specifically, the nurse recognizes that this problem is associated with a diet and sedentary lifestyle that are incongruent with the historical lifeways of this Native American culture. Assessment data collected during her interview with Mr. H. reveal that his lifestyle is sedentary and that he eats a diet high in saturated fat. Mr. H.'s blood pressure is also in a range that is slightly higher than normal.

The Sunrise Enabler will be a useful tool for the nurse as she continues to systematically explore the components of the patient's culture during the process of planning care. During the planning phase, the nurse develops a plan of care based on the data gathered and presents the plan to Mr. H. and his wife for review and modification. This process should result in culture care preservation or maintenance, accommodation, and repatterning as the nurse implements the plan to promote health and well-being of Mr. H. and his family in a way that is both congruent with the lifeways of the Choctaw and congruent with current best practices. Evaluation is based on the nurse's observation that the process has resulted in culturally congruent nursing care for Mr. H. and his family.

Throughout this process, the model may be applied simultaneously to other problems as they are identified by Mr. H. and the nurse. Culturally congruent strategies will be planned to address those issues that are also compatible with current best clinical practices.

CLASSROOM ACTIVITY 15-1

Form small groups. Each group should add to the plan of care for Mr. H. in the preceding scenario based on other potential or actual nursing problems typical for a patient with the same medical diagnosis or symptoms and demographics. Each group should develop a plan for one additional nursing problem using Leininger's theory as the basis for practice. Each group should then share its plan with the class.

CLASSROOM ACTIVITY 15-2

Form small groups. Using a case study provided by the instructor, develop a plan of care using Leininger's nursing theory as the basis for practice. Each group should then share its plan of care with the class.

CLASSROOM ACTIVITY 15-3

Form small groups. Using a case study provided by the instructor, develop a plan of care using one of the theories as the basis for practice; each group should select a different nursing theory. Each group should then share its plan of care with the class and discuss the similarities and differences in care.

REFERENCES

Leininger, M. (1984). Care: The essence of nursing and health. In M. Leininger (Ed.), *Care: The essence of nursing and health* (pp. 3–16). Thorofare, NJ: Slack.

Leininger, M. (1985). Transcultural care diversity and universality: A theory of nursing. *Nursing and Health Care, 6*(4), 209–212.

Leininger, M. (1991). *Culture care diversity and universality: A theory of nursing.* New York: National League for Nursing Press.

Leininger, M. (1995). Transcultural nursing perspectives: Basic concepts, principles, and culture care incidents. In M. M. Leininger (Ed.), *Transcultural nursing: Concepts, theories, research, and practices* (2nd ed., pp. 57–92). New York: McGraw-Hill.

Leininger, M. (2001). *Culture care diversity and universality: A theory of nursing.* Sudbury, MA: Jones and Bartlett.

Leininger, M. (2002). Part I. The theory of culture care and the ethnonursing research method. In M. Leininger & M. R. McFarland (Eds.), *Transcultural nursing: Concepts, theories, research, and practice* (3rd ed., pp. 71–98). New York: McGraw-Hill Medical Publishing Division.

Leininger, M. M., & McFarland, M. R. (2006). *Culture care diversity and universality. A worldwide theory of nursing* (2nd ed.). Sudbury, MA: Jones and Bartlett.

Luna, L., & Cameron, C. (1989). Leininger's transcultural nursing. In J. J. Fitzpatrick & A. L. Whall (Eds.), *Conceptual models of nursing: Analysis and application* (2nd ed., pp. 227–239). Norwalk, CT: Appleton & Lange.

McFarland, M. R. (2010). Madeleine M. Leininger: Culture care theory of diversity and universality. In M. R. Alligood & A. M. Tomey (Eds.), *Nursing theorists and their work* (7th ed., pp. 454–479). Maryland Heights, MO: Mosby.

Morgan, M. G. (2010). Leininger's theory of culture care diversity and universality in nursing practice. In M. R. Alligood (Ed.), *Nursing theory: Utilization and application* (4th ed., pp. 411–428). Maryland Heights, MO: Mosby.

NURSING PROCESS THEORY:
Ida Jean Orlando (Pelletier)

LEARNING OBJECTIVES

After completing this chapter the student should be able to

1. Identify and describe the major concepts of the nursing process theory as proposed by Orlando

2. Explain the major concepts important to nursing as defined by Orlando

3. Plan nursing care for a patient scenario utilizing Orlando's nursing process theory

KEY TERMS

⦙ Nursing process discipline

BACKGROUND

IDA JEAN ORLANDO, BORN IN 1926, was a first-generation American of Italian descent. She received a diploma in nursing from New York Medical College, Flower Fifth Avenue Hospital School of Nursing, in 1947. By 1951, she had earned a bachelor of science degree in public health nursing from St. John's University in Brooklyn, New York; in 1954, she completed a master of arts degree in mental health consultation from Columbia University Teachers College. During these years, Orlando worked in various clinical nursing positions in obstetrical, medical, surgical, and emergency services. Eventually, she became assistant director of nursing and was responsible for teaching several courses in the hospital-based school of nursing (Schmieding, 2002).

Beginning in 1954, Orlando taught for eight years at Yale School of Nursing. While at Yale, she served as a research associate and principal investigator on a grant-funded project examining the integration of mental health concepts into the basic nursing curriculum. The study was carried out by observing and participating in experiences with patients, students, nurses, and instructors and was derived inductively from field notes by analysis of content of 2000 nurse–patient contacts (Schmieding, 1993). Orlando reported her findings in her first book, entitled *The Dynamic Nurse–Patient Relationship: Function, Process and Principles of Professional Nursing Practice* (1961). The ideas in this book provided the foundation for Orlando's theory of deliberative nursing process (Fawcett, 2005; Schmieding, 2002).

From 1962 through 1972, Orlando worked as a nursing clinical consultant at McLean Hospital in Massachusetts, during which time she continued to develop and refine her work. In her second book, *The Discipline and Teaching of Nursing Process: An Evaluative Study* (1972), she redefined and renamed the deliberative nursing process as the "nursing process discipline" (Pokorny, 2010). From 1972 until 1981, she continued to consult, lecture, and conduct workshops related to her theory. Orlando accepted a position as a nurse educator for Metropolitan State Hospital in Massachusetts in 1981. Between 1984 and 1987, she held a variety of administrative positions within the hospital before becoming Assistant

Director for Nursing Education and Research in 1987. She retired from nursing in 1992 (Schmieding, 2002).

Orlando credits her search for facts in observing nursing situations as the major influence in the development of her theory, noting that she derived the theory from the conceptualization of those facts. She rejected preexisting frameworks from psychology, social work, and other disciplines for the analysis of the research project data, preferring to find what was there in the data (Orlando, 1989). Her goal was to develop a theory of effective nursing practice that would identify a distinctive role for professional nursing and provide a foundation for the systematic study of nursing (Schmieding, 2002, p. 400).

ORLANDO WAS ONE OF THE first nursing authors to emphasize the elements of the nursing process and the importance of the patient's participation in the nursing process. Her nursing process theory stresses the reciprocal relationship between the patient and the nurse, noting that what the nurse and patient say and do during their interaction affects both of them (Schmieding, 2002, p. 400).

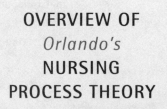

OVERVIEW OF
Orlando's
**NURSING
PROCESS THEORY**

In Orlando's view, the function of the professional nurse is to discover and meet the patient's immediate need for help. Her theory focuses on producing improvement in the patient's behavior. Thus evidence of relief of the patient's distress is seen as positive changes in the patient's observable behavior (Pokorny, 2010).

Persons become patients who require the care of a professional nurse when they have needs for help that cannot be met independently because of either physical limitations, negative reactions to the environment, or an experience that prevents them from communicating their needs. Patients may experience distress or feelings of helplessness as a result of unmet needs (Orlando, 1961). According to Orlando, a positive relationship exists between the time that the patient experiences unmet needs and the degree of distress; therefore, immediacy is stressed in the theory. When individuals are able to meet their own needs, they do not feel distressed and do not require the care of the nurse. It is imperative that nurses share

Orlando's nursing process theory stresses the reciprocal relationship between the patient and the nurse, noting that what the nurse and patient say and do during their interaction affects both of them.

MAJOR CONCEPTS OF NURSING ACCORDING TO *Orlando*

their perceptions with their patients to determine if their perception is congruent with the patient's perception of need (Orlando, 1961).

IN ADDITION TO THE CONCEPTS already presented, the four metaparadigm concepts of nursing are identified in Orlando's nursing process theory. These concepts are summarized in Table 16-1.

Person

Orlando defines the person in terms of the patient. According to Orlando (1961), persons become patients when they have needs that cannot be met independently because of either physical limitations, negative reactions to the environment, or an experience that prevents them from communicating their needs. She also states that each patient is unique.

Environment

Orlando does not define environment, but rather assumes that a nursing situation occurs when there is a nurse–patient contact. She does acknowledge the environment by warning that any aspect of the environment—even though it might be designed for therapeutic purposes—can cause the patient to become distressed (Orlando, 1961; Schmieding, 2002).

TABLE 16-1 Metaparadigm Concepts as Defined in Orlando's Theory

Person	Defines the person in terms of the patient or individual with unmet needs
Environment	Does not define environment but assumes that a nursing situation occurs when there is a nurse–patient contact
Health	Does not define health but assumes that feelings of adequacy and well-being from fulfilled needs contribute to health
Nursing	A distinct profession that functions autonomously, the function of which is to find out and meet the patient's immediate need for help

Health

Orlando does not define health, but rather assumes that freedom from mental or physical discomfort and feelings of adequacy and well-being from fulfilled needs contribute to health (Orlando, 1961; Schmieding, 2002).

Nursing

In Orlando's theory, nursing is a distinct profession that functions autonomously, the function of which is to find out and meet the patient's immediate need for help. The **nursing process discipline** is composed of three elements: the behavior of the patient; the reaction of the nurse; and the nursing actions, which are designed for the patient's benefit. The interaction of these three elements creates the nursing process (Orlando, 1961).

The nursing process discipline is composed of three elements: the behavior of the patient; the reaction of the nurse; and the nursing actions, which are designed for the patient's benefit.

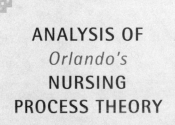

ANALYSIS OF *Orlando's* NURSING PROCESS THEORY

THE ANALYSIS PRESENTED HERE CONSISTS of an examination of assumptions and propositions as well as a brief critique of the nursing process theory.

Assumptions of Orlando's Nursing Process Theory

Nearly all of the assumptions in Orlando's theory are implicit and have been extrapolated by various authors. Schmieding (1993) derived assumptions from Orlando's writings in four areas. These assumptions are organized here based on categories and supporting evidence provided by Schmieding (2002, p. 402).

❖ Assumptions about nursing:

■ Nursing is a distinct profession, separate from other disciplines.

■ Professional nursing has a distinct function and product (outcome).

■ There is a difference between lay and professional nursing.

■ Nursing is aligned with medicine.

- ❖ Assumptions about patients:
  - ▪ Each patient's needs for help are unique.
  - ▪ Patients have an initial ability to communicate their needs for help.
  - ▪ When patients cannot meet their own needs, they become distressed.
  - ▪ The patient's behavior is meaningful.
  - ▪ Patients are able and willing to communicate verbally (and nonverbally when unable to communicate verbally).
- ❖ Assumptions about nurses:
  - ▪ The nurse's reaction to each patient is unique.
  - ▪ Nurses should not add to the patient's distress.
  - ▪ The nurse's mind is the major tool for helping patients.
  - ▪ The nurse's use of automatic responses prevents the responsibility of nursing from being fulfilled.
  - ▪ The nurse's practice is improved through self-reflection.
- ❖ Assumptions about the nurse–patient situation:
  - ▪ The nurse–patient situation is a dynamic whole.
  - ▪ The phenomenon of the nurse–patient encounter represents a major source of nursing knowledge.

Propositions of Orlando's Nursing Process Theory

Orlando did not formulate explicit propositions for the nursing process theory; nevertheless, propositional statements can be derived from concept relationships in the theory. Some authors have identified six propositions from the work of Orlando (Schmieding, 1995), whereas others have identified as many as nine (Fawcett, 2005). The six most commonly cited are listed here:

- ❖ There is a relationship between the patient's presenting behavior and the presence of patient distress (an immediate need for help).
- ❖ There is a relationship between a nurse's use of Orlando's distinct nursing function and the nurse's ability to recognize the need for inquiry (deliberative nursing process) into the meaning of the patient's presenting behavior.

❖ The more competent the nurse is in labeling his or her perceptions, thoughts, and feelings (immediate reaction), the more apt the nurse is to find out (deliberative nursing process) the nature of the patient's distress.

❖ If the nurse explores his or her immediate reaction with the patient, the patient's distress is lessened (improvement).

❖ The nurse's use of the deliberative nursing process will be less costly than the nurse's use of automatic personal responses (a secondary concept of the theory).

❖ Patients experiencing repeated improvement as the result of deliberative nursing will have positive cumulative effects (Schmieding, 1995).

Brief Critique of Orlando's Nursing Process Theory

Orlando's nursing process theory was developed inductively and is logical and applicable to nursing practice. The theory is considered simple because it includes few concepts and relationships. The theory is internally consistent and meets the criteria for testability for a middle-range theory. Orlando made a significant contribution to nursing knowledge by developing a middle-range predictive theory that specifies a nursing process that will meet a person's need for help (Fawcett, 2005, p. 525). According to Pokorny (2010, p. 66), Orlando's theory remains one of the most effective practice theories and is especially helpful to new nurses as they begin practice.

T HE FRAMEWORK FOR ORLANDO'S NURSING process theory consists of five interrelated concepts, as summarized by May (2010, p. 339):

❖ The organizing principle or professional nursing function

❖ The problematic situation or the patient's presenting behavior

❖ The internal response or immediate reaction

Orlando's
NURSING PROCESS THEORY AS A FRAMEWORK FOR NURSING PRACTICE

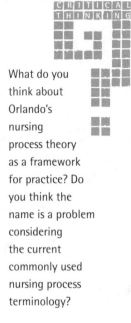

What do you think about Orlando's nursing process theory as a framework for practice? Do you think the name is a problem considering the current commonly used nursing process terminology?

❖ Reflective inquiry or deliberative nursing process

❖ Resolution or improvement

To elaborate briefly upon these concepts, Orlando believed that professional nursing practice was distinct and autonomous and that both the nurse and the patient participate in the exploratory process to identify the problem and the solution. Thus the nurse–patient situation is a dynamic process in which each party is affected by the behavior of the other. The patient's presenting behavior triggers an automatic and immediate reaction in the nurse based on the nurse's perceptions, past experiences, and knowledge. The deliberative (or disciplined) nursing process views the nurse–patient situation as a dynamic whole, and is a complex process in which observations are used to obtain facts. The nurse cannot assume that any of his or her perceptions are correct until they are validated through exploration with the patient. Nevertheless, the nurse's automatic thoughts, while less efficient, can be used if exploring perceptions does not prove successful. Once the patient's needs for help are discovered and met, the situation loses its problematic character and improvement occurs (May, 2010).

THE NURSING PROCESS AND *Orlando's* THEORY

ORLANDO'S NURSING PROCESS THEORY SHOULD not be confused with what is commonly known as the nursing process: They are not the same processes. In this section, however, nursing care using Orlando's theory will be considered in the context of the steps of the nursing process for the sake of discussion, consistency, and comparison.

Assessment

Information gathered through assessment is necessary to achieve an accurate understanding of the patient's presenting behavior and to determine if the patient is in need of the professional nurse's help. According to Orlando (1961, p. 26), the nurse should first take the initiative of helping the person express the specific meaning of the behavior in an effort to determine the source of his or her distress; next, the nurse should explore the distress to assess the help the person requires for the need to be met. The process used to share and validate the nurse's direct and indirect observations is known as the **deliberative nursing process**.

Planning

Planning occurs with participation from both the nurse and the patient.

Implementation

Two types of help are discussed by Orlando. Direct help occurs when the nurse meets the patient's need directly because the patient is unable to meet his or her own need and when the activity is confined to the nurse–patient contact. Indirect help occurs when the activity to meet the patient's need extends to arranging the services of a person, agency, or resource that the patient cannot contact by himself or herself (Fawcett, 2005, p. 523).

Evaluation

It is not the nurse's activity that is evaluated; rather, the focus is on whether the nurse's action helped the patient communicate his or her need for health and whether the need was met (Orlando, 1961). According to Orlando (1972), change will be observable in the patient's verbal and nonverbal behavior when improvement occurs. If the patient's behavior has not changed, then the function of nursing has not been met. In such a case, the nurse continues the process until improvement occurs.

T HE FOLLOWING SCENARIO ILLUSTRATES NURS- ING care of the patient relative to one identified nursing problem framed by Orlando's nursing process theory. This scenario is not intended to cover all aspects of care, but rather to stimulate thinking about how specific care might be approached using this theory as a framework for practice.

CRITICAL THINKING

Do you think that Orlando's nursing process theory allows the nurse to meet the standards of care practice requirements for assessment, planning, implementation, and evaluation?

SCENARIO ILLUSTRATING NURSING CARE FRAMED BY *Orlando's* **THEORY UTILIZING THE NURSING PROCESS**

Mrs. C. is an elderly home health patient. Her daughter phones the nurse on call one Saturday afternoon, saying that her mother is distressed because she has not had a bowel movement for several days and she will not come out of the bathroom. The nurse arrives to find Mrs. C. in tears. Mrs. C. has a standing order for an oil retention enema and cleansing enema as needed. After an initial assessment, the nurse shares with Mrs. C. her perception of the problem. Mrs. C. agrees that if she is able to have a bowel movement, her distress will be relieved; she also agrees to allow the nurse to administer the prescribed enemas. The nurse administers the oil retention enema followed by a cleansing enema and Mrs. C. is able to evacuate her bowels.

After Mrs. C. is able to evacuate her bowels, she thanks the nurse and is able to lie down and rest. Once the nurse assesses that the patient is no longer is distress, the nurse evaluates that the function of nursing has been met.

Throughout this process, the model may be applied simultaneously to other problems as they are identified by Mrs. C. and the nurse. If other issues arise during the nursing encounter, intervention strategies will be planned to address those issues that are also compatible with current best clinical practices.

CLASSROOM ACTIVITY 16-1

Form small groups. Each group should add to the plan of care for Mrs. C. in the preceding scenario based on other potential or actual nursing problems typical for a patient with the same medical diagnosis or symptoms and demographics. Each group should develop a plan for one additional nursing problem using Orlando's nursing process theory as the basis for practice. Each group should then share its plan with the class.

CLASSROOM ACTIVITY 16-2

Form small groups. Using a case study provided by the instructor, develop a plan of care using Orlando's nursing process theory as the basis for practice. Each group should then share its plan of care with the class.

CLASSROOM ACTIVITY 16-3

Form small groups. Using a case study provided by the instructor, develop a plan of care using one of the theories as the basis for practice; each group should select a different nursing theory. Each group should then share its plan of care with the class and discuss the similarities and differences in care.

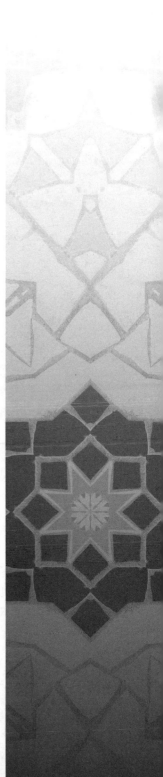

REFERENCES

Fawcett, J. (2005). *Contemporary nursing knowledge: Analysis and evaluation of nursing models and theories* (2nd ed.). Philadelphia: F. A. Davis.

May, B. A. (2010). Orlando's nursing process theory in nursing practice. In M. R. Alligood (Ed.), *Nursing theory: Utilization and application* (4th ed., pp. 337–357). Maryland Heights, MO: Mosby.

Orlando, I. J. (1961). *The dynamic nurse–patient relationship: Function, process and principles of professional nursing practice.* New York: G. P. Putman's Sons.

Orlando, I. J. (1972). *The discipline and teaching of nursing process: An evaluative study.* New York: G. P. Putman's Sons.

Orlando, I. J. (1989). *The nurse theorists: Portraits of excellence.* Athens, OH: Fuld Institute of Technology in Nursing Education.

Pokorny, M. E. (2010). Nursing theorists of historical significance. In A. M. Tomey & M. R. Alligood (Eds.), *Nursing theorists and their work* (7th ed., pp.54–68). Maryland Heights, MO: Mosby.

Schmieding, N. J. (1993). *Ida Jean Orlando: A nursing process theory.* Newbury Park, CA: Sage.

Schmieding, N. J. (1995). Ida Jean Orlando: A nursing process theory. In C. M. McQuiston & A. A. Webb (Eds.), *Foundations of nursing theory: Contributions of 12 key theorists* (pp. 561–620). Thousand Oaks, CA: Sage.

Schmieding, N. J. (2002). Ida Jean Orlando (Pelletier): Nursing process theory. In A. M. Tomey & M. R. Alligood (Eds.), *Nursing theorists and their work* (5th ed., pp. 399–417). St. Louis, MO: Mosby.

HEALTH AS EXPANDING CONSCIOUSNESS:
Margaret Newman

LEARNING OBJECTIVES

After completing this chapter the student should be able to

1. Identify and describe the major concepts of the health as expanding consciousness theory as proposed by Newman

2. Explain the major concepts important to nursing as defined by Newman

3. Plan nursing care for a patient scenario utilizing Newman's theory of health as expanding consciousness

KEY TERMS

Consciousness
Movement

Pattern
Time

BACKGROUND

MARGARET NEWMAN WAS BORN IN 1933 in Memphis, Tennessee. She earned a bachelor's degree in home economics and English from Baylor University and a second bachelor's degree in nursing from the University of Tennessee in Memphis. Newman earned a master's degree in medical–surgical nursing and teaching from the University of California, San Francisco. In 1971, she received her PhD in nursing science and rehabilitation nursing from New York University (Brown, 2010a, p. 480).

Newman held academic positions in four universities over her career: University of Tennessee, New York University, Pennsylvania State University, and University of Minnesota. Her theory of health as expanding consciousness was first published in 1979, and over the course of her career she published several books, chapters, and articles on the theory. She was invited to do presentations and consultations in numerous countries around the world and received many awards and honors for her contributions to the profession of nursing. Newman retired in 1996 with Professor Emeritus status (Brown, 2010a, p. 480–481).

Prior to studying nursing, Margaret Newman was the primary caregiver for her mother, who had amyotrophic lateral sclerosis (ALS). During this time, she became interested in nursing. She credits the work of Martha Rogers, one of her professors when she was a graduate student at New York University, and Rogers' science of unitary human beings as influencing her own work as Newman began exploring the relationships between time, movement, and space and thinking about how these concepts are related to health and illness. Other scholars also influenced her thinking, however (Brown, 2010b; Johnson & Webber, 2010, p. 159; Marchione, 1993; Newman, 1991; 1994/2000).

OVERVIEW OF Newman's THEORY OF HEALTH AS EXPANDING CONSCIOUSNESS

FROM THE EARLY DEVELOPMENT OF the theory, the major concepts specific to Newman's theory have been consciousness, pattern, movement, space, and time. Movement, space, and time have been viewed as dimensions of pattern and consciousness. Over time, these concepts have been synthesized and the theory has evolved so that now it includes the major concepts of health, consciousness, and patterns of movement and space–time (Brown, 2010b).

Newman's health as expanding consciousness theory proposes a view of health that is a unidirectional, unitary process of development (Newman, 1991)—an expansion of consciousness that is seen as the ability of the person to interact with the environment (Newman, 1994/2000). Newman considers health and illness to be components of a unitary process that she refers to as a pattern of wholeness. She posits not only that health is a process, but also that health and illness are a single process. She likens this process to rhythmic phenomena "manifest in ups and down, peaks and troughs, moving through varying degrees of organization and disorganization, but all as one unitary process" (Newman, 1986).

According to Newman, the "process of the evolution of consciousness is the process of health" (1994/2000, p. 43), in which human beings come from a state of potential consciousness into the world with the capacity for understanding that enables them to gain insight into their patterns. It is this insight that provides the turning point in evolving consciousness (Newman, 1994/2000, p. 43).

Consciousness is the system's ability to interact with the environment (Newman, 1990a). It includes the cognitive and affective awareness as well as the "interconnectedness of the entire living system" (Newman, 1990a, p. 38). According to Newman, the person does not just possess consciousness; rather, the person *is* consciousness.

Newman also asserts that the highest level of consciousness is absolute consciousness, which has been equated with love and is a state where all opposites are reconciled. According to Newman, "This kind of love embraces all experience equally and unconditionally: pain as well as pleasure, failure as well as success, ugliness as well as beauty, disease as well as non-disease" (Newman, 1994/2000, p. 48).

Pattern is the "information that depicts the whole and understanding of the meaning of all of the relationships at once" (Brown, 2010a, p. 485). Pattern is constantly moving unidirectionally and evolving, and it includes the dimensions of movement and time–space (Brown, 2010b, p. 462). **Movement** is a reflection of consciousness that indicates inner

Newman considers health and illness to be components of a unitary process that she refers to as a pattern of wholeness.

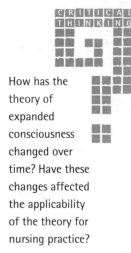

How has the theory of expanded consciousness changed over time? Have these changes affected the applicability of the theory for nursing practice?

organization or disorganization of persons; it communicates the harmony or a person's pattern with the environment (Newman, 1994/2000). **Time** is considered an index of consciousness. As consciousness expands, space–time transcends limitations of the linear and physical boundaries to extend beyond the present (Brown, 2010b, p. 462). However, Newman explains, it is important that one is fully present in the moment because all experiences are manifestations of the process of evolution to higher consciousness (Brown, 2010b; Newman, 1994/2000). The dimensions of space–time–movement are complementary and linked to one another (Brown, 2010b, p. 463). Thus, as consciousness expands, the distinction between self and the world becomes blurred, with the recognition that essence extends "beyond the physical boundaries" (Brown, 2010b, p. 463; Newman, 1994/2000). Newman believes that it is "important to examine movement–time–space together as dimensions of emerging patterns of consciousness rather than in isolation as separate concepts of the theory" (Brown, 2010a, p. 485).

MAJOR CONCEPTS OF NURSING ACCORDING TO *Newman*

IN ADDITION TO THE CONCEPTS already presented, the four metaparadigm concepts of nursing are identified in Newman's health as expanding consciousness theory. These concepts are summarized in Table 17-1.

Person

The person is defined as a "center of consciousness within an overall pattern of expanding consciousness" (Newman, 1986, p. 31). Patients are identified by their individual patterns of consciousness and are viewed by Newman as participants in the transformative process (Newman, 1986). Since the theory's inception, the definition of person has been expanded by Newman to include family and community (Newman, 1994/2000).

Environment

Although environment is not explicitly defined by Newman, interactions between the person and the environment are key processes. Environment is

▦ TABLE 17-1 Metaparadigm Concepts as Defined in Newman's Theory	
Person	A "center of consciousness within an overall pattern of expanding consciousness" (p. 31), identified by individual patterns of consciousness, and viewed as a participant in the transformative process (Newman, 1986)
Environment	An energy field; a universe of open systems; an event, situation, or phenomenon interacting with the person
Health	A synthesis that occurs due to the fusion of disease and nondisease that forms health. Health as a concept is a "pattern of the whole" (Newman, 1986, p. 12).
Nursing	Within the nurse–patient interaction, the nurse is seen as a "caring, pattern-recognizing presence" (Newman, 2008, p. 16) and the nursing process is a process of pattern recognition.

viewed as an energy field, as a universe of open systems, and as an event, situation, or phenomenon interacting with the person (Marchione, 1993, p. 39). Newman views health as the interaction pattern of a person with the environment; thus disease as a human energy field is a manifestation of a pattern of person–environment interactions (Brown, 2010a, p. 483).

Health

Health is the major concept of Newman's theory of expanding consciousness. Health is formed through a synthesis that occurs due to the fusion of disease and nondisease (Newman, 1979), where disease and nondisease are reflections of the larger whole. The concept of the health is described as a "pattern of the whole and wholeness *is*" (Newman, 1999, p. 228). Wholeness cannot be gained or lost; therefore, becoming ill does not diminish wholeness but rather causes wholeness to take on a different form (Brown, 2010, p. 483–484).

Nursing

In the context of Newman's theory, the nurse, within the nurse–patient interaction, is seen as a "caring, pattern-recognizing presence" (Newman, 2008, p. 16). The nurse functions to recognize patterns in patients by forming of relationships with patients and connecting with patients in an authentic way. The nurse–patient relationship is characterized by a "rhythmic coming together and moving apart as patients encounter disruption of their organized, predictable state" (Newman, 1999, p. 228), with the nurse continuing to connect with the patient as the pair move through periods of disorganization and unpredictability to arrive a higher, organized state (Newman, 1999).

ANALYSIS OF THE HEALTH AS EXPANDING CONSCIOUSNESS THEORY

THE ANALYSIS PRESENTED HERE CONSISTS of an examination of assumptions and propositions as well as a brief critique of Newman's health as expanding consciousness theory.

Assumptions of the Health as Expanding Consciousness Theory

Explicit assumptions of the health as expanding consciousness theory are considered by Newman to be basic to the theory:

❖ Health encompasses disease as a meaningful aspect of health, as a manifestation of the underlying pattern of person–environment interaction (Newman, 1990b, p. 133).

❖ Pathological conditions can be considered manifestations of the total pattern of the individual.

❖ The pattern of the individual that eventually manifests itself as pathology is primary and exists prior to structural or functional changes.

❖ Removal of the pathology in itself will not change the pattern of the individual.

❖ If becoming "ill" is the only way an individual's pattern can manifest itself, then that is health for that person.

❖ Health is the expression of consciousness (Newman, 1979, p. 56–58).

This last explicit assumption is the explanatory idea of Newman's entire theory—that is, the idea of health as expanding consciousness (Newman, 1986).

Implicit in the health as expanding consciousness theory are the following assumptions:

❖ Humans are open energy systems.

❖ Humans are in continual interconnectedness with a universe of open systems.

❖ Humans are continuously active in evolving their own pattern of the whole.

❖ Humans are intuitive as well as cognitive and affective beings.

❖ Humans are capable of abstract thinking and sensation.

❖ Humans are more than the sum of their parts (Marchione, 1993, p. 6).

Many of these assumptions, although implicit, were derived from Rogers' theory of unitary human beings (Marchione, 1993).

Propositions of the Health as Expanding Consciousness Theory

According to Newman, the explicit assumptions of her theory flowed from her proposition that health is a synthesis of disease and nondisease (Newman, 1979). Other propositions include the following ideas:

❖ Patterning of human health experiences occurs within the context of the environment.

❖ Consciousness is a manifestation of an evolving pattern of person–environment interaction (Newman, 1990a, p. 38).

❖ The evolving pattern of person–environment interaction can be viewed as a process of expanding consciousness (Newman, 1994/2000, p. 33).

❖ Movement is a pivotal choice point in the evolution of human consciousness (Newman, 1994/2000, p. 56).

❖ When we reach the choice point when movement is no longer an option, we learn to transcend the limitations of time–space–movement so as to reach higher levels of consciousness (Newman, 1994/2000, p. 57).

❖ Movement is a reflection of consciousness (Newman, 1979, p. 60).

❖ The consciousness that characterizes any form of life is expressed in its movement (Newman, 1994/2000, p. 57).

❖ Time is a measure of consciousness (Newman, 1979, p. 60).

❖ Manifestations of space–time–movement are indicators of consciousness (Newman, 1994/2000, p. 63).

❖ A person comes into being from the ground of consciousness and loses freedom as he or she is bound in time and finds his or her identity in space. Through movement, a person discovers the world of time–space and establishes personal territory (Newman, 1994/2000, p. 39).

❖ The rhythm of living phenomena is a vivid portrayal of the embeddedness of matter (consciousness) in space–time (Newman, 1994/2000, p. 53).

These relational propositions provide linkages between the various concepts in the theory of health as expanding consciousness (Fawcett, 2005, p. 456–457).

Brief Critique of the Health as Expanding Consciousness Theory

Newman's THEORY OF HEALTH AS EXPANDING CONSCIOUSNESS AS A FRAMEWORK FOR NURSING PRACTICE

Newman's theory of health as expanding consciousness was derived from both inductive and deductive forms of logic. The concepts are clearly defined and used consistently throughout the theory. The theory is broad in scope and has been used in several different cultures. However, it is complex and must be understood as a whole rather than by superficially examining the individual concepts in an attempt to use the theory in research or practice (Brown, 2010a).

In Newman's theory, the goal of the nurse is to care for the patient in the human health experience. To accomplish this goal, the nurse establishes a nurse–patient relationship so as to identify patterns and facilitate the patient's action potential and decision-making ability. The nurse's presence helps the patient to recognize his or her own patterns of interacting with the environment. This understanding is important because insight into these patterns clarifies for patients action possibilities and, therefore, brings the opportunity for transformation and evolution of consciousness (Brown, 2010b; Newman, 1990a).

When pattern recognition occurs, the nurse is able to assist the patient to facilitate a desired change. The patient resonates with the nurse through the time of disequilibrium until a new rhythm emerges from the patient's center of consciousness. At that point, the nurse and the patient move apart, both having been transformed by the process (Brown, 2010b, p. 467).

THE NURSING PROCESS FRAMED IN the theory of health as expanding consciousness is a process of pattern recognition that occurs as a function of the evolving fields of the nurse, the patient, and the environment. Newman outlined five steps involved in the application of the theory to practice: (1) engagement with the patient, (2) development of the narrative, (3) follow-up meetings, (4) application of the theory, and (5) family and community patterns (Newman, 2008).

THE NURSING PROCESS AND *Newman's* THEORY OF HEALTH AS EXPANDING CONSCIOUSNESS

Engagement with the Patient

The nurse recognizes disequilibrium in a patient and prepares for interaction with the patient. During this step, the nurse also shares his or her perception of the need for interaction and relationship with the patient. The nurse shows unconditional acceptance of the patient experience, becomes truly present with the patient, and grows with the patient (Brown, 2010b, p. 466).

Development of Narrative

During this step, the nurse examines the patient's story in terms of patterns of relating at critical points in time and diagrams the pattern to facilitate pattern identification (Brown, 2010b, p. 466).

The nursing process framed in the theory of health as expanding consciousness is a process of pattern recognition that occurs as a function of the evolving fields of the nurse, the patient, and the environment.

Follow-up Meetings

During follow-up meetings, the nurse facilitates the patient's recognition of patterns by sharing perceptions, supports the patient as insight into patterns occurs, and respects the patient's choices and response to pattern recognition. In addition, the nurse provides assistance to the patient in the implementation of choices, gauging support based on the level of independence that the patient has gained (Brown, 2010b, p. 466).

Application of the Theory

During this post-encounter analysis portion of the process, the nurse revisits data from the encounter in relation to the theory. The nurse also notes transformational changes that occurred for both the patient and the nurse (Brown, 2010b, p. 466).

Family and Community Pattern

The nurse recognizes and identifies individual patterns and their reciprocal patterns in the environment, including in relation to the family and community (Brown, 2010b, p. 466).

SCENARIO ILLUSTRATING NURSING CARE FRAMED BY *Newman's* THEORY OF HEALTH AS EXPANDING CONSCIOUSNESS UTILIZING THE NURSING PROCESS

THE FOLLOWING SCENARIO ILLUSTRATES NURSING care of the patient relative to one identified nursing problem framed by Newman's theory of health as expanding consciousness. This scenario is not intended to cover all aspects of care, but rather to stimulate thinking about how specific care might be approached using this theory as a framework for practice.

Ms. P. is a single mother of two who is currently pregnant with her third child. She has a history of alcohol dependency, which puts her pregnancy in a high risk category. Because of this risk, she has been assigned the services of a visiting nurse. The nurse's initial point of contact with Ms. P. will be focused on engagement with the patient. The nurse shows unconditional acceptance of the Ms. P. and her experiences, becomes truly present with the Ms. P., and grows with Ms. P.

The nurse recognizes that pregnancy is a time of disequilibrium for Ms. P., so it is important to examine Ms. P.'s story in terms of patterns of relating at critical points in time. As the nurse develops the narrative, she diagrams the patterns to facilitate pattern identification. During follow-up meetings, the nurse facilitates Ms. P.'s recognition of pattern by sharing perceptions and supporting Ms. P.'s insight into her personal patterns. The nurse provides assistance to the Ms. P. in the implementation of her choices as she is able to see a pattern to her alcohol abuse in relation to life stressors. The nurse gauges the amount of support that Ms. P. will need based on the level of independence that she has gained. Just as the nurse recognizes and identifies individual patterns, so she also identifies reciprocal patterns in the environment and incorporates these data in the encounter, as such patterns will also affect the patterns of Ms. P. in her effort to remain sober during her pregnancy.

Throughout this process, the theory may be applied simultaneously to other problems as they are identified by Ms. P. and the nurse. If other issues arise during the nursing encounter, intervention strategies will be planned to address those issues that are also compatible with current best clinical practices.

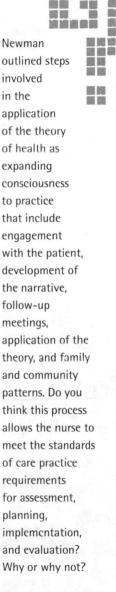

CRITICAL THINKING

Newman outlined steps involved in the application of the theory of health as expanding consciousness to practice that include engagement with the patient, development of the narrative, follow-up meetings, application of the theory, and family and community patterns. Do you think this process allows the nurse to meet the standards of care practice requirements for assessment, planning, implementation, and evaluation? Why or why not?

CLASSROOM ACTIVITY 17-1

Form small groups. Each group should add to the plan of care for Ms. P. in the preceding scenario based on other potential or actual nursing problems typical for a patient with the same medical diagnosis or symptoms and demographics. Each group should develop a plan for one additional nursing problem using Newman's theory of health as expanding consciousness as the basis for practice. Each group should then share its plan with the class.

CLASSROOM ACTIVITY 17-2

Form small groups. Using a case study provided by the instructor, develop a plan of care using Newman's theory of health as expanding consciousness as the basis for practice. Each group should then share its plan of care with the class.

CLASSROOM ACTIVITY 17-3

Form small groups. Using a case study provided by the instructor, develop a plan of care using one of the theories as the basis for practice; each group should select a different nursing theory. Each group should then share its plan of care with the class and discuss the similarities and differences in care.

REFERENCES

Brown, J. W. (2010a). Margaret Newman: Health as expanding consciousness. In M. R. Alligood & A. M. Tomey (Eds.), *Nursing theorists and their work* (7th ed., pp. 480–502). Maryland Heights, MO: Mosby.

Brown, J. W. (2010b). Newman's theory of health as expanding consciousness in nursing practice. In M. R. Alligood (Ed.), *Nursing theory: Utilization and application* (4th ed., pp. 457–493). Maryland Heights, MO: Mosby.

Johnson, B. M., & Webber, P. B. (2010). *An introduction to theory and reasoning* (3rd ed.). Philadelphia: Lippincott Williams & Wilkins.

Marchione, J. (1993). *Margaret Newman: Health as expanding consciousness.* Newbury Park, CA: Sage.

Newman, M. A. (1979). *Theory development in nursing.* Philadelphia: F. A. Davis.

Newman, M. A. (1986). *Health as expanding consciousness.* St. Louis, MO: Mosby.

Newman, M. A. (1990a). Newman's theory of health as praxis. *Nursing Science Quarterly, 3,* 37–41.

Newman, M. A. (1990b). Shifting to a higher consciousness. In M. E. Parker (Ed.), *Nursing theories in practice* (pp. 129–139). New York: National League for Nursing.

Newman, M. A. (1991). Health conceptualizations. In *Annual review of nursing research* (Vol. 9, pp. 221–243). New York: Springer.

Newman, M. A. (1994/2000). *Health as expanding consciousness* (2nd ed.). Sudbury, MA: Jones and Bartlett.

Newman, M. A. (1999). *The rhythm of relating in a paradigm of wholeness.* Image: The Journal of Nursing Scholarship, 31, 227–230.

Newman, M. A. (2008). *Transforming presence: The difference that nursing makes.* Philadelphia: F. A. Davis.

THE HEALTH PROMOTION MODEL:
Nola J. Pender

18

LEARNING OBJECTIVES

After completing this chapter the student should be able to

1. Identify and describe the major concepts of the health promotion model as proposed by Pender

2. Explain the major concepts important to nursing as defined by Pender

3. Plan nursing care for a patient scenario utilizing Pender's health promotion model

KEY TERMS

- Activity-related affect
- Behavior-specific cognitions and affect
- Perceived barriers to action
- Perceived benefits of action
- Perceived self-efficacy

BACKGROUND

NOLA J. PENDER WAS BORN in 1941 in Lansing, Michigan. She graduated in 1962 with a diploma in nursing. In 1964, Pender completed her BSN at Michigan State University. By 1969, she had earned a PhD in psychology and education. During this time in her career, Pender began looking at health and nursing in a broader way, including defining the goal of nursing care as optimal health.

In 1975, Pender published a conceptual model for preventive health behavior. Her health promotion model initially appeared in the first edition of the text *Health Promotion in Nursing Practice* in 1982. Pender's health promotion model has its roots in Albert Bandura's social learning theory (which postulates that cognitive processes affect behavior change) and is influenced by Fishbein's theory of reasoned action (which asserts that personal attitudes and social norms affect behavior).

OVERVIEW OF *Pender's* HEALTH PROMOTION MODEL

THE HEALTH PROMOTION MODEL IS an attempt to portray the multidimensionality of persons interacting with their interpersonal and physical environments as they pursue health while integrating constructs from expectancy-value theory and social cognitive theory with a nursing perspective of holistic human functioning (Pender, 1996, p. 53). With the third edition of *Health Promotion in Nursing Practice* (1996), Pender revised the health promotion model significantly; this revised model is addressed in this chapter.

There are three major categories to consider in Pender's health promotion model: (1) individual characteristics and experiences, (2) behavior-specific cognitions and affect, and (3) behavioral outcome. Each of these categories will be considered separately here.

Each person has unique personal characteristics and experiences that affect actions. Significant to this category are prior related behavior and personal factors. Prior related behavior is important in influencing future behavior. Pender proposes that prior behavior has both direct and indirect effects on the likelihood of engaging in health-promoting behaviors. The direct effect of past behavior on the current health-promoting behavior is due to habit formation, with habit strength increasing each time a behavior occurs. Prior behavior indirectly influences health-promoting behavior through perceptions of self-efficacy, benefits, barriers, and activity-related affect or emotions (Pender, Murdaugh, & Parsons, 2006, p. 51–52).

Personal factors include personal biological factors such as age, body mass index, pubertal status, menopausal status, aerobic capacity, strength, agility, or balance. Personal psychological factors include factors such as self-esteem, self-motivation, and perceived health status; personal sociocultural factors include factors such as race, ethnicity, acculturation, education, and socioeconomic status. Some personal factors are amenable to change, whereas others cannot be changed (Pender, Murdaugh, & Parsons, 2006, p. 52).

Behavior-specific cognitions and affect are behavior-specific variables within the health promotion model. Such variables are considered to have motivational significance. In the health promotion model, these variables are the target of nursing intervention because they are amenable to change. The behavior-specific cognitions and affect identified in the health promotion model include (1) perceived benefits of action, (2) perceived barriers to action, (3) perceived self-efficacy, and (4) activity-related affect.

> Prior behavior indirectly influences health-promoting behavior through perceptions of self-efficacy, benefits, barriers, and activity-related affect or emotions.

❖ **Perceived benefits of action** are the anticipated positive outcomes resulting from health behavior.

❖ **Perceived barriers to action** are the anticipated, imagined, or real blocks or personal costs of a behavior.

❖ **Perceived self-efficacy** refers to the judgment of personal capability to organize and execute a health-promoting behavior. It influences the perceived barriers to actions, such that higher efficacy results in lower perceptions of barriers.

❖ **Activity-related affect** refers to the subjective positive or negative feelings that occur before, during, and following behavior based on the stimulus properties of the behavior. Activity-related affect influences perceived self-efficacy, such that the more positive the subjective feeling, the greater the perceived of efficacy (Pender, Murdaugh, & Parsons, 2006; Sakraida, 2010, p. 438).

CRITICAL
THINKING

Can you think
of any specific
variables that
might be
perceived as
barriers to health-
promoting actions
or behaviors?

Other cognitions fall into the category of interpersonal influences and situational influences. Sources of interpersonal influences on health-promoting behaviors include family, peers, and healthcare providers; the influences themselves include norms, social support, and modeling. Situational influences on health-promoting behavior include perceptions of available options, demand characteristics, and aesthetic features of the environment. Nursing plans are tailored to meet the needs of diverse patients based on assessment of prior behavior, behavior-specific cognitions and affect, interpersonal factors, and situational factors (Pender, Murdaugh, & Parsons, 2006, p. 54–56).

The third category of the model is the behavioral outcome. Commitment to a plan of action marks the beginning of a behavioral event. This commitment propels the person into the behavior unless it is countermanded by a competing demand that cannot be avoided or a competing preference that is not resisted. Interventions in the health promotion model focus on raising consciousness related to health-promoting behaviors, promoting self-efficacy, enhancing the benefits of change, controlling the environment to support behavior change, and managing the barriers to change. Health-promoting behavior, which is ultimately directed toward attaining positive health outcomes, is the product of the health promotion model (Pender, Murdaugh, & Parsons, 2006, p. 56–63).

MAJOR CONCEPTS OF NURSING ACCORDING TO *Pender*

IN ADDITION TO THE CONCEPTS already presented, the four metaparadigm concepts of nursing are identified in Pender's model. These concepts are summarized in Table 18-1.

Person

The person in the health promotion model refers to the individual who is the primary focus of the model. In Pender's model, each person has unique personal characteristics and experiences that affect subsequent actions. It is recognized that individuals learn health behaviors within the context of the family and the community; thus the model includes components for

▦ TABLE 18-1 Metaparadigm Concepts as Defined in Pender's Theory	
Person	The individual, who is the primary focus of the model
Environment	The physical, interpersonal, and economic circumstances in which persons live
Health	A positive high-level state
Nursing	The role of the nurse includes raising consciousness related to health-promoting behaviors, promoting self-efficacy, enhancing the benefits of change, controlling the environment to support behavior change, and managing barriers to change

assessment and interventions at the family and community levels as well as at the individual level (Pender, Murdaugh, & Parsons, 2002; 2006).

Environment

The environment refers to the physical, interpersonal, and economic circumstances in which persons live. The quality of the environment depends on the absence of toxic substances, the availability of restorative experiences, and the accessibility of human and economic resources needed for healthful living. Socioeconomic conditions such as unemployment, poverty, crime, and prejudice have adverse effects on health, while environmental wellness is manifested by balance between human beings and their surroundings. (Pender, Murdaugh, & Parsons, 2006, p. 9).

Nursing plans are tailored to meet the needs of diverse patients based on assessment of prior behavior, behavior-specific cognitions and affect, interpersonal factors, and situational factors.

Health

Health is viewed as a positive high-level state. According to Pender, the person's definition of health for himself or herself is more important than any general definition of health (Pender, Murdaugh, & Parsons, 2006; Sakraida, 2010).

Nursing

Although Pender does not specifically define nursing as a metaparadigm concept, she does describe the expected role of the nurse within the context of the health promotion model. The role of the nurse in her model revolves around raising consciousness related to health-promoting behaviors, promoting self-efficacy, enhancing the benefits of change, controlling the environment to support behavior change, and managing the barriers to change (Pender, Murdaugh, & Parsons, 2006, p. 57–63).

ANALYSIS OF THE HEALTH PROMOTION MODEL

THE ANALYSIS AND CRITIQUE PRESENTED here consist of an examination of assumptions and propositions as well as an analysis of the clarity, simplicity, generality, empirical precision, and derivable consequences of Pender's health promotion model.

Assumptions of the Health Promotion Model

Assumptions of the health promotion model reflect both nursing and behavioral science perspectives and emphasize the active role of the patient in shaping and maintaining health behaviors and in modifying the environment context for health behaviors. These assumptions include the following ideas:

❖ Persons seek to create conditions of living through which they can express their unique human potential.

❖ Persons have the capacity for reflective self-awareness, including assessment of their own competencies.

❖ Persons value growth in directions viewed as positive and attempt to achieve a personally acceptable balance between change and stability.

❖ Persons seek to actively regulate their own behavior.

❖ Persons, in all their biopsychosocial complexity, interact with the environment progressively, transforming the environment and being transformed themselves over time.

❖ Health professionals constitute a part of the interpersonal environment, which influences persons throughout their life span.

❖ Self-initiated reconfiguration of person–environment interactive patterns is essential for behavior change (Pender, Murdaugh, & Parsons, 2002, p. 63).

CRITICAL THINKING

How has Pender's model and view of health influenced the practice of the nurse? How does Pender's definition of health compare to other theorists' conceptualizations of health?

Propositions of the Health Promotion Model

The health promotion model is based on 14 theoretical propositions. These theoretical relationship statements provide a basis for research related to health behaviors:

1. Prior behavior and inherited and acquired characteristics influence health beliefs, affect, and enactment of health-promoting behavior.

2. Persons commit to engaging in behaviors from which they anticipate deriving personally valued benefits.

3. Perceived barriers can constrain commitment to action, mediators of behavior, and actual behavior.

4. Perceived competence or self-efficacy to execute a given behavior increases the likelihood of commitment to action and actual performance of behavior.

5. Greater perceived self-efficacy results in fewer perceived barriers to a specific health behavior.

6. Positive affect toward a behavior results in greater perceived self-efficacy, which can, in turn, result in increased positive affect.

7. When positive emotions or affect is associated with a behavior, the probability of commitment and action are increased.

8. Persons are more likely to commit to and engage in health-promoting behaviors when significant others model the behavior, expect the behavior to occur, and provide assistance and support to enable the behavior.

9. Family, peers, and healthcare providers are important sources of interpersonal influence that can either increase or decrease commitment to and engagement in health-promoting behavior.

10. Situational influences in the external environment can either increase or decrease commitment to or participation in health-promoting behavior.

11. The greater the commitment to a specific plan of action, the more likely that health-promoting behaviors will be maintained over time.

12. Commitment to a plan of action is less likely to result in the desired behavior when competing demands over which persons have little control require immediate attention.

13. Commitment to a plan of action is less likely to result in the desired behavior when other actions are more attractive and preferred over the target behavior.

14. Persons can modify cognitions, affect, and the interpersonal and physical environments to create incentives for health actions (Pender, Murdaugh, & Parsons, 2002, p. 63–64).

Brief Critique of the Health Promotion Model

Pender's model was formulated using inductive reasoning and existing research, which is a common approach when building middle-range theories. The research used to derive the model was based on adult samples that included male, female, young, old, well, and ill samples, allowing the model to easily be generalized to broader adult populations (Sakraida, 2010).

The health promotion model is simple to understand, using language that is well understood by nurses. The concept of health promotion is also a popular concept in nursing practice. The relationships among the various factors are linked and relationships are identified and consistently defined. Considering all of these factors, it is not difficult to see why Pender's model is popular with practicing nurses and is frequently used as a tool in research. The model has not, however, been used extensively in nursing education, where the emphasis is on illness care in acute care settings (Sakraida, 2010).

Pender identified health promotion as a goal for the twenty-first century and, through her development of the health promotion model, has assisted in the delineation of the role of nursing in meeting that goal. Although Pender has now retired, work continues on the health promotion model, which is more important than ever in the current healthcare system. The current scenario—characterized by increasing costs of health care associated with episodic illness treatment; increases in chronic, preventable conditions within the population; and a focus on managing health care costs—provides ample incentives to further explore the concepts of the health promotion model.

THE HEALTH PROMOTION MODEL IS useful in practice when the focus of nursing care includes promoting behaviors to enhance health. The role of the nurse in the health promotion model revolves around raising consciousness related to health-promoting behaviors, promoting self-efficacy, enhancing the benefits of change, controlling the environment to support behavior change, and managing the barriers to change (Pender, Murdaugh, & Parsons, 2006, p. 57–63).

> *Pender's*
> **HEALTH PROMOTION MODEL AS A FRAMEWORK FOR NURSING PRACTICE**

WHILE THE NURSING PROCESS IS not explicitly mentioned in Pender's theory, the various phases known as the nursing process can be easily identified and incorporated for the sake of discussion, consistency, and comparison.

> **THE NURSING PROCESS AND** *Pender's* **HEALTH PROMOTION MODEL**

Assessment

During the assessment phase of the nursing process, the nurse gathers data on prior related behavior of the person, personal factors (biological, psychological, and sociocultural), and the patient's perceptions of benefits from actions, barriers to action, efficacy, and any activity-related effects and competing demands.

Planning

Based on the data collected, the nurse and the patient work together to develop a health promotion plan that addresses and accounts for past experiences, personal factors, perceived barriers, efficacy issues, and affect issues, and that takes advantage of the perceived benefits identified. Plans should also include measures to address competing demands. The patient commits to the plan of action.

Implementation

The implementation phase includes the actual incorporation of the health-promoting behavior into the patient's routine and life. Examples of health-promoting behaviors that the nurse might work with the patient to incorporate include exercising regularly, eating a healthy diet, and achieving adequate rest and recreation.

Evaluation

Evaluation is based on the achievement of the action outcome or the incorporation of a health-promoting behavior that is directed toward the ultimate goal of attaining positive health outcomes such as optimal well-being.

SCENARIO ILLUSTRATING NURSING CARE FRAMED BY *Pender's* HEALTH PROMOTION MODEL

THE FOLLOWING SCENARIO ILLUSTRATES NURSING care of the patient relative to one identified nursing problem framed by Pender's health promotion model. This scenario is not intended to cover all aspects of care, but rather to stimulate thinking about how specific care might be approached using this theory as a framework for practice.

Mrs. H. is a 52-year-old, married, Caucasian female who has spent the last 20 years working in a sedentary job and raising children. She admits that she has taken little time for herself during the previous two decades. Mrs. H. is not obese but she has gained approximately 10 pounds over the past five years. She is consulting with the clinic nurse because she wants to lose weight.

During the assessment, the nurse gathers data on Mrs. H.'s prior health-related behaviors such as diet and exercise, her personal health history, Mrs. H.'s perceptions of the benefits and barriers to a health promotion plan, her efficacy, and any activity-related effects or competing demands in Mrs. H.'s life. Based on the data collected, the nurse and Mrs. H. work together to develop a health promotion plan that addresses and accounts for Mrs. H.'s experiences, personal factors, perceived barriers, efficacy issues, and affect issues, and that takes advantage of the perceived benefits identified. Mrs. H. is in good health with no known disease processes, she does not take any prescription medications, and she does not currently have any exercise or diet limitations. For Mrs. H., the proposed regimen includes cardiovascular and muscle building exercises. The nurse and Mrs. H. determine what Mrs. H. believes is the best time of day for her to stick to an exercise routine. Mrs. H. states that she is committed to the plan.

During follow-up meetings, reassessment occurs to determine if alterations need to be made in the plan. Ultimately, evaluation is based on Mrs. H.'s incorporation of the planned exercise behavior into her lifestyle and her success in meeting her goal of attaining optimal well-being.

Throughout this process, the health promotion theory may be applied simultaneously to other issues as they are identified by Mrs. H. and the nurse. If other issues arise during the nursing encounter, intervention strategies will be planned to address those health promotion issues that are also compatible with current best clinical practices.

CLASSROOM ACTIVITY 18-1

Form small groups. Each group should add to the plan of care for Mrs. H. in the preceding scenario based on other potential or actual nursing problems typical for a patient with the same medical diagnosis or symptoms and demographics. Each group should develop a plan for one additional issue amenable to a health promotion intervention using Pender's model as the basis for practice. Each group should then share its plan with the class.

CLASSROOM ACTIVITY 18-2

Form small groups. Using a case study provided by the instructor, develop a plan of care using Pender's health promotion model as the basis for practice. Each group should then share its plan of care with the class.

CLASSROOM ACTIVITY 18-3

Form small groups. Using a case study provided by the instructor, develop a plan of care using one of the theories as the basis for practice; each group should select a different nursing theory. Each group should then share its plan of care with the class and discuss the similarities and differences in care.

REFERENCES

Pender, N. J. (1982). *Health promotion in nursing practice.* Norwalk, CT: Appleton Century Crofts.

Pender, N. J. (1996). *Health promotion in nursing practice* (3rd ed.). Stamford, CT: Appleton and Lange.

Pender, N. J., Murdaugh, C. L., & Parsons, M. A. (2002). *Health promotion in nursing practice* (4th ed.). Upper Saddle River, NJ: Prentice Hall.

Pender, N. J., Murdaugh, C. L., & Parsons, M. A. (2006). *Health promotion in nursing practice* (5th ed.). Upper Saddle River, NJ: Prentice Hall.

Sakraida, T. J. (2010). The health promotion model. In A. M. Tomey & M. R. Alligood (Eds.), *Nursing theorists and their work* (7th ed., pp. 434–453). St. Louis, MO: Mosby.

THEORY OF HUMANBECOMING:
Rosemarie Rizzo Parse

19

LEARNING OBJECTIVES

After completing this chapter the student should be able to

1. Identify and describe the concepts specific to the theory of humanbecoming as identified by Parse

2. Explain the major concepts important to nursing as defined by Parse

3. Plan nursing care for a patient scenario utilizing Parse's theory of humanbecoming

KEY TERMS

Humanbecoming	Rhythmicity
Meaning	Transcendence

BACKGROUND

ROSEMARY RIZZO PARSE GRADUATED FROM Duquesne University in Pittsburg. She received her master's degree and doctorate from the University of Pittsburg. Since then, she has been a nursing professor at the University of Pittsburg, Hunter College of City University of New York, and Loyola University Chicago, as well as Dean of the School of Nursing at Duquesne University. She is currently Distinguished Professor Emeritus at Loyola University in Chicago (Mitchell & Bournes, 2010).

Parse is the author of numerous books and articles, many of which have been translated into multiple languages. Her research method methodologies and theory have been used by nurse scholars around the world to guide practice (Mitchell & Bournes, 2010). In addition, Parse is the founder and editor of *Nursing Science Quarterly* and founder of the *Institute of Humanbecoming*.

The humanbecoming school of thought is grounded in human science and is consistent with the principles and postulates about unitary human beings as proposed by Martha Rogers (Mitchell & Bournes, 2010, p. 504). It is also "consistent with major tenets and concepts from existential–phenomenological thought, but it is a new product, a different conceptual system" (Parse, 1998, p. 4).

OVERVIEW OF *Rosemary Parse's* HUMANBECOMING THEORY

PARSE'S THEORY WAS ORIGINALLY CALLED *man–living–health* (1981). The name was changed by Parse in 1992 to *human becoming* and then changed again in 2007 to *humanbecoming* (Mitchell & Bournes, 2010) to coincide with Parse's evolution of thought relative to the theory. Parse has identified four essential ideas that are reflected in the concepts, assumptions, and propositions of her theory:

- ❖ The human–universe mutual process
- ❖ The coconstitution of health
- ❖ The multidimensional meanings the indivisible human gives to being and becoming

❖ The human's freedom in each situation to choose alternative ways of becoming (Fawcett, 2005, p. 475)

Parse uses terminology in her theory that may be unfamiliar, as well as terminology that she has created, thus making it important to examine some basic definitions of concepts as we begin discussing the theory. The central concept of her theory is **humanbecoming**, which refers to the human being's living health (Parse, 1997, p. 32). Parse uses the verb form of the word "become" (*becoming*) to emphasize the ongoing and changing nature of the process (Parse, 1998, p. 34).

The humanbecoming theory consists of three major themes: meaning, rhythmicity, and transcendence (Parse, 1998). **Meaning** is the linguistic and imagined content of something and the interpretation that one gives to something (Parse, 1998, p. 29). Meaning is further defined by the concepts of imaging, valuing, and languaging (Fawcett, 2005, p. 476). **Rhythmicity** is the cadent, paradoxical patterning of the human–universe mutual process (Parse, 1998, p. 29). Rhythmicity is further defined by the concepts of revealing–concealing, enabling–limiting, and connecting–separating (Fawcett, 2005, p. 476). **Transcendence** is the third major theme, and it is defined by Parse as reaching beyond with possibles—the "hopes and dreams envisioned in multidimensional experiences powering the originating of transforming" (1998, p. 30). Transcendence is further defined by the concepts of powering, originating, and transforming (Fawcett, 2005, p. 476).

The three major principles of the humanbecoming theory flow from the themes. The first principle of the humanbecoming theory states, "Structuring meaning multidimensionally is cocreating reality through the languaging of valuing and imaging" (Parse, 1998, p. 35). This principle proposes that persons structure or choose the meaning of their realities and that the choosing occurs at levels that are not always known explicitly (explicit–tacit knowing) (Mitchell, 2006). In other words, the way a person sees the world, or the person's imaging of it, is the person's reality. Persons create this reality with others, and they show or "language" their reality in the ways they speak, remain silent, and in the ways they move or stay still. Moreover, when people language their reality, they also language their value and priorities and meanings (Mitchell & Bournes, 2010, p. 507). As a consequence, one person cannot decide the significance of

The humanbecoming theory consists of three major themes: meaning, rhythmicity, and transcendence.

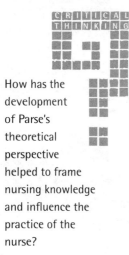

CRITICAL
THINKING

How has the
development
of Parse's
theoretical
perspective
helped to frame
nursing knowledge
and influence the
practice of the
nurse?

something for another person and does not even understand the meaning of the event unless that person shares the meaning through the expression of his or her views, concerns, and dreams.

The second principle in the theory of humanbecoming states, "Cocreating rhythmical patterns of relating is living the paradoxical unity of revealing–concealing and enabling–limiting while connecting–separating" (Parse, 1998, p. 42). This principle means that persons create patterns in life, and these patterns reveal something about their personal meanings and values. The patterns of relating that persons create involve freedoms and restrictions as well as complex engagements and disengagements with other persons, ideas, and preferences (Mitchell, 2006). According to Parse (1998), the second principle has three associated concepts: revealing–concealing, enabling–limiting, and connecting–separating. All of these concepts contain rhythmical paradoxes. Persons change their patterns as they integrate new priorities, ideas, hopes, and dreams.

The third principle of the humanbecoming theory posits that "Cotranscending with the possibles is powering unique ways of originating in the process of transforming" (Parse, 1998, p. 46). This principle means that persons are always engaging with and choosing from infinite possibilities. The choices made by a person reflect that person's ways of moving and changing in the process of becoming (Mitchell, 2006). The three concepts associated with this principle include powering, originating, and transforming. *Powering* conveys meaning about struggle and the will to persevere despite hardship; it is always happening and affirms our being in the light of the possibility of nonbeing (Parse, 1998, p. 47). *Originating* deals with uniqueness and refers to inventing new ways of conforming or nonconforming in the certainty–uncertainty (Parse, 1998, p. 49). *Transforming* refers to shifting the view of the familiar–unfamiliar, the changing of change in coconstituting anew in a deliberate way (Mitchell & Bournes, 2010, p. 509–510; Parse, 1998, p. 51).

MAJOR CONCEPTS OF NURSING ACCORDING TO *Parse*

IN ADDITION TO THE CONCEPTS already presented, the four metaparadigm concepts of nursing are identified in Parse's theory of humanbecoming. These concepts are summarized in Table 19-1.

⊞ TABLE 19-1 Metaparadigm Concepts as Defined in Parse's Theory	
Person	An open being, more than and different from the sum of parts, in mutual simultaneous interchange with the environment, who chooses from options and bears responsibility for choices (Parse, 1987, p. 160)
Environment	Coexists in mutual process with the person
Health	Continuously changing process of becoming
Nursing	A learned discipline; the nurse uses true presence to facilitate the becoming of the participant

Person

Humanbecoming reflects the unity of the constructs of man–living–health. Thus the theory lacks references to particular aspects of human beings, such as the biological, psychological, or spiritual (Parse, 1992, p. 37). Parse further conceptualizes human beings as open beings who mutually cocreate with the rhythmical patterns of the universe, who are recognized by patterns of relating, and who freely choose in situations (Parse, 1998).

Environment

The environment (universe) is not described separately from the person because, according to Parse (1998), the environment coexists in mutual process with the person.

Health

For Parse, the concept of health is synonymous with what she has named humanbecoming. She stresses that the concepts of human, universe, and health are inseparable and irreducible. To emphasize this inseparability, she has unified the words "human" and "universe" into "humanuniverse" and the words "human" and "becoming" into "humanbecoming" (Mitchell & Bournes, 2010, p. 514). Health is structuring meaning, configuring rhythmical patterns of relating, and cotranscending with possibles. It is also linked to personal commitment: An individual's way of becoming is cocreated by that individual based on his or her value priorities (Parse, 1990, p. 136). Health is not a linear entity and cannot be qualified by terms such as "good" or "bad"; it is not man adapting or coping; it is not the opposite of disease or a state; but rather it is a synthesis of values, a way of living (Parse, 1987, p. 160).

Nursing

As part of a learned discipline, the nurse uses true presence to help human beings move toward becoming through choosing ways of cocreating their own health and finding meaning in situations.

Parse does not write about nursing as a concept in the metaparadigm of the discipline. She does, however, write about nursing as a basic science, a learned discipline in which nursing theories guide practice and research activities (Mitchell & Bournes, 2010). As part of a learned discipline, the nurse uses true presence to help human beings move toward becoming through choosing ways of cocreating their own health and finding meaning in situations. The goal of nursing is to improve quality of life (Parse, 1998). Parse believes that nursing is a service to humankind and, more specifically, that "nursing is a science, the practice of which is performing art" (Parse, 1992, p. 35).

ANALYSIS OF *Parse's* THEORY OF HUMANBECOMING

THE ANALYSIS PRESENTED HERE CONSISTS of an examination of the assumptions and propositions as well as a brief critique of the theory of humanbecoming.

Assumptions of the Theory of Humanbecoming

According to Mitchell and Bournes (2010, p. 512), Parse synthesized principles, tenets, and concepts from drawn from Rogers' work as well as from existential phenomenology (Parse, 1998, p. 19), thereby building on the work of other theorists to create a solid foundation for the humanbecoming school of thought. The assumptions of the humanbecoming theory focus on beliefs about humans and about health:

❖ The human is coexisting while coconstituting rhythmical patterns with the universe (coexistence, coconstitution, and pattern).

❖ The human is open, freely choosing meaning with situation, bearing responsibility for decisions (situated freedom, openness, and energy field).

❖ The human is continuously coconstituting patterns of relating (energy field, pattern, and coconstitution).

❖ The human is transcending illimitably with possibles (pandimensionality, openness, and situated freedom).

❖ Becoming is human–living–health (openness, situated freedom, and coconstitution).

❖ Becoming is rhythmically coconstituting with humanuniverse (coconstitution, pattern, and pandimensionality).

❖ Becoming is the human's patterns of relating value priorities (situated freedom, pattern, and openness).

❖ Becoming is intersubjective transcending with possibles (openness, situated freedom, and coexistence).

❖ Becoming is the human's emerging (coexistence, energy field, and pandimensionality) (Mitchell & Bournes, 2010, p. 512; Parse, 1998).

Parse synthesized these original assumptions about humans and becoming into three assumptions about humanbecoming:

❖ Humanbecoming is freely choosing personal meaning with situation, intersubjectively living value priorities.

❖ Humanbecoming is configuring rhythmical patterns of relating with the humanuniverse.

❖ Humanbecoming is cotranscending illimitably with emerging possibles (Mitchell & Bournes, 2010, p. 513; Parse, 1998).

Propositions of the Theory of Humanbecoming

The relational propositions of the theory of humanbecoming are listed below. The propositions, while relational, are nondirectional and noncausal (Parse, 1992).

❖ Humanbecoming is structuring meaning multidimensionally in cocreating paradoxical rhythmical patterns of relating while cotranscending with the possibles (Parse, 1998, p. 34).

❖ Humanbecoming is the day-to-day creating of reality through the languaging of valuing and imaging as the paradoxical rhythmical patterns of revealing–concealing, enabling–limiting, and connecting–separating are powering ways of originating transforming (Parse, 1998, p. 55).

❖ Powering emerges with the revealing–concealing of imaging (p. 55).

❖ Originating emerges with the enabling–limiting of valuing (p. 55).

❖ Transforming emerges with the languaging of connecting–separating (p. 55).

According to Fawcett (2005, p. 478), the first two propositions listed link concepts, whereas the third, fourth, and fifth propositions are what Parse (1998) refers to as theoretical structures. The definitions of the theory provided earlier in the chapter represent the nonrelational propositions of the theory (Fawcett, 2005, p. 476).

Brief Critique of the Theory of Humanbecoming

Parse's theory of humanbecoming is internally consistent and is congruent with its conceptual and philosophical origins (Fawcett, 2005). The theory is highly abstract and complex. While the concepts in the theory are defined, the vocabulary of the theory presents a barrier to use because most nurses are unfamiliar with the terminology. For those nurses who do take the time to understand the theory and use it in either research or practice, Parse's theory has been shown to be supported by evidence and has been used in a variety of settings with individuals, families, and communities throughout the world (Mitchell & Bourne, 2010).

Parse's THEORY OF HUMANBECOMING AS A FRAMEWORK FOR NURSING PRACTICE

NURSING IS PRACTICED IN RELATIONSHIP with humans in their processes of becoming. Nursing care will initially be explored here based on the three principles of the theory of humanbecoming.

The first principle involves the use of imaging, valuing and languaging. The nurse cannot completely know another's imaging, but using the theory of humanbecoming, the nurse explores, respects, and bears witness as people struggle with the processes.

The nurse learns about the person's perspectives and confirms values by asking the person what is most important. In addition, the nurse witnesses languaging, although he or she cannot know the meaning of the languaging without asking people the meaning of their words, actions, and gestures (Mitchell & Bournes, 2010, p. 507–508).

The second principle involves the paradoxical concepts of revealing–concealing, enabling–limiting, and connecting–separating. People disclose differently in different situations and with different people. In choosing how to be with others, nurses cocreate what happens when they are with persons through processes that include revealing–concealing. Although one cannot know all of the consequences of all choices, every choice has the possibilities of opportunity and restriction. Nurses can assist persons through the rhythmical process of enabling–limiting in relation to opportunities. They can also help persons as they contemplate options and anticipated consequences of difficulty choices. Nurses learn about a person's patterns of connecting–separating by asking about relationships and projects (Mitchell & Bournes, 2010, p.508–509).

The third principle involves the concepts of powering, originating, and transforming. Conflict presents opportunities to clarify meanings and values. Powering becomes manifest as nurses enhance the process by being present with persons who are exploring issues, conflicts, and options. Nurses are witnesses to originating with persons who are in the process of choosing how they are going to be with their changing health patterns. Nurses, in the way they are present with persons, may help or hinder persons' efforts to clarify their hopes, dreams, and desired directions. This is the manifestation of the concept of transforming (Mitchell & Bournes, 2010, p. 509–510).

According to Parse (1989, p. 11), certain skills are necessary for practicing effective nursing:

❖ Know and use nursing frameworks and theories.

❖ Be available to others.

❖ Value the other as a human presence.

❖ Respect differences in view.

❖ Own what you believe and be accountable for your actions.

❖ Move on to the new and untested.

❖ Connect with others.

❖ Take pride in self.

❖ Like what you do.

❖ Recognize the moments of joy in the struggles of living.

❖ Appreciate mystery and be open to new discoveries.

❖ Be competent in your chosen area.

❖ Rest and begin anew.

THE NURSING PROCESS AND *Parse's* THEORY OF HUMANBECOMING

THREE PROCESSES FOR PRACTICE HAVE been developed from the concepts and principles in the humanbecoming theory (Parse, 1998, p. 69, 70):

❖ *Illuminating meaning* is explicating what was, is, and will be. "Explicating" is making clear what is appearing now through speech, silence, movement, and stillness of languaging.

❖ *Synchronizing rhythms* is dwelling with the pitch, yaw, and roll of the humanuniverse process. "Dwelling with" is immersing with the flow of connecting–separating.

❖ *Mobilizing transcendence* is moving beyond the meaning moment with what is not yet. "Moving beyond" is propelling with envisioned possibles of transforming.

These dimensions and processes happen all at once. In practice, nurses guided by the theory of humanbecoming prepare to be truly present with others through focused attentiveness on the moment at hand through immersion (Parse, 1998). Nurses have opportunities to be with others and participate with them during times of change, uncertainty, recovery, and hope. During these times, as the nurse and the person engage in dialogue, persons speak about their situations to nurses. In the telling, there are moments of clarification, discovery, and change as people begin to see themselves and their situations in a new light (Mitchell, 2010, p. 441).

According to Parse (1981, 1998), persons cannot be assessed, controlled, or manipulated. The nurse respects that every person is already living a process of complex unfolding as he or she structures meaning while configuring rhythmical patterns of relating and cotranscending with possibles. The nurse has the privilege of serving others through being present, and this participation through true presence that makes a difference is the outcome of practice as guided by the theory of humanbecoming (Mitchell, 2010, p. 441).

Assessment and Planning

The practice dimensions and processes guide the nurse to be present as the person speaks about his or her meanings, concerns, and issues as the person perceives them. The nurse is present as the person explores his or her situation and considers options. For the nurse whose practice is guided by the theory of humanbecoming, the information provided by the person would be explored from the perspective of the person by asking questions such as the following. What is this situation like for you? What is most important to you at this time? What do you hope happens? Based on the person's descriptions, a plan of care based upon his or her priorities is designed (Mitchell, 2010, p. 445).

Implementation

Nursing practice guided by the theory of humanbecoming complements the medically driven care for which the nurse is responsible. The nurse, as always, is expected to practice according to current best clinical practices. However, completing the tasks to care for a patient that require physical, skill-based nursing practices does not detract from the opportunity to practice nursing in relationship with persons and families (Mitchell, 2010).

Evaluation

As with the assessment, the evaluation phase of care focuses on the outcomes from the perspective of the person. The nurse must accept the outcome with respect for the person and without judgment.

CRITICAL THINKING

What do you think about the three processes for practice developed by Parse—illuminating meaning, synchronizing rhythms, and mobilizing transcendence? Do these processes allow the nurse to meet the standards of care practice requirements for assessment, planning, implementation, and evaluation, particularly in light of Parse's view that persons cannot be assessed?

SCENARIO ILLUSTRATING NURSING CARE FRAMED BY *Parse's* THEORY OF HUMANBECOMING

THE FOLLOWING SCENARIO ILLUSTRATES NURSING care of the patient relative to one identified nursing problem framed by Parse's theory of humanbecoming. This scenario is not intended to cover all aspects of care, but rather to stimulate thinking about how specific care might be approached using this theory as a framework for practice.

Mrs. Q. is a 58-year-old, African American patient with diabetes and renal failure who has just undergone her first week of hemodialysis. The nurse caring for Mrs. Q. during this time of change plans to be truly present through focused attentiveness on the moment at hand through immersion as Mrs. Q. speaks about concerns and issues as she perceives them. The nurse is present as Mrs. Q. explores her situation and considers options. To facilitate the exploration, the nurse may ask Mrs. Q., "What is this situation like for you?" or "What is most important to you at this time?" or "What do you hope happens?" Based on Mrs. Q.'s descriptions, a plan of care is designed based on Mrs. Q.'s priorities that will complement the required medically driven care.

During the evaluation phase of the process, the nurse focuses on outcomes related to the three principles of structuring meaning, configuring rhythmical patterns, and cotranscending with possibles. This evaluation is undertaken from the perspective of Mrs. Q.

Throughout this process, the theory of humanbecoming may be applied simultaneously to other issues as they are identified by Mrs. Q. and the nurse. As always, if problems arise that require additional medically driven care, intervention strategies are planned to address those issues that are congruent with current best clinical practices.

CLASSROOM ACTIVITY 19-1

Form small groups. Each group should add to the plan of care for Mrs. Q. in the preceding scenario based on other potential or actual nursing problems typical for a patient with the same medical diagnosis or symptoms and demographics. Each group should develop a plan for one additional nursing problem using Parse's theory of humanbecoming as the basis for practice. Each group should then share its plan with the class.

CLASSROOM ACTIVITY 19-2

Form small groups. Using a case study provided by the instructor, develop a plan of care using Parse's theory of humanbecoming as the basis for practice. Each group should then share its plan of care with the class.

CLASSROOM ACTIVITY 19-3

Form small groups. Using a case study provided by the instructor, develop a plan of care using one of the theories as the basis for practice; each group should select a different nursing theory. Each group should then share its plan of care with the class and discuss the similarities and differences in care.

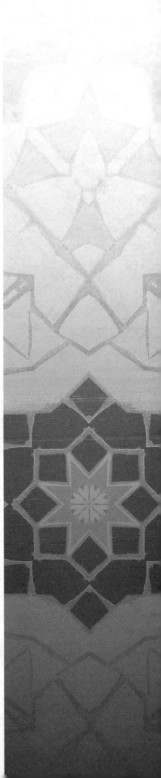

REFERENCES

Fawcett, J. (2005). *Contemporary nursing knowledge: Analysis and evaluation of nursing models and theories* (2nd ed.). Philadelphia: F. A. Davis.

Mitchell, G. J. (2006). Rosemarie Rizzo Parse: Human becoming. In A. M. Tomey & M. R. Alligood (Eds.), *Nursing theorists and their work* (6th ed., pp. 522–559). St. Louis, MO: Mosby.

Mitchell, G. J., & Bournes, D. A. (2010). Rosemarie Rizzo Parse: Humanbecoming. In M. R. Alligood & A. M. Tomey (Eds.), *Nursing theorists and their work* (7th ed., pp. 503–535). Maryland Heights, MO: Mosby.

Parse, R. R. (1981). *Man–living–health: A theory of nursing.* New York: John Wiley & Sons.

Parse, R. R. (1987). *Nursing science: Major paradigms, theories, and critiques.* Philadelphia: Saunders.

Parse, R. R. (1990). Health: A personal commitment. *Nursing Science Quarterly, 3,* 136–140.

Parse, R. R. (1992). Human becoming: Parse's theory of nursing. *Nursing Science Quarterly, 5,* 35–42.

Parse, R. R. (1997). The human becoming theory: The was, is, and will be. *Nursing Science Quarterly, 10,* 32–38.

Parse, R. R. (1998). *The human becoming school of thought: A perspective for nurses and other health professionals.* Thousand Oaks, CA: Sage.

Parse, R. R. (2007). The humanbecoming school of thought in 2050. *Nursing Science Quarterly, 20,* 308–311.

THE THEORY OF NURSING AS CARING: A MODEL FOR TRANSFORMING PRACTICE:
Anne Boykin and Savina O. Schoenhofer

20

LEARNING OBJECTIVES

After completing this chapter the student should be able to

1. Identify and describe the major concepts of the theory of nursing as caring

2. Explain the major concepts important to nursing as defined in the theory of nursing as caring

3. Plan nursing care for a patient scenario utilizing the theory of nursing as caring

KEY TERMS

Caring

BACKGROUND

ANNE BOYKIN BEGAN HER NURSING career after graduation from Alverno College in Milwaukee, Wisconsin, in 1966. She earned a master's degree in nursing from Emory University in Atlanta, Georgia, and a doctorate from Vanderbilt University in Nashville, Tennessee. Boykin is the dean and professor of the College of Nursing at Florida Atlantic University and is Director for the Christine E. Lynne Center for Caring. The Center was created to humanize care through the integration of teaching, research, and service.

Boykin's scholarly work has centered on caring as the grounding for nursing. This focus is evidenced in her book, chapter, and journal publications. Boykin's initial publication on caring was the book she coauthored with Savina Schoenhofer, *Nursing as Caring: A Model for Transforming Practice* (1993); a revised edition was published in 2001. Boykin's commitment to caring is also evidenced by her long-standing service as an officer (including president) of the International Association of Human Caring and co-editor of the journal *International Association for Human Caring* (Boykin & Schoenhofer, 2006, p. 335).

Savina Schoenhofer earned both undergraduate and graduate degrees in nursing, psychology, and counseling from Wichita State University. She then completed a PhD in educational foundations and administration at Kansas State University in 1983. Schoenhofer is currently Professor of Graduate Nursing at the Cora S. Balmat School of Nursing at Alcorn State University in Natchez, Mississippi, and Professor at the University of Mississippi's School of Nursing in Jackson, Mississippi. In addition, she manages the website and discussion forum that she created on the theory of nursing as caring.

In 1990, Schoenhofer cofounded *Nightingale Songs*, a venue for communicating the beauty of nursing via poetry and prose. In 1993, she coauthored the book *Nursing as Caring: A Model for Transforming Practice* with Anne Boykin; the revised edition was published in 2001. In addition to her publications related to caring, Schoenhofer has published widely on nursing values, primary care, nursing education, support, touch, personnel management in nursing homes, and mentoring (Boykin & Schoenhofer, 2006, p. 335).

Schoenhofer credits three colleagues for significantly influencing her career in nursing. The first was Lt. Col. Ann Ashjian (now retired), whose community nursing practice in Brazil presented an inspiring model of nursing to a young Schoenhofer, who spent three years in the Amazon region of Brazil during the 1960s (Purnell, 2010). A second influence was Marilyn E. Parker, a faculty colleague who mentored Schoenhofer in the idea of nursing as a discipline, the role of higher education, and the world of nursing theories and theorists. Finally, Anne Boykin introduced Schoenhofer to caring as a substantive field of nursing study (Boykin & Schoenhofer, 2006, p. 335).

The theory of nursing as caring was actually developed as a part of curriculum development work in the College of Nursing at Florida Atlantic University. Boykin and Schoenhofer were among the faculty group responsible for revising their caring-based curriculum. When the new curriculum was instituted, they both realized the significance of continuing to develop the ideas underlying it. The pair worked to develop the ideas into a comprehensive conceptual framework that expressed the meaning and purpose of nursing as a discipline and as a profession. What made their framework different from the traditional ideas related to caring was the expression of caring as the end—rather than the means—of nursing and the definition of caring as the intention of nursing, rather than merely an instrument of nursing (Boykin & Schoenhofer, 2006, p. 338).

Several theoretical works significantly influenced the initial development of the theory of nursing as caring. Notably, Paterson and Zderad's (1988) existential phenomenological theory of humanistic nursing served as a substantive and structural base for the conceptualization of Boykin and Schoenhofer's own theory. Roach's (2002) thesis that caring is the human mode of being is expressed in the assumptions of the theory of nursing as caring. Mayeroff's (1971) work provided language for the theory that facilitated the description and expression of living as caring. Boykin and Schoenhofer's work continues on this theory in collaboration with graduate students, nursing faculties, and healthcare agencies that are using the theory to ground research, teaching, and practice (Boykin & Schoenhofer, 2006, p. 339).

OVERVIEW OF THE THEORY OF NURSING AS CARING

AN OVERVIEW OF THE THEORY of nursing as caring is presented here in terms the concepts of the theory. The primary concepts of this theory include caring, focus and intention of nursing, nursing situation, personhood, call for nursing, nursing response, and the "caring between" (Boykin & Schoenhofer, 2006, p. 337).

Caring is not unique to the discipline of nursing. Nevertheless, as a discipline, nursing uniquely focuses on caring as its central value, primary interest, and the direct intention of practice. According to these theorists, **caring** is an expression of nursing and is the "intentional and authentic presence of the nurse with another who is recognized as living in caring and growing in caring" (Boykin & Schoenhofer, 1993, p. 24). More recently, the theorists have defined caring is an "altruistic, active expression of love [that] is the intentional and embodied recognition of value and connectedness," adding that the full meaning of caring cannot be restricted to a definition but is illuminated in the experience of caring and in the reflection on that experience (Boykin & Schoenhofer, 2006, p. 335–336).

The general intention of nursing is to know persons as caring and to support and sustain them as they live caring (Boykin & Schoenhofer, 2006). This intention is expressed when the nurse enters into a relationship with the person with the intention of knowing the other as a caring person, and affirming and celebrating the person as caring.

The practice of nursing lives in the context of person-with-person caring. The nursing situation involves the values, intentions, and actions of two or more persons choosing to live a nursing relationship. In this theory, the nursing situation is understood to mean the shared lived experience in which caring between the nurse and the nursed enhances personhood. Nursing is created in the "caring between," and all knowledge of nursing is created and understood within the nursing situation (Boykin & Schoenhofer, 2006, p. 336). An extension of the nursing situation introduced by Boykin and Schoenhofer (2001), known as direct invitation, clarifies the role of the nurse in initiating and sustaining caring responses. The nurse risks entering the world of the other person in an effort to come to know what is meaningful to that person. An example of direct invitation

CRITICAL THINKING

Is the definition of the concept of caring as presented in the theory of nursing as caring congruent with your own conceptual definition of caring? What is it about the definition that is different? What is it about the definition that is similar?

to share what really matters may include the nurse saying, "How might I nurse you in ways that are meaningful to you?" The power of the direct invitation reaches deep into the nursing situation, uniting and guiding the intention of both the nurse and the nursed (Purnell, 2010, p. 397).

The caring between is the source and ground of nursing. Without the loving relation of the caring between, unidirectional activity or reciprocal exchange can occur but nursing in its fullest sense does not happen because it is within the context of the caring between that personhood is enhanced (Boykin & Schoenhofer, 2006, p. 337).

Personhood is a universal human call that is understood within the context of the theory of nursing as caring to mean living grounded in caring. Personhood is being authentic and demonstrating congruence between beliefs and behaviors. It is living out the meaning of one's life. Personhood acknowledges the potential for unfolding caring possibilities from moment to moment (Boykin & Schoenhofer, 2001). An understanding of the concept of personhood simultaneously communicates the paradox of person-as-person and person-in-communication (Boykin & Schoenhofer, 2006, p. 336).

Calls for nursing are calls for nurturance through personal expressions of caring that originate within persons as they live out caring. Calls for nursing are unique situated personal expressions; as such, they cannot be predicted in a nursing diagnosis. Nurses develop sensitivity and expertise in hearing calls for nursing through intention, experience, study, and reflection in a broad range of situations (Boykin & Schoenhofer, 2006, p. 336).

The nursing response is a specific expression of caring nurturance to sustain and enhance the person as he or she lives caring and grows in caring in the situation of concern. Nurses' responses to calls for nursing evolve as nurses clarify their own understandings of calls through presence and dialogue. The response of each nurse is uniquely created for the moment and cannot be predicted or applied from a preplanned protocol (Boykin & Schoenhofer, 2006, p. 336).

Also introduced in 2001, a visual representation of Boykin and Schoenhofer's model entitled "The Dance of Caring Persons" illustrates the interrelated meanings of the major concepts and assumptions of their theory. In this illustration, dancers enter the circle of caring, and each brings special gifts as the nursing situation evolves. The dancers move

> The caring between is the source and ground of nursing.

freely, but all move in relation to one another and to the circle. Personal knowing of self and other leads to connectedness of persons, and all persons in the nursing situation are energized and sustain the dance (Boykin & Schoenhofer, 2001).

MAJOR CONCEPTS OF NURSING BASED ON THE THEORY OF NURSING AS CARING

IN ADDITION TO THE CONCEPTS already presented, the four metaparadigm concepts of nursing are identified in the theory of nursing as caring. These concepts are summarized in Table 20-1.

Person

Persons are viewed as caring by virtue of their humanness. Persons are not viewed as segmented into parts, but rather as a whole or complete—without insufficiency, brokenness, or absence of anything. Within the context of the theory, to view a person as less than whole fails to truly encounter the person.

Environment

Although not explicitly defined, the environment is referred to in the writing of Boykin and Schoenhofer (2006, p. 337) in relation to environmental pressures in the roles of nurse researchers, administrators, practitioners, and educators.

TABLE 20-1 Metaparadigm Concepts as Defined in the Theory of Nursing as Caring	
Person	Persons are viewed as caring by virtue of their humanness. Persons are not viewed as segmented into parts but rather as a whole.
Environment	Not explicitly defined, but "environmental pressures" are mentioned in relation to nursing roles (Boykin & Schoenhofer, 2006, p. 337).
Health	Nursing is concerned with the broad spectrum of human living rather than the narrow concept of health.
Nursing	Nursing is viewed as both a discipline and a profession. The intention of nursing is "nurturing persons living caring and growing in caring" (Boykin & Schoenhofer, 2006, p. 336).

Health

The notion of nursing as primarily concerned with the concept of health seemed limiting to these theorists. After refinement of the theory, they proposed that nursing is concerned with the broad spectrum of human living rather than the narrow concept of health (Purnell, 2010, p. 395).

Nursing

Nursing is viewed as both a discipline and a profession (Boykin & Schoenhofer, 2006, p.335). As a discipline, nursing attends to the discovery, creation, development, and refinement of knowledge needed for the practice of nursing; in contrast, the profession of nursing focuses on the application of that knowledge in response to human needs (Purnell, 2010, p. 400). The focus of nursing, from the perspective of the theory of nursing as caring, is the person as living in caring and growing in caring; the general intention of nursing as a practiced discipline is "nurturing persons living caring and growing in caring" (Boykin & Schoenhofer, 2006, p. 336).

> The focus of nursing, from the perspective of the theory of nursing as caring, is the person as living in caring and growing in caring.

ANALYSIS OF THE THEORY OF NURSING AS CARING

THE ANALYSIS PRESENTED HERE CONSISTS of an examination of assumptions and propositions as well as a brief critique of Boykin and Schoenhofer's theory of nursing as caring.

Assumptions of the Theory of Nursing as Caring

Boykin and Schoenhofer (2006, p. 335) identify six assumptions about what it means to be human that provide a foundation for the theory of nursing as caring. These fundamental beliefs are as follows:

- ❖ Persons are caring by virtue of their humanness. This assumption does not require that each act of a person be caring, but it does require acceptance that "fundamentally, potentially, and actually, each person is caring" (Boykin & Schoenhofer, 2001, p. 2).

- ❖ Persons are whole and complete in the moment. This assumption communicates respect for the total person.

❖ Persons live caring from moment to moment. This assumption expresses the belief that caring is a lifetime process that is lived from moment to moment and is constantly unfolding (Purnell, 2010, p. 399).

❖ Personhood is a way of living grounded in caring.

❖ Personhood is enhanced through participation in nurturing relationships with caring others.

❖ Nursing is both a discipline and a profession.

Propositions of the Theory of Nursing as Caring

The theoretical assertions within the theory of nursing as caring include (1) that to be human is to be caring and (2) the purpose of the discipline and profession is to come to know persons and nurture them as persons living caring and growing in caring. These assertions lead to the notion of respect for persons and for what is important to them. The notion of respect characterizes relationships and is the starting place for all nursing activities (Purnell, 2010, p. 400).

Brief Critique of the Theory of Nursing as Caring

The theory of nursing as caring is presented in a logical format. The concepts and assumptions of the theory are presented in everyday language that is clear and easy to understand. The theory of nursing as caring is a general theory that offers a broad framework for transforming practice. It is applicable for use at the individual level or within organizations. This theory offers an excellent example of the growth of theory through the further development of existing theories (Purnell, 2010, p. 396).

THE THEORY OF NURSING AS CARING AS A FRAMEWORK FOR NURSING CARE

THE COMMITMENT OF THE NURSE practicing as caring is to "nurture persons living caring and growing in caring" (Boykin & Schoenhofer, 2006, p. 339). According to these theorists, this commitment implies that the nurse comes to know the other person as a caring person in the moment. The role of the nurse in practice is not to discover what is missing, weakened, or needed in the other person, but rather to come to know the other person as a caring person; to nurture that person in situation-specific, creative ways; and to acknowledge, support, and celebrate the caring. The nurse practicing within the caring context will most often be interacting with the healthcare system in two ways: (1) communicating nursing so that it is understood with clarity and richness, and (2) articulating nursing service as a unique contribution within the system in such a way that the system grows to support nursing (Boykin & Schoenhofer, 2006, p. 339–340).

THE NURSING PROCESS AS IT is understood in the discipline of nursing is a linear process with an endpoint. The theory of nursing as caring views nursing as an ongoing process that is dynamic and unfolding; although guided by intentionality, this process is not directed by a preenvisioned outcome or product (Boykin & Schoenhofer, 2006, p. 343). In this section, the theory will, however, be examined in light of the components of the nursing process for the sake of comparison and discussion because the standards of nursing care are presented based on the components of the nursing process.

THE NURSING PROCESS AND THE THEORY OF NURSING AS CARING

Assessment and Planning

Initially, the nurse prepares to enter the nursing relationship with the formed intention of offering caring through authentic presence. The call for nursing will emerge as the nurse begins to understand that the person in a particular moment is seeking to be known as a caring person of value.

Implementation

The nurse listens intently and responds with presence and caring communicated in the nurse's way of being and of doing. The caring between develops and personhood is enhanced as growing in caring is realized.

Evaluation

The concepts of predictable and evidence-based outcomes of care are incompatible with the values-oriented experience in caring nursing. Rather, outcomes of nursing care are conceptualized from values experienced in the nursing relationship (Purnell, 2010, p. 401). Thus evaluation will be based on the nurse and the nursed moving forward, newly affirmed and celebrated as caring persons.

SCENARIO ILLUSTRATING NURSING CARE FRAMED BY THE THEORY OF NURSING AS CARING UTILIZING THE NURSING PROCESS

THE FOLLOWING SCENARIO ILLUSTRATES NURSING care of the patient relative to one identified nursing problem framed by the theory of nursing as caring. This scenario is not intended to cover all aspects of care, but rather to stimulate thinking about how specific care might be approached using this theory as a framework for practice.

You are the nurse assigned to care for Mrs. M. You have just received a report on her from the day-shift nurse, who states that Mrs. M. has been very demanding during the day shift. As you ready yourself to enter Mrs. M.'s room, you prepare to enter the nursing relationship with the formed intention of offering caring through authentic presence.

Clarity of the call for nursing begins to emerge as you begin to understand that Mrs. M. in a particular moment is seeking to be known as a caring person of value, who is worthy of respect. You listen intently to her statements and begin to understand that the anger and demanding behavior of Mrs. M. are actually a reflection of her desire to be truly known and worthy of care. You respond with presence and caring that is communicated in your way of being and of doing. Hope is drawn forth, and Mrs. M. softens. The caring between develops and personhood is enhanced as growing in caring is realized. Both the nurse and the nursed move forward, newly affirmed and celebrated as caring persons, and the nursing situation continues to be a source of inspiration for living in caring and growing in caring (Boykin & Schoenhofer, 2006, p. 337–338).

Throughout this process, the theory of nursing as caring may be applied simultaneously as other issues are identified by Mrs. M. and the nurse. If other issues arise during the nursing encounter that are outside the focus of the theory, nursing interventions will be planned to address those issues using strategies that are congruent with current best clinical practices.

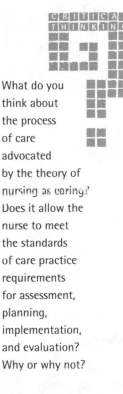

CRITICAL THINKING

What do you think about the process of care advocated by the theory of nursing as caring? Does it allow the nurse to meet the standards of care practice requirements for assessment, planning, implementation, and evaluation? Why or why not?

CLASSROOM ACTIVITY 20-1

Form small groups. Each group should add to the plan of care for Mrs. M. in the preceding scenario based on other potential or actual nursing problems typical for a patient with the same medical diagnosis or symptoms and demographics. Each group should develop a plan for one additional nursing problem using the theory of nursing as caring as the basis for practice. Each group should then share its plan with the class.

CLASSROOM ACTIVITY 20-2

Form small groups. Using a case study provided by the instructor, develop a plan of care using the theory of nursing as caring as the basis for practice. Each group should then share its plan of care with the class.

CLASSROOM ACTIVITY 20-3

Form small groups. Using a case study provided by the instructor, develop a plan of care using one of the theories as the basis for practice; each group should select a different nursing theory. Each group should then share its plan of care with the class and discuss the similarities and differences in care.

REFERENCES

Boykin, A., & Schoenhofer, S. O. (1993). *Nursing as caring: A model for transforming practice.* New York: National League for Nursing Press.

Boykin, A., & Schoenhofer, S. O. (2001). *Nursing as caring: A model for transforming practice.* Sudbury, MA: Jones and Bartlett.

Boykin, A., & Schoenhofer, S. O. (2006). Anne Boykin and Savina O. Schoenhofer's nursing as caring theory. In M. E. Parker (Ed.), *Nursing theories and nursing practice* (2nd ed., pp. 334–348). Philadelphia: F. A. Davis.

Mayeroff, M. (1971) *On caring.* New York: Harper Collins.

Paterson, J. G., & Zderad, L. T. (1988). *Humanistic nursing.* New York: National League for Nursing Press.

Purnell, M. J. (2010). The theory of nursing as caring: A model for transforming practice. In M. R. Alligood & A. M. Tomey (Eds.), *Nursing theorists and their work* (7th ed., pp. 395–415). Maryland Heights, MO: Mosby.

Roach, M. S. (2002). *Caring, the human mode of being* (2nd ed.). Ottawa, Ontario, Canada: CHA Press.

MODELING AND ROLE-MODELING:

Helen C. Erickson, Evelyn M. Tomlin, Mary Ann P. Swain

LEARNING OBJECTIVES

After completing this chapter the student should be able to

1. Identify and describe the major concepts of the modeling and role-modeling theory

2. Explain the major concepts important to nursing as defined in the modeling and role-modeling theory

3. Plan nursing care for a patient scenario utilizing the modeling and role-modeling theory

KEY TERMS

Modeling

Nurturance

Role-modeling

Self-care knowledge

Self-care resources

BACKGROUND

HELEN C. ERICKSON RECEIVED HER initial nursing education at Saginaw General Hospital in Michigan. After graduating with a nursing diploma in 1957, she worked for many years in various professional roles and settings, including in emergency rooms as a staff nurse and head nurse, as night supervisor in a hospital for mentally impaired and handicapped patients, as Director of Health Services in Puerto Rico, and as a psychiatric nurse consultant. In 1974, Erickson completed a baccalaureate degree; in 1976, she earned dual master's degrees in psychiatric nursing and medical–surgical nursing from the University of Michigan. In 1984, she received a doctor of educational psychology degree from the University of Michigan.

Erickson's academic career began at the University of Michigan, where she served in various positions ranging from assistant instructor to dean for undergraduate studies. In 1986, she left the University of Michigan to go to the University of South Carolina, where she served as an associate professor and administrator responsible for academic programs and academic affairs. In 1988, Erickson moved to the University of Texas at Austin, where she served as Professor and Chair of Adult Health as well as Special Assistant to the Dean of Graduate Programs. She retired from academia in 1997 and has been Professor Emeritus at the University of Texas at Austin; in addition, she has maintained an independent nursing practice since her retirement (Erickson, 2010a, p. 537).

Erickson has received numerous awards for her contributions to the profession of nursing over her career. She continues to actively research the modeling and role-modeling theory and makes presentations on the theory at seminars, at conferences, and through papers nationally and internationally. In addition, she serves as a consultant to organizations related to the implementation of the theory in practice (Erickson, 2010a, p. 538).

Evelyn M. Tomlin began her nursing education at Pasadena City College, Los Angeles County General Hospital School of Nursing, and the University of Southern California, where she received her bachelor's of science degree in nursing. In 1976, Tomlin earned a master of science degree in psychiatric nursing from the University of Michigan. Her professional experiences are numerous and varied. Tomlin began as a clinical instructor in surgical nursing and maternal and premature infant nursing. In addition, she has served as a school nurse, family nurse, home visiting nurse, coronary care unit nurse, respiratory intensive care unit nurse, head nurse in an emergency room, and mental health consultant, and she has taught English in Afghanistan. All of this experience came before she began her career in academia at the University of Michigan's School of Nursing. Tomlin is currently retired but remains active as a volunteer in her community, where she teaches and counsels homeless women (Erickson, 2010a, p. 538–539).

Mary Ann P. Swain's educational background is in psychology rather than nursing. She earned a bachelor of arts degree in psychology from DePauw University and master of science and doctoral degrees in psychology from the University of Michigan. She accepted a position as lecturer and Professor of Psychology and Nursing Research at the University of Michigan, where she later served as the Director of the Doctoral Program in Nursing. Swain also served as the chairperson of nursing research from 1977 until 1982, when she became Associate Vice President for Academic Affairs. During her tenure at the University of Michigan, Swain developed and taught courses in nursing research and collaborated with nursing faculty on research projects; one of those collaborations included work with Erickson on a model that is significant to the modeling and role-modeling theory (Erickson, 2010a, p. 538). Swain is currently Provost and Vice President for Academic Affairs at Binghamton University.

The modeling and role-modeling theory was derived inductively from Erickson's clinical and personal life experiences. At the same time, the work of Maslow, Erikson, Piaget, Engel, Selye, and others was integrated to label, articulate, and refine the theory (Erickson, 2010a, p. 540). Erickson's initial theoretical work, called the adaptive potential assessment model, focused on the individual's ability to mobilize resources when confronted with stressors (Erickson & Swain, 1982).

OVERVIEW OF THE MODELING AND ROLE-MODELING THEORY

To UNDERSTAND THE MODELING AND role-modeling theory, it is necessary to have a clear understanding of the definitions of the concepts used in the theory. Throughout this overview of the theory, definitions will be provided as new concepts are discussed.

The first terms requiring a definition are the concepts of modeling and role-modeling. **Modeling** is "the process used by the nurses as she develops an image and understanding of the client's world, as the client perceives it" (Erickson, Tomlin, & Swain, 1983/2009, p. 254). **Role-modeling** is "the facilitation and nurturance of the individual in attaining, maintaining or promoting health through purposeful interventions" (Erickson, Tomlin, & Swain, 1983/2009, p. 254). In defining the concept of **nurturance**, these authors explain that within the context of their theory, it is "the fusing and integrating of cognitive, physiological, and affective processes with the aim of assisting a client to move toward holistic health" (Erickson, Tomlin, & Swain, 1983/2009, p. 254).

When using the modeling and role-modeling theory, the nurse attempts to understand the "client's personal model of his or her world and to appreciate its value and significance for the client from the client's perspective" (Erickson, Tomlin, & Swain, 1983/2009, p. 49). "The way that an individual communicates, thinks, feels, acts, and reacts—all of these factors—comprise the individual's *model of his or her world*. Each person's model is unique" (Erickson, Tomlin, & Swain, 1983/2009, p. 84). After the patient's world has been modeled, the nurse facilitates and nurtures the individual through role-modeling. In role-modeling the client's world, the nurse plans interventions that identify mutual nurse–client goals; promote client strengths, control, and positive orientation; and build trust. During this process, the nurse assists the client in identifying, developing, and mobilizing internal and external resources in an effort to cope with stressors. Essential to this process is the nurse's unconditional acceptance of the client (Erickson, 2010b, p.365). The ultimate goal of interventions is to help the client "achieve an optimal state of perceived health and contentment (Erickson, Tomlin, & Swain, 1983/2009, p. 49).

Nursing interventions are designed in cooperation with the client, based on the belief that individuals know what has altered their health status and know what they need to improve and optimize their health status, promote their growth and development, and maximize their quality of life. This knowledge is referred to as **self-care knowledge** (Erickson, 2010b, p. 365). According to the theory, all individuals also have internal **self-care resources**. Self-care resources are mobilized through self-care action to help the person gain, maintain, and promote the optimal level of holistic health (Erickson, Tomlin, & Swain, 1983/2009, p. 254–255). Internal self-care resources refer to all of the "internal resources that an individual can use to promote health and growth (Erickson, Tomlin, & Swain, 1983/2009, p. 128). These self-strengths can be defined in terms of attitudes, endurance, patterns, or any other way that the client chooses to define them. In addition, internal resources may be characterized as mobilizing resources.

Within Erickson, Tomlin, and Swain's framework, a major focus is adaptation—that is, the client's ability to respond to internal and external stressors and to mobilize resources for coping in a way that promotes health and growth. These resources may be both physiological and psychosocial (Erickson, Tomlin, & Swain, 1983/2009, p. 128). External self-care resources may also affect the health of the client, including aspects of the client's social network and support systems.

The development and utilization of self-care knowledge and mobilization self-care resources is collectively known as self-care action (Erickson, Tomlin, & Swain, 1983/2009, p. 128). The ability to mobilize resources is depicted by the adaptive potential assessment model, which identifies three potential coping states: arousal, equilibrium, and impoverishment. Each of these states represents a different potential to mobilize self-care resources in response to stress (Erickson, 2010b, p. 543).

Nursing interventions are designed to help clients use self-care actions to meet their physiological, psychological, social, cognitive, and spiritual needs; however, basic needs are met only when the individual perceives that they are met (Erickson, Tomlin, & Swain, 1983/2009, p. 57). An important concept in the theory related to nursing intervention is the concept of holism. Because human beings are viewed in the modeling and role-modeling theory as holistic persons who have multiple

When using the modeling and role-modeling theory, the nurse attempts to understand the "client's personal model of his or her world and to appreciate its value and significance for the client from the client's perspective."

Nursing interventions are designed to help clients use self-care actions to meet their physiological, psychological, social, cognitive, and spiritual needs.

interacting systems and who are more than the sum of their parts, it is important that nursing interventions take into account these interactions so that the effect of the intervention is not just shifting energy among the various subsystems. When there is merely a shifting of energy, problems may be resolved in one subsystem at the cost of creating another problem within the same or another subsystem. No subsystem is left in jeopardy if adaptation occurs (Erickson, Tomlin, & Swain, 1983/2009, p. 129).

MAJOR CONCEPTS OF NURSING BASED ON THE MODELING AND ROLE-MODELING THEORY

IN ADDITION TO THE CONCEPTS already presented, the four metaparadigm concepts of nursing are identified in the modeling and role-modeling theory. These concepts are summarized in Table 21-1.

Person

Human beings are viewed in terms of how people are alike and how they are different. All human beings are seen as holistic persons who have multiple interacting subsystems, including biophysical, cognitive, psychological, and social subsystems. Intersecting these subsystems and permeating these subsystems are the genetic base and the spiritual drive (Erickson, Tomlin, & Swain, 1983/2009, p. 44). All persons also engage in a lifetime of development that is reflected in their passage through various developmental stages and cognitive stages. All persons also have an instinctual need for *affiliated-individuation*—that is, "the need to be able to be dependent on support systems while simultaneously maintaining independence from these support systems" (Erickson, Tomlin, & Swain, 1983/2009, p. 252). Persons differ because of variations in their inherent endowment, which includes their genetic makeup and inherited characteristics and their ability to adapt.

Throughout the modeling and role-modeling theory, its authors draw a clear distinction between the terms "patient" and "client." According to these theorists, a patient is given a treatment and instruction. By comparison, a client participates in his or her own care, making the client a "legitimate member of the decision-making team, who always has some control over the planned regimen, and who is incorporated into the

TABLE 21-1 Metaparadigm Concepts as Defined in the Modeling and Role-Modeling Theory	
Person	Human beings are seen as holistic persons who have multiple interacting subsystems, including biophysical, cognitive, psychological, and social subsystems. Intersecting these subsystems and permeating these subsystems are the genetic base and the spiritual drive (Erickson, Tomlin, & Swain, 1983/2009, p. 44).
Environment	The client's environment consists of internal and external stressors as well as internal and external resources.
Health	Health is viewed as a state of physical, mental, and social well-being, and not merely as the absence of disease or infirmity.
Nursing	Nursing is assisting persons holistically to use their adaptive strengths to attain and maintain optimum bio-psycho-social-spiritual functioning (Erickson, Tomlin, & Swain, 1983/2009, p. 50).

planning and implementation of his or her own care as much as possible" (Erickson, Tomlin, & Swain, 1983/2009, p. 253).

Environment

The client's environment consists of internal and external stressors as well as internal and external resources. In addition, the environment is viewed in the context of social subsystems and as the interaction between self and other (Erickson, 2010a, p. 547).

Health

Health is viewed as a state of physical, mental, and social well-being, and not as merely the absence of disease or infirmity. Health is also viewed as a state of dynamic equilibrium among the various subsystems that make up the person and the environment (Erickson, Tomlin, & Swain, 1983/2009, p. 46).

Nursing

According to Erickson, Tomlin, and Swain (1983/2009), nursing is the holistic helping of persons with their self-care activities in relation to

CRITICAL THINKING

How is the concept of adaptation in the modeling and role-modeling theory similar or dissimilar to definitions of adaptation proposed by other nurse theorists?

their health. This interactive, interpersonal process nurtures strengths to enable development, release, and channeling of resources for coping with one's circumstances and environment. The goal of nursing intervention is for the recipient of care to achieve a state of perceived optimal health and contentment. These theorists point out that their definition of nursing does not specify the tasks of nursing, because they believe that tasks are merely a means to an end (Erickson, Tomlin, & Swain, 1983/2009, p. 49). The five aims of nursing interventions are to build trust, to affirm and promote client strengths, to promote positive orientation, to facilitate perceived control, and to set health-directed mutual goals (Erickson, Tomlin, & Swain, 1983/2009, p. 170).

ANALYSIS OF THE MODELING AND ROLE-MODELING THEORY

THE ANALYSIS PRESENTED HERE CONSISTS of an examination of assumptions and propositions as well as a brief critique of the modeling and role-modeling theory as proposed by Erickson, Tomlin, and Swain.

Assumptions of the Modeling and Role-Modeling Theory

Five assumptions are presented; in addition, many of the statements included in the definitions of the metaparadigm concepts are, in fact, assumptions. The additional five assumptions listed here are directly related to the five aims of nursing interventions:

❖ The nursing process requires that a trusting and functional relationship exist between the nurse and the client.

❖ Affiliated-individuation depends on the individual's perceiving that he or she is an acceptable, respectable, and worthwhile human being.

❖ Human development depends on the individual's perceiving that he or she has some control over his or her life, while concurrently sensing a state of affiliation.

❖ There is an innate drive toward holistic health that is facilitated by consistent and systematic nurturance.

❖ Human growth depends on satisfaction of basic needs and is facilitated by growth–need satisfaction (Erickson, Tomlin, & Swain, 1983/2009, p. 170).

Propositions of the Modeling and Role-Modeling Theory

Three theoretical relationship statements have been identified by Erickson (2010a, p. 547):

❖ "The degree to which developmental tasks are resolved is dependent on the degree to which human needs are satisfied" (Erickson, Tomlin, & Swain, 1983/2009, p. 87).

❖ "The degree to which needs are satisfied by object attachment depends on the availability of those objects and the degree to which they provide comfort and security as opposed to threat and anxiety" (Erickson, Tomlin, & Swain, 1983/2009, p. 90).

❖ An individual's potential for mobilizing resources—the person's state of coping according to the adaptive potential assessment model—is directly associated with the person's need satisfaction level (Erickson, Tomlin, & Swain, 1983/2009, p. 91).

Additional theoretical propositions that have been identified include the following:

❖ An individual's ability to contend with new stressors is directly related to his or her ability to mobilize the resources needed.

❖ An individual's ability to mobilize resources is directly related to his or her need deficits and assets.

❖ Distressors are related to unmet basic needs; stressors are related to unmet growth needs.

❖ Objects that repeatedly facilitate the individual in need satisfaction take on significance for the individual. When this occurs, attachment to the objects results.

❖ Secure attachment produces feelings of worthiness.

❖ Feelings of worthiness result in a sense of futurity.

❖ Real, threatened, or perceived loss of the attachment object results in the grief process.

❖ Basic-need deficits coexist with the grief process.

❖ An adequate alternative object must be perceived to be available for the individual to resolve the grief process.

❖ Prolonged grief due to an unavailable or inadequate object results in morbid grief.

❖ Unmet basic and growth needs interfere with growth processes.

❖ Repeated satisfaction of basic needs is a prerequisite to working through developmental tasks and resolution of related developmental crisis.

❖ Morbid grief is always related to need deficits (Schultz, 2004, p. 245–246).

Brief Critique of the Modeling and Role-Modeling Theory

The modeling and role-modeling theory is presented clearly, and concepts are defined and used consistently throughout the theory. The concepts are operationally defined, and the theorists provide guidelines for data collection, analysis, and synthesis as well as guidelines for implementation. The theory is presented in language that is understandable to the practicing nurse; examples are provided to illustrate its meaning. The theory is based on concepts that have a broad range of applicability to various settings and populations, making it generalizable for professional nursing practice (Erickson, 2010a, p. 549–550).

THE MODELING AND ROLE-MODELING THEORY AS A FRAMEWORK FOR NURSING CARE

THE MODELING AND ROLE-MODELING THEORY is guided by the five intervention aims, five principles, and outcome goals for the nursing process. Interview guidelines are provided that influence the categories of data collected. The data collected are interpreted, analyzed, and synthesized, and strategies are planned to facilitate growth and healing. The primary data source is the patient. Secondary sources include the views of the family and the observations of the nurse. All other sources of data are considered tertiary (Erickson, 2010b, p. 369).

T HE MODELING AND ROLE-MODELING THEORY is presented by the theorists within the framework of the nursing process, thereby emphasizing the importance of the interactive and interpersonal nature of nursing as well as the theoretical and scientific bases of nursing practice (Schultz, 2004, p. 246).

THE NURSING PROCESS AND THE MODELING AND ROLE-MODELING THEORY

Assessment

During the assessment phase of the nursing process, data are collected and organized in a manner consistent with developing an overview of the client's perspective of the situation, determining the client's expectations for the future, determining the internal and external resources available to the client, and determining the client's developmental status and personal model of the world (Erickson, Tomlin, & Swain, 1983/2009).

Planning

Planning occurs in partnership with the client. The theory provides a structure for the general aims of interventions that are associated with the theoretical principles, thereby assisting the nurse in planning for systematic interventions within the framework of the theory (Schultz, 2004, p. 246).

Implementation

During the implementation phase of the nursing process, the nurse's goal is to carry out one intervention that reflects each aim during every contact with the client, although a single intervention can meet more than one of the general aims (Schultz, 2004, p. 246). While the use of standardized interventions is not consistent with the theory, Erickson, Tomlin, and Swain (1983/2009) do provide suggested guidelines in each of the "aims of intervention" categories to assist the nurse in providing care.

Evaluation

Evaluation is closely tied to the perception of the client. Basic needs—whether they are developmental, cognitive, physiological, or psychosocial—are met only when the individual client perceives that they are met.

SCENARIO ILLUSTRATING NURSING CARE FRAMED BY THE MODELING AND ROLE-MODELING THEORY UTILIZING THE NURSING PROCESS

THE FOLLOWING SCENARIO ILLUSTRATES NURSING care of the patient relative to one identified nursing problem framed by the modeling and role-modeling theory. This scenario is not intended to cover all aspects of care, but rather to stimulate thinking about how specific care might be approached using this theory as a framework for practice.

Mr. P. is an African American male who has recently been diagnosed with hypertension and is at the clinic for a follow-up visit. Mr. P. is accompanied by his wife. Initially, after establishing a relationship with the Mr. P., the nurse begins to gather data to determine Mr. P.'s perspective on the situation, his expectations for the future, and the internal and external resources available to Mr. P. This information allows the nurse to gain a perspective on and of understanding of Mr. P.'s world.

Based on the assessment data collected through observations and interviews with Mr. P. and his wife, the nurse has the impression that Mr. P. believes that he has no control over his high blood pressure due to his family history and the prevalence of high blood pressure among African American men. Mr. P. and the nurse plan strategies in partnership for each of the five aims for interventions to facilitate growth and healing. For example, to promote a positive orientation for Mr. P., the nurse refers to the future and to a time when his blood pressure will be controlled. To encourage Mr. P.'s perception that he does have some control over his life, the nurse encourages Mr. P. by asking what he believes he can do to help himself and then urging him to set goals to achieve the desired behavior change. To affirm Mr. P.'s strengths, the nurse mirrors his statements related to identified strengths and points out her perception of his strengths, such as a supportive wife and extended family. The evaluation for this encounter is based on the perception of Mr. P. that he does have the internal and external resources necessary for adaptation and on his perception that he does have some control related to his blood pressure.

Throughout this process, the theory is applied simultaneously to other issues as they are identified by Mr. P. and the nurse. If other issues arise during the nursing encounter that are outside of the focus of the theory, nursing interventions are planned to address those issues using strategies that are congruent with current best clinical practices.

CLASSROOM ACTIVITY 21-1

Form small groups. Each group should add to the plan of care for Mr. P. in the preceding scenario based on other potential or actual nursing problems typical for a patient with the same medical diagnosis or symptoms and demographics. Each group should develop a plan for one additional nursing problem using Erickson, Tomlin, and Swain's modeling and role-modeling theory as the basis for practice. Each group should then share its plan with the class.

CLASSROOM ACTIVITY 21-2

Form small groups. Using a case study provided by the instructor, develop a plan of care using Erickson, Tomlin, and Swain's modeling and role-modeling theory as the basis for practice. Each group should then share its plan of care with the class.

CLASSROOM ACTIVITY 21-3

Form small groups. Using a case study provided by the instructor, develop a plan of care using one of the theories as the basis for practice; each group should select a different nursing theory. Each group should then share its plan of care with the class and discuss the similarities and differences in care.

REFERENCES

Erickson, H. C., & Swain, M. A. (1982). A model for assessing potential adaptation to stress. *Research in Nursing and Health, 5,* 93–101.

Erickson, H. C., Tomlin, E. M., & Swain, M. A. P. (1983/2009). *Modeling and role modeling: A theory and paradigm for nursing.* Charleston, SC: Booksurge.

Erickson, M. E. (2010a). Helen C. Erickson, Evelyn M. Tomlin, and Mary Ann P. Swain: Modeling and role-modeling. In M. R. Alligood & A. M. Tomey (Eds.), *Nursing theorists and their work* (7th ed., pp. 536–559). Maryland Heights, MO: Mosby.

Erickson, M. E. (2010b). Modeling and role-modeling theory in nursing practice. In M. R. Alligood (Ed.), *Nursing theory: Utilization and application* (4th ed., pp. 359–388). Maryland Heights, MO: Mosby.

Schultz, E. D. (2004). Modeling and role-modeling. In S. J. Peterson & T. S. Bredow (Eds.), *Middle range theories: Application to nursing research* (pp. 235–254). Philadelphia: Lippincott Williams & Wilkins.

MIDDLE-RANGE
THEORIES

PARENT–CHILD INTERACTION MODEL:
Kathryn E. Barnard

LEARNING OBJECTIVES

After completing this chapter the student should be able to

1. Identify and describe the major concepts proposed in the parent–child interaction model

2. Explain the major concepts important to nursing as defined by Barnard

3. Plan nursing care for a patient scenario utilizing Barnard's parent–child interaction model

BACKGROUND

KATHRYN E. BARNARD WAS BORN in 1938 in Omaha, Nebraska. She received a baccalaureate degree in nursing in 1960 from the University of Nebraska. She earned in master's degree in nursing from Boston University in 1962, along with a certificate of Advanced Graduate Specialization in Nursing Education. After receiving these academic credentials, she accepted a position to teach maternal and child nursing at the University of Washington in Seattle. In 1971, Barnard became project director for a research study to develop a method of nursing child assessment. A year later, Barnard received a PhD in the ecology of early childhood development from the University of Washington and then accepted a position as professor in parent–child nursing at the University of Washington (Fine, 2002, p. 484).

Barnard has served as project director or principal investigator for more than 22 research grants and projects. In addition, she has provided consultation, presented lectures, and numerous published articles and books related to child health assessment, teaching mentally retarded and developmentally delayed children, and working with families of vulnerable infant and children. Barnard has received many honors during her career as a result of her contributions to the profession, including induction into the American Academy of Nursing in 1975 (Fine, 2002, p. 485).

Barnard credits various nursing theorists such as Florence Nightingale, Virginia Henderson, and Martha Rogers as influencing her work. However, more direct influence came from the Neal nursing construct and its four expressions of health and illness: cognition, sensation, motion, and affiliation. Barnard also credits Florence Blake for elucidating the beliefs and values making up the foundation of nursing practice, which include turning nurses' minds toward an orientation on the patient rather than the procedure and acknowledging the importance of family and Reva Rubin for her work with interventions during pregnancy. Barnard was also influenced by the writings of child development theorists and general systems theory (Fine, 2002).

B ARNARD DID NOT SET OUT to develop a theory of nursing. Her research in child health assessment provided the basis for the original child health assessment interaction model, which visually displays three overlapping circles, with interaction occurring in the segment of the circle where the overlap exists (Pokorny, 2010). Barnard (1978) proposed in this model that individual characteristics of each of the participants influence the parent–infant system and that adaptive behavior modifies those characteristics to meet the needs of the system. Participants in the interaction include the child, the caregivers, and the environment. Characteristics of the child include physical appearance, temperament, feeding and sleeping patterns, and self-regulation. Characteristics of the caregiver include variables such as psychosocial assets, physical health, mental health, coping skills, life changes, expectations and concerns about the child, caregiving style, adaptation skills, and educational level. Environmental characteristics include factors such as social support, financial resources, safe housing, adequate food, and community involvement. The Barnard parent–child interaction model focuses on the mother–child–environment interactive process—that is, the area in the model where all three of the circles overlap.

Other caregiver/parent characteristics and infant/child characteristics affect the interaction of parent and child as well. These characteristics include the caregiver/parent's sensitivity to cues, ability to alleviate distress, and ability to provide a growth-fostering situation. Sensitivity to cues reflects the parent's ability to both recognize and respond to the infant's cues. In measurable terms, how do parents modify their behavior related to timing, force, rhythm, and duration to set the tone of the interaction as they respond to the cues of the child? In looking at the parent's ability to alleviate the infant's distress, does the parent recognize the distress cues, select appropriate action, and respond with the appropriate action? Finally, does the parent use voice, tone, touch, and movement to communicate and provide a supportive environment that fosters social and emotional growth? What about fostering cognitive growth activities?

OVERVIEW OF THE PARENT–CHILD INTERACTION MODEL

The Barnard parent–child interaction model focuses on the mother–child–environment interactive process—that is, the area in the model where all three of the circles overlap.

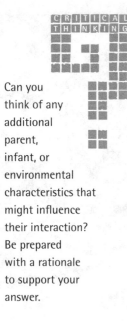

CRITICAL THINKING

Can you think of any additional parent, infant, or environmental characteristics that might influence their interaction? Be prepared with a rationale to support your answer.

For example, do the parent's verbalizations encourage the child's response or allow exploration?

The corresponding characteristics of the infant/child include the clarity of cues and the child's responsiveness to the parent. Clear cues from the infant make it easier for the parent to interpret and modify behavior, whereas ambiguous cues can interrupt a parent or caregiver's adaptive abilities. The infant's ability to respond by smiling or vocalizing rather than crying serves to reinforce the caregiving behaviors of the parent.

This interaction is illustrated by Barnard by two boxes: one labeled caregiver/parent characteristics and one labeled infant/child characteristics. The boxes are connected by two arrows: one from the caregiver/parent box to the infant/child box and one from the infant/child box to the caregiver/parent box. Each of the arrows has a double line intersecting it, representing an interruption of the adaptive process that causes the interaction to break down. This interaction breakdown can originate in the parent, the child, or the environment.

MAJOR CONCEPTS OF NURSING BASED ON THE PARENT–CHILD INTERACTION MODEL

IN ADDITION TO THE CONCEPTS already presented, the four metaparadigm concepts of nursing are identified in Barnard's parent–child interaction model. These concepts are summarized in Table 22-1.

Person

Barnard defines a person in relation to human beings having the ability to take part in an interaction to which both parts of the dyad bring qualities, skills, and responses that affect the interaction (Fine, 2002).

Environment

The concept of environment is an essential aspect of the parent–child interaction model. According to Barnard, the environment includes all experiences encountered by the child—people, objects, places, sounds, visual, and tactile sensations (Barnard & Eyres, 1979), as well as social

TABLE 22-1	Metaparadigm Concepts as Defined in Barnard's Model
Person	Human beings having the ability to take part in an interaction to which both parts of the dyad bring qualities, skills, and responses that affect the interaction (Fine, 2002).
Environment	All experiences encountered by the child: people, objects, places, sounds, visual, and tactile sensations, as well as social and financial resources, other persons, and adequacy of home and community (Barnard, 1986).
Health	A dynamic state of being in which the developmental and behavioral potential of an individual is realized to the fullest extent possible; health is viewed as a continuum that includes wellness and illness (American Nurses Association, Division of Maternal and Child Health Nursing Practice, 1980, p. 5).
Nursing	The "process by which the patient is assisted in maintenance and promotion of his independence. This process may be educational, therapeutic, or restorative; it involves facilitation of change, most preferably a change in the environment" (Barnard, 1966, p. 629).

support and resources, financial resources, other persons, and adequacy of home and community (Barnard, 1986). The environment affects both the child and the caregiver.

Health

While not defined specifically in any publication related to her theory, Barnard as one of the members of the Executive Committee of the American Nurses Association Maternal and Child Nursing Division in 1980 helped to define health for that organization's scope of practice statement (Fine, 2002). According to this document, health is viewed as a "dynamic state of being in which the developmental and behavioral potential of an individual is realized to the fullest extent possible . . . health is viewed as a continuum that includes wellness and illness. Each being possesses various strengths and limitations resulting from the interaction of environmental and hereditary factors. The relative dominance of the strengths and limitations determines an individual's place on the health continuum from wellness to illness" (American Nurses Association, Division of Maternal and Child Health Nursing Practice, 1980, p. 5).

CRITICAL THINKING

Does the definition of nursing proposed by Barnard remind you of any definitions proposed by theorists that you have already studied? Which theorist or theory? What similarities and differences do you see, if any?

Nursing

Nursing, according to Barnard is a "process by which the patient is assisted in maintenance and promotion of his independence. This process may be educational, therapeutic, or restorative; it involves facilitation of change, most preferably a change in the environment" (Barnard, 1966, p. 629). In the context of family care, the role of the nurse is to assist families in providing conditions that promote growth and development of individual members (Thomas, Barnard, & Summer, 1993, p. 127).

ANALYSIS OF THE PARENT–CHILD INTERACTION MODEL

THE ANALYSIS PRESENTED HERE CONSISTS of an examination of assumptions and propositions as well as a brief critique of the parent–child interaction model as proposed by Barnard.

Assumptions of the Parent–Child Interaction Model

The following assumptions are included in the parent–child interaction model:

❖ The term "person" includes infants, children, and adults (Fine, 2002).

❖ Nursing is a process (Barnard, 1966).

❖ The environment includes all experiences encountered by the child (Barnard, 1986).

Propositions of the Parent–Child Interaction Model

Relational theoretical statements of the parent–child interaction model include the following:

❖ The ultimate goal in child assessment is to identify problems at a point before they develop and when intervention would be most effective.

❖ Social–environmental factors are important for determining child health outcomes.

❖ Brief observations of caregiver–infant interaction can provide a valid sample of ongoing experiences and expectations.

❖ Each adult caregiver brings to caregiving a basic personality and skill level that is the foundation upon which his or her caregiving skill is built. The enactment of caregiving depends on these characteristics as well as the characteristics of the child and of the environment.

❖ Through interaction, caregivers and children modify one another's behaviors.

❖ The process of adaptation of caregiver to infant, or infant to caregiver, is more modifiable than the basic characteristics of either party.

❖ An important way to promote learning is to respond and elaborate on child-initiated behaviors and reinforce the child's attempt to try new things.

❖ A major task for the helping profession is to promote a positive early learning environment that includes a nurturing relationship.

❖ Assessing the child's social environment is important in any comprehensive child healthcare model.

❖ Assessing the child's physical environment is equally important in any child health assessment model (Summer & Spietz, 1994, as cited in Fine, 2002, p. 488–489).

Brief Critique of the Parent–Child Interaction Model

Barnard's parent–child interaction model (referred to in some references as the child health assessment interaction theory) was derived inductively from research with all of the theoretical assertions supported by evidence from research. The theory is clear and easy to understand. Its terminology is familiar and defined consistently. The theory remains population specific; although it was originally designed to be applicable to interactions between the caregiver and the child in the first year of the child's life, it has since been expanded to the three years of life. Although it was developed specifically for nursing, this model has also been used by other professionals concerned with parent–child interactions. An additional facet of this model is the many scales and subscales that have been developed with established reliability and validity, because the model was actually generated through extensive research.

THE PARENT–CHILD INTERACTION MODEL AS A FRAMEWORK FOR NURSING PRACTICE

NURSING SERVICES ARE REQUIRED BY the parent–infant dyad when an interruption or potential interruption of the adaptive process causes interactions to break down. This interaction breakdown can originate in the parent, the child, or the environment. The process of facilitating change that the nurse will employ to assist the dyad maintain healthy interactions may be educational, therapeutic, or restorative and will preferably focus on environmental change.

The Nursing Process and the Parent–Child Interaction Model

Although Barnard does not specifically address the nursing process, for the sake of discussion, consistency, and comparison, the parent–child interaction model is described here within the context of the steps of the nursing process.

Assessment

The assessment phase of the nursing process using Barnard's theory will involve assessment of the caregiver, child, and environment interaction and the characteristics that affect that interaction. This can be accomplished through observation as well as the use of instruments or tools developed to measure these characteristics.

Planning

Based on the analysis of data, the nurse plans for the facilitation of change so as to address the breakdown in interactions or the potential for breakdown in interactions. Planning for change in the environmental characteristics is the first choice.

Implementation

The nurse's interventions focus on restoration and maintenance of interaction that promotes social, emotional, and cognitive growth-fostering activities for the child. In addition, the nurse assists families in providing conditions that promote growth and development of all individual members. These interventions may be educative, therapeutic, or restorative in nature.

Evaluation

Evaluation is based on the restoration of parent, child, and environment interaction that promotes the social, emotional, and cognitive growth for the child. Data to validate this interaction will include continued assessment of the characteristics of each participant that influence the interaction.

T HE FOLLOWING SCENARIO ILLUSTRATES NURS-ING care of the patient relative to one identified nursing problem framed by Barnard's parent–child interaction model. This scenario is not intended to cover all aspects of care, but rather to stimulate thinking about how specific care might be approached using this theory as a framework for practice.

> **SCENARIO ILLUSTRATING NURSING CARE FRAMED BY THE PARENT–CHILD INTERACTION MODEL UTILIZING THE NURSING PROCESS**

Ms. P. was a single mother of two who was pregnant with her third child when you began visiting her more than a year ago. She had a history of alcohol dependency that placed her unborn child at risk. Because of that risk, she had been assigned the services of a visiting nurse. Ms. P. did not consume alcohol during the pregnancy, and she had a good outcome with the pregnancy, delivering a healthy infant girl at full term.

Since the nurse has been visiting this family, she has determined that the home is safe and that Ms. P. has adequate financial resources and social support in her family and local community. On this visit, the nurse will assess the interaction of Ms. P. and infant K. as well as the characteristics that affect their interaction. This will be accomplished through observation as well as the use of instruments developed to measure interaction characteristics. The nurse will observe specifically if Ms. P. is sensitive to and responsive to infant K.'s cues and if Ms. P. is able to soothe infant K. when she cries. The nurse will also assess the clarity of infant K.'s cues and determine whether infant K. responds to Ms. P.'s attempts to communicate. In addition, the nurse will assess the tone of voice, touch, and verbalizations of Ms. P. as she interacts with infant K.

Based on these observations, the nurse will plan to address any breakdown in interactions or the potential for breakdown in interactions between Ms. P. and infant K. The nurse's interventions will focus on restoration and maintenance of interaction that promotes social, emotional, and cognitive growth-fostering activities for the infant K. as well as the toddler and other young child living in the home. Ms. P. and infant K. initially interacted without problems during the nurse's visit. When the other children in the home grew bored with the visit and Ms. P. became distracted by the other children, the nurse observed a decline in Ms. P.'s sensitivity to the infant's cues. The interventions planned by the nurse for Ms. P. are educative in nature. Evaluation will be based on the interaction of Ms. P., infant K., and the environment in promoting social, emotional, and cognitive growth for the infant K. and the other children in the home.

Throughout this process, the parent–child interaction model may be applied simultaneously to other issues as they are identified by Ms. P. and the nurse—for instance, issues with adequate food or safe housing. If other issues arise during the nursing encounter that are outside of the interaction focus of the theory, nursing interventions will be planned to address those issues using strategies that are congruent with current best clinical practices.

CLASSROOM ACTIVITY 22-1

Form small groups. Each group should add to the plan of care for Ms. P. and infant K. in the preceding scenario based on other potential or actual nursing problems typical for a patient with the same medical diagnosis or symptoms and demographics. Each group should develop a plan for one additional nursing problem using Barnard's theory as the basis for practice. Each group should then share its plan with the class.

CLASSROOM ACTIVITY 22-2

Form small groups. Using a case study provided by the instructor, develop a plan of care using Barnard's nursing model as the basis for practice. Each group should then share its plan of care with the class.

CLASSROOM ACTIVITY 22-3

Form small groups. Using a case study provided by the instructor, develop a plan of care using one of the theories as the basis for practice; each group should select a different nursing theory. Each group should then share its plan of care with the class and discuss the similarities and differences in care.

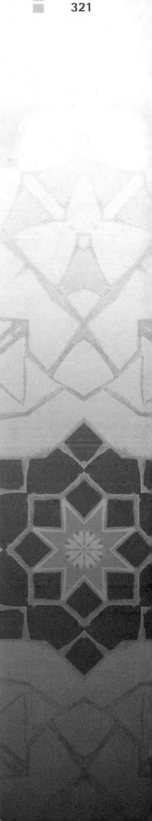

REFERENCES

American Nurses Association, Division of Maternal and Child Health Nursing Practice. (1980). *Standards of maternal and child health nursing practice.* Kansas City, MO: Author.

Barnard, K. E. (1966). Symposium on mental retardation. *Nursing Clinics of North America, 1,* 629–630.

Barnard, K. E. (1978). *Nursing child assessment and training: Learning resource manual.* Seattle, WA: University of Washington.

Barnard, K. E. (1986). *Nursing child assessment satellite training: Learning resource training manual.* Seattle, WA: NCAST Publications, University of Washington.

Barnard, K. E. & Eyres, S. J. (1979). *Child health assessment, part 2: The first year of life.* Hyattsville, MD: U.S. Department of Health, Education, and Welfare, Public Health Service, HRA, Bureau of Health Manpower.

Fine, J. M. B. (2002). Parent–child interaction model. In A. M. Tomey & M. R. Alligood (Eds.), *Nursing theorists and their work* (5th ed., pp. 484–500). St. Louis, MO: Mosby.

Pokorny, M. E. (2010). Nursing theorists of historical significance. In A. M. Tomey & M. R. Alligood (Eds.), *Nursing theorists and their work* (7th ed., pp. 54–68). Maryland Heights, MO: Mosby.

Thomas, R. B., Barnard, K. E., & Summer, G. A. (1993). Family nursing diagnosis as a framework for family assessment. In S. L. Feetham, S. B. Meister, J. M. Bell, & C. L. Gilliss (Eds.), *The nursing of families: Theory, research, education, practice* (pp. 127–136). Newbury Park, CA: Sage.

MATERNAL ROLE ATTAINMENT— BECOMING A MOTHER:
Ramona T. Mercer

After completing this chapter the student should be able to

1. Identify and describe the major concepts of the maternal role attainment—becoming a mother theory as proposed by Mercer

2. Explain the major concepts important to nursing as defined by Mercer

3. Plan nursing care for a patient scenario utilizing Mercer's model

KEY TERMS

Anticipatory stage

Formal stage

Informal stage

Macrosystem (exosystem)

Maternal identity

Maternal role attainment

Mesosystem

Microsystem

Role identity stage

BACKGROUND

RAMONA T. MERCER WAS BORN in 1929. She received a diploma in nursing from St. Margaret's School of Nursing in Montgomery, Alabama, where she earned the L. L. Hill Award for Highest Academic Standing. She earned a bachelor's degree in nursing in 1962 from the University of New Mexico, Albuquerque, and a master's degree in maternal–child nursing from Emory University in 1964. Mercer completed a PhD in maternity nursing from the University of Pittsburg in 1973 (Meighan, 2010a, p. 581).

Mercer accepted a position teaching in the Department of Family Health Care Nursing at the University of California, San Francisco, where she retired at the rank of professor in 1987. Mercer published her first book, *Nursing Care for Parents at High Risk,* in 1977; it was followed by a second book, *Perspectives in Adolescent Health Care,* in 1979 that focused on teenage mothers in the first year of motherhood. Both books received *American Journal of Nursing* "Book of the Year" awards. Other books that resulted from research conducted during Mercer's career were published in 1986, 1990, and 1995. In addition, Mercer authored numerous journal articles.

During her career, Mercer received many awards and honors for her work, including being honored by the prestigious American Academy of Nursing as a Living Legend. Currently, she is Professor Emeritus in Family Health Nursing at the University of California, San Francisco (Meighan, 2010a, p. 581–582).

Mercer's theory of maternal role attainment was based on her extensive research, which began in the late 1960s and early 1970s. Her earliest research focused on a mother's ability to cope with an infant having a congenital defect. She also studied the needs and concerns of breastfeeding mothers, adolescent mothers, mothers with postpartum illness, and the response of fathers to stress and complications during the childbearing process. In 1981, Mercer introduced a framework for studying factors that affect maternal role. Ten years later, in 1991, she introduced her maternal role attainment theory and descriptive model (Meighan, 2010b, p. 391).

In addition to incorporating her own research, Mercer's theory was influenced by her professor and mentor at the University of Pittsburg, Reva Rubin. Mercer's research was initially based on Rubin's concepts and assertions about the variables influencing maternal role attainment. Whereas Rubin's work focused on maternal role attainment during pregnancy and the first month after birth, however, Mercer's work expanded the concepts to include the first year after birth and to include the parents, the influence of high-risk pregnancy, and maternal illness in the theory (Meighan, 2010b, p. 391). Mercer's work was also influenced by role and developmental theories put forth by such luminaries as Mead, Turner, Thornton and Nardi, and Werner. In addition, her model was influenced by von Bertalanffy's general systems theory and Brontenbrenner's conceptual model of the ecological environment (Meighan, 2010a, p. 581–582).

B ASED ON RECENT RESEARCH FINDINGS, Mercer (2004a) supports retiring the term "maternal role attainment" in favor of "becoming a mother" given that maternal role attainment has a connotation of an end point rather than emphasizing the continuous growth and change that occurs throughout life in the role of mother. In looking at the overview of the model, we will first briefly examine the original model and then consider the revision of the theory.

> ## OVERVIEW OF THE MATERNAL ROLE ATTAINMENT— BECOMING A MOTHER MODEL

> Mercer supports retiring the term "maternal role attainment" in favor of "becoming a mother" given that maternal role attainment has a connotation of an end point rather than emphasizing the continuous growth and change that occurs throughout life in the role of mother.

Overview of Mercer's Original Theory of Maternal Role Attainment

According to Mercer (1986), **maternal role attainment** is an interactional and developmental process that occurs over time in which the mother becomes attached to her infant, acquires competence in caretaking tasks involved in the role, and expresses pleasure and gratification in the role. Embedded in this definition are the major components of the mothering role: "attachment to the infant, gaining competence in mothering behaviors, and expressing gratification in maternal–infant interactions (Mercer, 1986, p. 6; 1995, p.13). **Maternal identity** occurs as an end point of maternal role attainment, when the mother experiences a sense of harmony, confidence, and competence in how she performs the role (Mercer, 1981, p. 74).

CRITICAL
THINKING

Can you
think of any
additional
factors
that might
affect maternal
role identity? Be
prepared with
a rationale to
support your
answer.

According to Mercer (1986, p. 14), a woman who becomes a mother must first recognize the permanency of the required change, and then seek out information, seek role models, and test herself for competency. These tasks are accomplished through four stages of maternal role attachment: (1) anticipatory stage, (2) formal stage, (3) informal stage, and (4) personal stage.

❖ The **anticipatory stage** begins during pregnancy and includes commitment and preparation. During this stage, there is initial social and psychological adjustment to pregnancy and expectations of the maternal role are learned by seeking information and visualizing oneself as a mother (Mercer, 1981).

❖ The **formal stage** begins with the birth of the infant and continues through physical restoration (about two weeks). During this stage, maternal behavior is learned from others, including professionals, and the new mother replicates and practices the behaviors.

❖ The next stage, the **informal stage**, occurs at two weeks through about four months after the birth of the child and is characterized by approaching normalization. During this stage, the mother learns infant cues and develops her own style of mothering.

❖ In the final stage, the personal or **role identity stage**, an internalization of maternal role identity occurs and the mother views herself as competent. This stage generally begins approximately four months post birth of the infant (Mercer, 1981).

Factors that can affect maternal role identity either directly or indirectly include stress, social support, family functioning, the mother's relationship with the infant's father, maternal age, childbearing attitudes, personality traits, early separation from the infant, birth experience, the infant's temperament, the infant's health status, and self-concept (Mercer, 1986). Desired outcomes for the infant include cognitive development, health, attachment, and social competence.

It is within the context of the ecological environment—represented graphically by nested circles that include the macrosystem, mesosystem, and microsystem—that maternal role attainment develops. The mother's **microsystem** includes the mother, the infant, her partner, and close relationships within the family; it is the microsystem that is the most influential in maternal role attainment. The **mesosystem** includes the extended family, school, work, church, and other systems in the community that influence the microsystem. The **macrosystem** (**exosystem**) represents relationships between two or more mesosystem factors (Meighan, 2010b).

Overview of the Revised Theory of Becoming a Mother

The revised version of the theory also includes four stages to becoming a mother, but Mercer updates these stages by using words and expressions taken from studies of women in the process of becoming a mother (Meighan, 2010b):

❖ Stage 1 begins during pregnancy and includes the social and psychological adjustments to pregnancy. During this stage, expectations of the maternal role are explored and the woman visualizes herself as a mother.

❖ Stage 2 begins with the birth of the infant and includes recovery from the birth process. During this role-taking stage, the new mother learns from others, replicates behaviors, and gains competence through practicing behaviors.

❖ During stage 3, the mother structures the role that fits based on her past experiences and future goals. The mother learns infant cues and develops her own style of mothering.

❖ Stage 4 begins as the new mother integrates mothering into her self-system, internalizes the role, and views herself as a competent mother (Mercer, 2004a).

In the revision, Mercer also updates the environment by replacing the terminology of "microsystem," "mesosystem," and "macrosystem" ("exosystem") with the labels *family and friends, community,* and *society at large,* respectively (Mercer & Walker, 2006). In the current model, the mother–infant–father (or significant other) remain at the center, with the interacting environments of *family and friends, community,* and *society at large* surrounding them. Environmental factors that influence becoming a mother are included in the model. The factors within the family and friends environment that influence becoming a mother include family functioning, family values, stressors, social support, and cultural guidelines for parenting. Community factors that influence becoming a mother include day care, school, work setting, places of worship, recreational facilities, hospitals, and cultural centers. Transmitted cultural consistencies, laws, national healthcare programs, and evolving reproductive and neonatal science are included in the environment labeled "society at large" (Meighan, 2010b, p 398).

MAJOR CONCEPTS OF NURSING BASED ON *Mercer's* MATERNAL ROLE ATTAINMENT— BECOMING A MOTHER MODEL

IN ADDITION TO THE CONCEPTS already presented, the four metaparadigm concepts of nursing are identified in Mercer's maternal role attainment— becoming a mother model. These concepts are summarized in Table 23-1.

Person

Mercer refers to the person as the self or the core self that is separate from roles, although she does not specifically define the term "person" (Mercer, 1985a). The core self evolves from the cultural context and determines how situations are defined and shaped. The mother as a separate self or person interacts with her infant and with her significant other; however, she both influences and is influenced by both the infant and the significant other (Mercer, 1995). Through maternal individuation, a woman may regain her own personhood as she extrapolates self from the mother–infant dyad (Mercer, 1985b).

Environment

Mercer's conceptualization of the environment is drawn from Bronfenbrenner's conceptual model of the ecological environment, represented by nested circles that include the macrosystem, mesosystem, and microsystem. It is within the ecological interacting environments that

TABLE 23-1 Metaparadigm Concepts as Defined in Mercer's Model	
Person	A person is the self or the core self that is separate from roles (Mercer, 1986).
Environment	"Development of a role/person cannot be considered apart from the environment; there is a mutual accommodation between the developing person and the changing properties of the immediate settings, relationships between settings, and the larger context in which the settings are embedded" (Mercer, 2003, as cited in Meighan, 2010a, p. 587).
Health	Health is based on the mother's and father's perception of their prior health status, current health, health outlook, resistance or susceptibility to illness, health worry or concern, sickness orientation, and rejection of the sick role (Mercer, 1986).
Nursing	Nursing is a dynamic profession with three major foci: health promotion and prevention of illness, providing care for those who need professional assistance to achieve their optimal level of health and functioning, and research to enhance the knowledge base for providing excellent nursing care (Mercer, 2004b, as cited in Meighan, 2010a, pp. 586–587).

maternal role attainment develops. According to Mercer (2003, as cited in Meighan, 2010a, p. 587), "Development of a role/person cannot be considered apart from the environment; there is a mutual accommodation between the developing person and the changing properties of the immediate settings, relationships between settings, and the larger context in which the settings are embedded." Stressors and supports within the environment also influence maternal role attainment and the developing child (Meighan, 2010a, p. 587).

Health

Health as defined by Mercer is based on the mother's and father's perceptions of their prior health status, current health, health outlook, resistance or susceptibility to illness, health worry or concern, sickness orientation, and rejection of the sick role. The health status of the newborn reflects the extent of disease present and infant health status by parental rating of overall health and is a desired outcome for the infant (Mercer, 1986).

Nursing

Nurses are the healthcare professionals with the "most sustained and intense interaction with women in the maternity cycle" (Mercer, 1995, p. xii). According to Mercer:

> Nursing is a dynamic profession with three major foci: health promotion and prevention of illness, providing care for those who need professional assistance to achieve their optimal level of health and functioning, and research to enhance the knowledge base for providing excellent nursing care. Nurses provide health care for individuals, families, and communities. Following assessment of the client's situation and environment, the nurse identifies goals with the client, provides assistance to the client through teaching, supporting, providing care the client is unable to provide for self, and interfacing with the environment and the client. (Mercer, 2004b, as cited in Meighan, 2010a, p. 586–587)

ANALYSIS OF THE MATERNAL ROLE ATTAINMENT— BECOMING A MOTHER MODEL

THE ANALYSIS PRESENTED HERE CONSISTS of an examination of assumptions and propositions as well as a brief critique of the maternal role attainment—becoming a mother model as proposed by Mercer.

Assumptions of the Maternal Role Attainment—Becoming a Mother Model

Assumptions related to maternal role attainment include the following statements by Mercer (Meighan, 2010a, p. 586):

❖ A relatively stable core self, acquired through lifelong socialization, determines how a mother defines and perceives an event; her perceptions of her infant's and others' responses to her mothering, with her life situation, are the real world to which she responds (Mercer, 1986).

❖ In addition to the mother's socialization, her developmental level and innate personality characteristics influence her behavioral responses (Mercer, 1986).

- The mother's role partner, her infant, will reflect the mother's competence in the mothering role through growth and development (Mercer, 1986).

- The infant is considered an active partner in the maternal role-taking process, affecting and being affected by role enactment (Mercer, 1981).

- The father's or mother's intimate partner contributes to role attainment in a way that cannot be duplicated by any other supportive person (Mercer, 1995).

- Maternal identity develops concurrently with maternal attachment, and each depends on the other (Mercer, 1995).

Propositions of the Maternal Role Attainment— Becoming a Mother Model

Relational propositional statements include the following:

- Health is influenced by both maternal and infant variables (Mercer, 1995).

- Antepartum stress negatively affects the health of the family (Mercer, Ferketich, DeJoseph, May, & Sollid, 1988; Mercer, May, Ferketich, & DeJoseph, 1986).

- Health status has indirect influence on satisfaction with relationships in childbearing families (Mercer, 1995).

- Stresses and social support within the environment influence maternal role attainment.

Brief Critique of the Maternal Role Attainment— Becoming a Mother Model

Mercer used deductive and inductive forms of logic in the development of her theory. Her model is logical, and adaptations to the model based on recent research findings have improved the clarity and increased the usefulness of the model for practice. The concepts in the theory are defined consistently, with concepts, assumptions, and goals being organized into a coherent and understandable whole. The theory can be generalized to all women during pregnancy through the first year after birth, regardless

CRITICAL THINKING

Do you see overlap in the definition of nursing proposed by Mercer and any definitions proposed by theorists whom you have already studied? Which similarities and differences do you see if any? Do you see overlap between Mercer's theory and any other theory you have already studied? What similarities and differences do you see if any?

THE MATERNAL ROLE ATTAINMENT— BECOMING A MOTHER MODEL AS A FRAMEWORK FOR NURSING PRACTICE

of age, parity, or environment. The theory is specific to parent–child nursing practice, research and education, although it has been used by other disciplines interested in mothering and parenting (Meighan, 2010a).

THE NURSE USING MERCER'S THEORY in practice will consider the various factors that influence maternal role identity. These factors are assessed in relation to the stage of maternal role identity and in relation to the three environments (*family and friends, community,* and *society at large*). Interventions provided by the nurse will address those factors in one of the environments and in relation to the stage of maternal role identity that may impede the achievement of maternal role identity or affect infant outcomes.

THE NURSING PROCESS AND THE MATERNAL ROLE ATTAINMENT— BECOMING A MOTHER MODEL

USE OF THE NURSING PROCESS along with Mercer's theory of becoming a mother incorporates assessment of the interacting environments, the stages of maternal role identity, and factors that influence maternal role identity. Nursing goals and outcomes are included as a part of the maternal role identity and child outcome in Mercer's model, and nursing care is evaluated based on achievement of maternal role identity and infant outcomes.

Assessment and Planning

During the assessment of the family and friends environment, the nurse examines both the health and the responses of the mother, infant, and the father. Has the mother recovered from childbirth? Is the infant free from illness? Is the father involved with the mother and the infant? If other family members need to be included in teaching, then they should also be included in the assessment. Issues the nurse will consider include whether the family members are supportive and whether they live nearby (Meighan, 2010b, p. 400).

In addition, assessment will address factors in the community environment. These factors may be assessed by ascertaining which resources are available in the local community for the new family and whether the mother will return to a work environment outside the home. To assess the influence of the society at large environment, the nurse will determine if cultural influences related to childbirth or childcare need to be addressed or if issues related to access to services should be considered (Meighan, 2010b, p. 401).

Stages of maternal role identity also need to be assessed by the nurse. The nurse will ask about attendance at prenatal classes, the mother's need for information or assistance with nourishment for the infant, and the mother's role models. The nurse will observe the mother for behavior that shows empathy toward or attachment to the infant as well as for evidence that the mother is committed to the child and sees herself as a mother (Meighan, 2010b, p. 400).

Implementation

Nursing interventions will vary depending on the data collected during the assessment phase of the nursing process. Moreover, they will vary with each stage of maternal role identity and with the assessment findings related to factors influencing maternal role identity within the interacting environments.

Evaluation

Nursing care is evaluated based on the achievement of maternal role identity and infant outcomes. Maternal role identity is evaluated by identifying the woman's feelings of confidence and competence in her role, her satisfaction with her role, and her attachment to her child. These feelings are validated based on the woman's statements related to her mothering role, her ability to provide care to the infant, and her behavior toward the infant, such as demonstrating affection and showing concern. Infant outcomes to be evaluated by the nurse include cognitive development, attachment behaviors, health state, and social competence (Meighan, 2010b, p. 402–403).

Nursing care is evaluated based on the achievement of maternal role identity and infant outcomes.

SCENARIO ILLUSTRATING NURSING CARE FRAMED BY THE MATERNAL ROLE ATTAINMENT— BECOMING A MOTHER MODEL UTILIZING THE NURSING PROCESS

THE FOLLOWING SCENARIO ILLUSTRATES NURSING care of the patient relative to one identified nursing problem framed by maternal role attainment—becoming a mother model. This scenario is not intended to cover all aspects of care, but rather to stimulate thinking about how specific care might be approached using this theory as a framework for practice.

Mrs. M. is a 28-year-old woman who delivered her first baby 1 week ago. She is free from illness, and her infant girl is healthy. The father is in the military and is deployed overseas in a combat zone. Mrs. M. lived on base until Mr. M. was deployed three months ago. She is now living with her parents so they can help her with the infant R. and with living expenses, because she is not planning to return to work for several months. Her parents are supportive and want to be included in the care of the new mother and baby.

After gathering the initial data, the nurse turns her attention to issues related to stages of maternal role identity. The nurse finds that Mrs. M. did attend prenatal classes and that Mr. M. attended until he was deployed overseas, at which time her mother took his place in the class. Mrs. M. is breastfeeding the infant R. Mrs. M. states that at first she had some difficulty with feeding the baby, but after a couple of days and some assistance from her mother, she has not had any further difficulties. The nurse observes that Mrs. M. is responsive to the cues of infant R. and displays attachment and concern for the infant. All of the assessment data and observations gathered by the nurse indicate that Mrs. M. is committed to the infant R. and sees herself as a mother who is satisfied with her role as a mother and who is growing in confidence in the mothering role. The nurse's role with Mrs. M. will be to provide education and encouragement.

The maternal role attainment—becoming a mother theory is a middle-range theory that has a specific focus. Throughout the nursing process, if other issues arise during the nursing encounter that are outside the focus of this theory, the nurse will intervene to provide nursing care using strategies that are congruent with current best clinical practices.

CLASSROOM ACTIVITY 23-1

Form small groups. Each group should add to the plan of care for Mrs. M. in the preceding scenario based on other potential or actual nursing problems typical for a patient with the same medical diagnosis or symptoms and demographics. Each group should develop a plan for one additional nursing problem using Mercer's theory as the basis for practice. Each group should then share its plan with the class.

CLASSROOM ACTIVITY 23-2

Form small groups. Using a case study provided by the instructor, develop a plan of care using Mercer's nursing theory as the basis for practice. Each group should then share its plan of care with the class.

CLASSROOM ACTIVITY 23-3

Form small groups. Using a case study provided by the instructor, develop a plan of care using one of the theories as the basis for practice; each group should select a different nursing theory. Each group should then share its plan of care with the class and discuss the similarities and differences in care.

REFERENCES

Meighan, M. (2010a). Maternal role attainment—becoming a mother. In M. R. Alligood & A. M. Tomney (Eds.), *Nursing theorists and their work* (7th ed., pp. 581–598). Maryland Heights, MO: Mosby.

Meighan, M. (2010b). Mercer's becoming a mother theory in nursing practice. In M. R. Alligood (Ed.), *Nursing theory: Utilization and application* (4th ed., pp. 389–410). Maryland Heights, MO: Mosby.

Mercer, R. T. (1977). *Nursing care for parents at risk*. Thorofare, NJ: Charles B. Slack.

Mercer, R. T. (1979). *Perspectives on adolescent health care*. Philadelphia: J. B. Lippincott.

Mercer, R. T. (1981). A theoretical framework for studying factors that impact on the maternal role. *Nursing Research, 30*, 73–77.

Mercer, R. T. (1985a). The process of maternal role attainment over the first years. *Nursing Research, 34*, 198–204.

Mercer, R. T. (1985b). The relationship of age and other variables to gratification in mothers. *Health Care for Women International, 6*, 295–308.

Mercer, R. T. (1986). *First-time motherhood: Experiences from teens to forties*. New York: Springer.

Mercer, R. T. (1990). *Parents at risk*. New York: Springer.

Mercer, R. T. (1995). *Becoming a mother: Research on maternal identity from Rubin to the present*. New York: Springer.

Mercer, R. T. (2003, September 3). Personal correspondence with M. Meighan.

Mercer, R. T. (2004a). Becoming a mother versus maternal role attainment. *Journal of Nursing Scholarship, 36*(3), 226–232.

Mercer, R. T. (2004b, March 21). Personal correspondence with M. Meighan.

Mercer, R. T., Ferketich, S. L., DeJoseph, J., May, K. A., & Sollid, D. (1988). Effects of stress on family functioning during pregnancy. *Nursing Research, 37*, 268–275.

Mercer, R. T., May, K. A., Ferketich, S., & DeJoseph, J. (1986). Theoretical models for studying the effect of antepartum stress on the family. *Nursing Research, 35*, 339–346.

Mercer, R. T., & Walker, L. O. (2006). A review of nursing interventions to foster becoming a mother. *Journal of Obstetric, Gynecologic, and Neonatal Nurses, 35*(5), 568–582.

SELF-TRANSCENDENCE THEORY:
Pamela G. Reed

LEARNING OBJECTIVES

After completing this chapter the student should be able to

1. Identify and describe the major concepts of the self-transcendence theory

2. Explain the major concepts important to nursing as proposed by Reed in the self-transcendence theory

3. Plan nursing care for a patient scenario utilizing Reed's self-transcendence theory

KEY TERMS

: Moderating-mediating factors   : Self-transcendence

BACKGROUND

Pamela G. Reed was born in Detroit, Michigan. She graduated with a baccalaureate degree from Wayne State University in 1974. Reed earned her master of science degree in psychiatric–mental health of children and adolescents and in nursing education in 1976. She received her PhD, with a concentration in nursing theory and research and a minor in adult development and aging, in 1982. Reed's dissertation research focused on the relationship between well-being and spiritual perspectives on life and death in terminally ill and well individuals (Coward, 2010, p. 618).

Reed is currently on the faculty at the University of Arizona College of Nursing in Tucson. During her career in academia, she has taught, directed thesis and dissertations, conducted research, and served in administration positions. Reed's major areas of research have included well-being and spirituality, and she has developed two widely used research instruments related to these areas of research: the Spiritual Perspectives Scale and the Self-Transcendence Scale. Her current areas of research and scholarship focus on family caregiver wisdom in palliative care, and she maintains a continuing focus on knowledge development and theory in nursing. Reed has published several book chapters and numerous journal articles related to her theory and research and served on editorial review boards for several journals. She has also received many awards and honors over the course of her career, including induction as a fellow in the American Academy of Nursing (Coward, 2010, p. 618–619).

Reed (2008) describes her theory as originating from three primary sources. First, the life span movement in the field of developmental psychology during the 1970s provided a philosophic awareness and empirical evidence that development did continue beyond adolescence, into adulthood, and throughout the processes of aging and dying (Reed, 1983; 2008). A second source of influence was the early postulations of Martha Rogers (1970) related to the nature of change in human beings (Reed, 1997; 2008). Third, the theory of self-transcendence was influenced by clinical experiences in applying developmental theories in child and adolescent psychiatric–mental health care (Reed, 2008) as well as clinical experience and research with older adults that linked mental health and well-being to developmental resources (Reed, 1986).

THREE MAJOR CONCEPTS ARE CENTRAL to the theory of self-transcendence: self-transcendence, well-being, and vulnerability. Each is defined and briefly discussed in this section.

Self-transcendence is the capacity to expand self-boundaries intrapersonally, interpersonally, temporally, and transpersonally (Reed, 2008, p. 107). The capacity to expand self-boundaries intrapersonally refers to a greater awareness of one's philosophy, values, and dreams. The capacity to expand interpersonally relates to others and one's environment. The capacity to expand temporally refers to integration of one's past and future in a way that has meaning for the present. Finally, the capacity to expand transpersonally refers to the capacity to connect with dimensions beyond the typically discernable world (p. 107).

Self-transcendence is a characteristic of developmental maturity that is congruent with enhanced awareness of the environment and a broadened perspective on life. Notably, older adults and others facing end-of-life issues acquire an expanded awareness of self and environment. Older adults also use postformal patterns of thought in reasoning about the world. The person who uses postformal thinking does not seek absolute answers to questions about life, but rather seeks the meaning of life events and has an appreciation of the greater environment, things unseen, and an inner knowledge of self. Self-transcendence is conceptualized as a correlate of postformal thinking that is expressed through behaviors such as sharing wisdom with others, integrating physical changes of aging, accepting death as a part of life, and finding spiritual meaning in life (Reed, 2008, p. 107–108).

Well-being is the second major concept of Reed's theory. Well-being is a sense of feeling whole and healthy, according to one's own criteria for wholeness and health. The definition of well-being depends on the individual or population. Indeed, indicators of well-being are as diverse as human perceptions of health and wellness. Examples of indicators of well-being may include life satisfaction, positive self-concept, hopefulness, happiness, and having meaning in life. Well-being is viewed as a correlate and an outcome of self-transcendence (Reed, 2008).

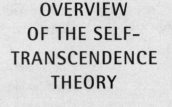

OVERVIEW OF THE SELF-TRANSCENDENCE THEORY

Self-transcendence is the capacity to expand self-boundaries intrapersonally, interpersonally, temporally, and transpersonally.

The third major concept, vulnerability, is the awareness of personal mortality and the likelihood of experiencing difficult life situations. Self-transcendence emerges naturally in health experiences when a person is confronted with mortality and immortality. Life events such as illness, disability, aging, childbirth, or parenting—all of which heighten a person's sense of mortality, inadequacy, or vulnerability—can trigger developmental progress toward a renewed sense of identity and expanded self-boundaries. According to Reed (2008, p. 108–109), self-transcendence is evoked through life events and may enhance well-being by transforming losses and difficulties into healing experiences.

Additional concepts in Reed's theory include moderating–mediating factors and points of intervention. **Moderating–mediating factors** are personal and contextual variables such as age, gender, life experiences, and social environment that can influence the relationships between vulnerability and self-transcendence and between self-transcendence and well-being. Nursing activities that facilitate self-transcendence are referred to as *points of intervention* (Coward, 2010, p. 623). Two points of intervention are intertwined with the process of self-transcendence: Nursing actions may focus either directly on a person's inner resource for self-transcendence or indirectly on the personal and contextual factors that affect the relationship between vulnerability and self-transcendence and the relationship between self-transcendence and well-being (p. 621).

MAJOR CONCEPTS OF NURSING BASED ON *Reed's* SELF-TRANSCENDENCE THEORY

IN ADDITION TO THE CONCEPTS already presented, the four metaparadigm concepts of nursing are identified in Reed's self-transcendence theory. These concepts are summarized in Table 24-1.

Person

Persons are viewed as human beings who develop over the life span through interactions with other persons and within an environment of changing complexity that could both positively and negatively contribute to health and well-being (Coward, 2010, p. 622).

⊞ TABLE 24-1 Metaparadigm Concepts as Defined in Reed's Self-Transcendence Theory	
Person	Persons are human beings who develop over the life span through interactions with other persons and within an environment.
Environment	The environment is composed of family, social networks, physical surroundings, and community resources.
Health	Well-being is a sense of feeling whole and healthy, according to one's own criteria for wholeness and health.
Nursing	The role of nursing activity is to assist persons through interpersonal processes and therapeutic management of their environment to promote health and well-being.

Environment

According to Reed's theory, the environment is composed of family, social networks, physical surroundings, and community resources, all of which make significant contributions to the health processes that nurses influence through their management of therapeutic interactions among people, objects, and nursing activities (Coward, 2010, p. 622).

Health

In the early work of Reed, health was the central concept, around which revolved the concepts of nursing activity, person, and environment. In that early model, health was defined implicitly as a life process of both positive and negative experiences from which individuals create unique values and environments that promote well-being (Coward, 2010, p. 622). In more recent publications, Reed has not defined health except in the context of well-being. Well-being is a sense of feeling whole and healthy, according to one's own criteria for wholeness and health (Reed, 2008).

Nursing

The role of the nurse is to assist persons through interpersonal processes and therapeutic management of their environment with the skills required for promoting health and well-being. Nursing is referred to in terms of nursing activity (Coward, 2010, p. 622).

ANALYSIS OF THE SELF-TRANSCENDENCE THEORY

THE ANALYSIS PRESENTED HERE CONSISTS of an examination of assumptions and propositions as well as a brief critique of the self-transcendence theory as proposed by Reed.

Assumptions of the Self-Transcendence Theory

One major assumption that Reed began with as she developed the theory of self-transcendence was that the focus of the discipline of nursing should be on building and engaging knowledge to promote health processes (Coward, 2010, p.622). Another key assumption was that persons are open systems who impose conceptual boundaries upon themselves to define their reality and to provide a sense of wholeness and connectedness within themselves and their environment. This assumption is based on assumptions found within Martha Rogers' science of unitary human beings (1970), which Reed identified as an initial inspiration for her own work. According to Reed, self-imposed conceptual boundaries fluctuate across the life span and are associated with health and development. Self-transcendence is an indicator of self-boundaries that may be assessed at specific times (Coward, 2010, p. 623).

In her later work, Reed noted that self-transcendence is a developmental imperative. Thus self-transcendence must be expressed, just as any other developmental imperative must be expressed, for a person to realize a sense of wholeness and connectedness (Reed, 2003).

Propositions of the Self-Transcendence Theory

Specific relationship statements of the theory of self-transcendence include the following:

❖ Self-transcendence is greater in persons facing end-of-own-life issues than in persons not facing these issues.

❖ Conceptual boundaries are related to well-being.

❖ Increased vulnerability is related to increased self-transcendence.

❖ Self-transcendence is positively related to well-being.

❖ Personal and contextual factors influence the relationship between vulnerability and self-transcendence.

❖ Personal and contextual factors influence the relationship between self-transcendence and well-being.

Brief Critique of the Self-Transcendence Theory

The theory of self-transcendence was derived using deductive reformulation. This technique calls for middle-range theory construction knowledge to be derived from non-nursing theory and then reformulated deductively from a nursing conceptual model. Reed used primarily life span theories, which were then reformulated using the nursing perspective proposed in Martha Rogers' science of unitary human beings.

Reed's theory is clear and easy to understand, and uses terms consistently throughout. With three major concepts and two additional concepts, the number of relationships generated is minimal, yet still meaningful and fairly comprehensive. The theory can be applied to a wide variety of situations. Although the major concepts are broad and abstract, empirical indicators have been identified and scales developed to facilitate research and the ongoing development of the theory for use in nursing practice (Coward, 2010, p. 627–628).

THE NURSE USING SELF-TRANSCENDENCE THEORY as a framework for nursing practice will incorporate nursing activities that will facilitate self-transcendence. Nursing practices that facilitate self-transcendence result in enhanced well-being and healing outcomes during health events (Reed, 2008, p. 122).

THE NURSING PROCESS IS NOT specifically addressed in the self-transcendence theory. Nevertheless, this theory will be examined within the context of the nursing process in this section for the sake of discussion, consistency, and comparison.

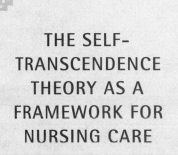

Nursing practices that facilitate self-transcendence result in enhanced well-being and healing outcomes.

THE SELF-TRANSCENDENCE THEORY AS A FRAMEWORK FOR NURSING CARE

THE NURSING PROCESS AND THE SELF-TRANSCENDENCE THEORY

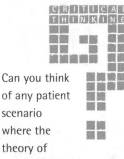

Can you think of any patient scenario where the theory of self–transcendence might not be appropriate in nursing practice? Briefly describe the scenario and explain the rationale.

Assessment and Planning

During the course of the nurse–patient relationship, the nurse will need to assess indicators of self-transcendence, well-being, and vulnerability as well as the moderating–mediating factors that can influence the relationships between vulnerability and self-transcendence and between self-transcendence and well-being.

Implementation

Nursing actions may focus on either or both points of intervention that intersect with the process of self-transcendence. Thus the focus may be directly on a person's inner resources for self-transcendence or indirectly on the personal and contextual factors that affect the relationship between vulnerability and self-transcendence and the relationship between self-transcendence and well-being (Coward, 2010, p. 621).

Intrapersonal strategies assist the person to look inward so as to clarify and expand knowledge about self and find or create meaning and purpose in the experience. Meditation, prayer, visualization, life review, and journaling are just some of the techniques of self-transcendence that nurses can incorporate as nursing activities (Reed, 2008, 122–123).

Interpersonal strategies for facilitating self-transcendence focus on connecting the person to others. Nursing strategies may include strengthening affiliations with civic groups or faith communities, formal support groups, nurse visits, peer counseling, and informal networks (Reed, 2008, p. 123).

Altruistic activities can also facilitate self-transcendence, as they provide a context for expanding awareness about oneself and one's world and enhance one's inner sense of worth and purpose. Connections between people are key strategies for enhancing self-transcendence, whether the person is providing service or receiving service; thus nursing activities that encourage connections can be useful in facilitating self-transcendence (Reed, 2008, p. 123).

Evaluation

Evaluation is based on the effectiveness of nursing activities to facilitate self-transcendence and well-being. Specific realms to consider include the enhanced capacity of the person to expand self-boundaries intrapersonally, interpersonally, temporally, and transpersonally.

T HE FOLLOWING SCENARIO ILLUSTRATES NURSING care of the patient relative to one identified nursing problem framed by the self-transcendence theory. This scenario is not intended to cover all aspects of care, but rather to stimulate thinking about how specific care might be approached using this theory as a framework for practice.

SCENARIO ILLUSTRATING NURSING CARE FRAMED BY THE SELF–TRANSCENDENCE THEORY UTILIZING THE NURSING PROCESS

Mr. M. is 34-year-old Caucasian male who presents to the mental health clinic with depression and complaints of fatigue. An interview reveals that his wife and both of his children were killed in a traffic accident six months ago. The nurse knows that Mr. M. is vulnerable due to the loss of his family, but that self-transcendence is evoked through life events and may enhance well-being by transforming losses and difficulties into healing experiences. Because well-being is a correlate of self-transcendence, the nurse assesses the well-being by assessing Mr. M.'s level of life satisfaction.

Based on the assessment, the nurse knows that her nursing activity should focus on facilitating self-transcendence in Mr. M. Nursing activities will begin with a focus on intrapersonal strategies to assist Mr. M. in looking inward to clarify and expand his knowledge about self and find or create meaning and purpose in the experience. Together, Mr. M. and the nurse choose the techniques of meditation, prayer, life review, and journaling.

During follow-up visits with Mr. M., interpersonal strategies for facilitating self-transcendence are added that focus on connecting to others. Nursing activities chosen at that time by the nurse and Mr. M. include strengthening affiliations with his faith community and connecting with service organizations in his community.

Evaluation is based on the effectiveness of nursing activities to facilitate self-transcendence and well-being in Mr. M. In this case, evaluation may include the measurement of specific indicators or changes in Mr. M.'s expressions related to the meaning of life.

The self-transcendence theory is a middle-range theory that has a specific focus. It is important to note that throughout the nursing process if other issues arise during the nursing encounter that are outside the focus of this theory, the nurse will intervene to provide nursing care using strategies that are congruent with current best clinical practices.

CLASSROOM ACTIVITY 24-1

Form small groups. Each group should add to the plan of care for Mr. M. in the preceding scenario based on other potential or actual nursing problems typical for a patient with the same medical diagnosis or symptoms and demographics. Each group should develop a plan for one additional nursing problem using Reed's theory as the basis for practice. Each group should then share its plan with the class.

CLASSROOM ACTIVITY 24-2

Form small groups. Using a case study provided by the instructor, develop a plan of care using Reed's self-transcendence theory as the basis for practice. Each group should then share its plan of care with the class.

CLASSROOM ACTIVITY 24-3

Form small groups. Using a case study provided by the instructor, develop a plan of care using one of the theories as the basis for practice; each group should select a different nursing theory. Each group should then share its plan of care with the class and discuss the similarities and differences in care.

REFERENCES

Coward, D. D. (2010). Self-transcendence theory: Pamela G. Reed. In M. R. Alligood & A. M. Tomey (Eds.), *Nursing theorists and their work* (7th ed., pp. 618–637). Maryland Heights, MO: Mosby.

Reed, P. G. (1983). Implications of the life-span developmental framework for well-being in adulthood and aging. *Advances in Nursing Science, 6,* 18–25.

Reed, P. G. (1986). Developmental resources and depression in the elderly. *Nursing Research, 35*(6), 368–374.

Reed, P. G. (1997). The place of transcendence in nursing's science of unitary human beings: Theory and research. In M. Madrid (Ed.), *Patterns of Rogerian knowing* (pp. 187–196). New York: National League for Nursing.

Reed, P. G. (2003). The theory of self-transcendence. In M. J. Smith & P. R. Liehr (Eds.), *Middle range theory for nursing* (2nd ed., pp. 145–165). New York: Springer.

Reed, P. G. (2008). Theory of self-transcendence. In M. J. Smith & P. R. Liehr (Eds.), *Middle range theory for nursing* (2nd ed., pp. 105–129). New York: Springer.

Rogers, M. E. (1970). *Introduction to the theoretical basis of nursing.* Philadelphia: F. A. Davis.

THEORY OF CHRONIC SORROW:
Georgene Gaskill Eakes, Mary Lermann Burke, and Margaret A. Hainsworth

25

LEARNING OBJECTIVES

After completing this chapter the student should be able to

1. Identify and describe the major concepts proposed in the theory of chronic sorrow

2. Explain the major concepts important to nursing as defined in the theory of chronic sorrow

3. Plan nursing care for a patient scenario utilizing the theory of chronic sorrow

KEY TERMS

⋮ Management methods ⋮ Trigger events

BACKGROUND

GEORGENE GASKILL EAKES ENTERED NURSING in 1966 after graduating from Watts Hospital School of Nursing in Durham, North Carolina, with a diploma in nursing. In 1977, she graduated from North Carolina Agricultural and Technical State University with a bachelor's degree in nursing. Eakes received a master's degree in the science of nursing in 1980 from the University of North Carolina at Greensboro; in 1988, she completed her EdD at North Carolina State University. Eakes practiced nursing in acute and community-based psychiatric and mental health settings early in her professional career, then joined the faculty at East Carolina University School of Nursing in 1980.

In the 1970s, Eakes sustained life-threatening injuries in an automobile accident. Her near-death experience heightened her awareness of how ill-prepared healthcare professionals are when it comes to dealing with individuals who are facing their mortality and the general lack of understanding of grief reactions experienced during loss. Motivated by these insights, Eakes' early research and scholarship interests were related to death, dying, grief, loss, death anxiety among nurses, grief resolution among hospice nurses, and grief reactions in patients with life-threatening, chronic illness. In 1989, she presented her dissertation research at the Sigma Theta Tau International Research Conference (Schreier & Droes, 2010, p. 657).

Mary Lermann Burke began her nursing career in 1962 after graduating with a diploma from Good Samaritan Hospital School of Nursing in Cincinnati, Ohio, followed later that same year by a postgraduate certification from Children's Medical Center in the District of Columbia. Burke later earned a bachelor's degree in nursing from Rhode Island College, Providence, and in 1982 she received a master's degree in parent–child nursing from Boston University. Burke earned her doctorate of nursing science in Family Studies Cognate from Boston University in 1989. During her early career, Burke practiced in pediatrics in both acute and primary care settings. In 1980, she joined the faculty of Rhode Island College's Department of Nursing, where she remained until her retirement in 2002 (Schreier & Droes, 2010, p. 658–659).

Burke's interest in the concept of chronic sorrow was inspired by her clinical practicum experiences working with children with spina bifida and their parents as part of her master's degree program. In the course of this work, she developed a hunch that the emotions displayed by the parents were consistent with the concept of chronic sorrow. Burkes pursued this line of thinking during her thesis work and again with the development of a research instrument in her doctoral dissertation research. She presented her dissertation research at the Sigma Theta Tau International Research Conference in 1989 (Schreier & Droes, 2010, p. 659).

Margaret A. Hainsworth began her nursing career in 1953 following graduation from Brockville General Hospital School of Nursing in Brockville, Ontario. She immigrated to the United States in 1959 to attend George Peabody College for Teachers in Nashville, Tennessee, from which she graduated with a diploma in public health nursing. Hainsworth stayed in the United State and attended Salve Regina College in Newport, Rhode Island, where she graduated in 1973 with a bachelor's degree in nursing. In 1974, she received a master's degree in psychiatric and mental health nursing from Boston College. In 1986, she earned a doctoral degree in education administration from the University of Connecticut; in 1988, she was board certified as a clinical specialist in psychiatric and mental health nursing. Hainsworth's nursing practice focused on public health nursing and mental health nursing. In 1974, she accepted a faculty position in the Department of Nursing at Rhode Island College. During her years in academia, Hainsworth also maintained her clinical practice (Schreier & Droes, 2010, p. 659–660).

Hainsworth's interest in chronic illness and sorrow was spurred by her practice as a facilitator for a support group for women with multiple sclerosis. This experience led to dissertation research, which she presented in 1989 at the same Sigma Theta Tau International Research Conference that was also attended by Burke and Eakes (Schreier & Droes, 2010, p. 660).

During the Sigma Theta Tau International Research conference, Eakes attended the presentation of Burke's dissertation research and immediately made a connection between the description of chronic sorrow and her observations of grief reactions. After the conference, Eakes contacted Burke to explore the possibility of collaboration. They met together with Hainsworth and a colleague of Hainsworth, Carolyn Lindgren, and formed the Nursing Consortium for Research on Chronic Sorrow (NCRCS) to expand the understanding of chronic sorrow (Schreier & Droes, 2010, p. 657, 660).

The theory of chronic sorrow has two theoretical origins. Olshansky (1962) is credited as the source for the original concept of chronic sorrow (Eakes, Burke, & Hainsworth, 1998), and the stress and adaptation model of Lazarus and Folkman (1984) formed the foundation for the conceptualization of how persons cope with chronic sorrow. Thus what began as a theory that examined the experience of chronic sorrow was eventually expanded to include the coping responses to chronic sorrow (Schreier & Droes, 2010, p. 660–661).

OVERVIEW OF THE THEORY OF CHRONIC SORROW

THE THEORY OF CHRONIC SORROW was first documented in the literature in 1998 by Eakes, Burke, and Hainsworth, who positioned their work as a middle-range theory for nursing that offered an alternative view of the experience of grief and a framework for explaining how persons respond to ongoing and single-loss events (Eakes, 2004, p. 165). Chronic sorrow is conceptualized as "the periodic recurrence of permanent, pervasive sadness or other grief-related feelings associated with ongoing disparity resulting from a loss experience" (Eakes, Burke, & Hainsworth, 1998, p. 180). It is characterized as pervasive, permanent, periodic, and potentially progressive in nature. The theory of chronic sorrow proposes that the periodic return of grief among persons and caregivers whose anticipated life course has been interrupted continues throughout one's lifetime as long as the disparity created by the loss remains (Lindgren, Burke, Hainsworth, & Eakes, 1992). Thus chronic sorrow is viewed as a normal response to the void created by ongoing disparity or a loss, although it is important to note that normalization of the experience does not diminish the validity or the intensity of the feelings (Eakes, 2004, p. 167).

An experience of significant loss is a necessary antecedent to the development of chronic sorrow. This loss may be a loss with no predicable

> Chronic sorrow is conceptualized as "the periodic recurrence of permanent, pervasive sadness or other grief-related feelings associated with ongoing disparity resulting from a loss experience."

end, such as the birth of a disabled child or the diagnosis of a chronic disease, or it may be a clearly defined loss event, such as the death of a loved one. The second necessary element is ongoing disparity resulting from the loss—in other words, a gap exists between the desired state and the actual reality. The lack of closure associated with the ongoing disparity sets the stage for chronic sorrow (Eakes, 2004, p. 167).

Trigger events or milestones are those situations or circumstances that bring the disparity created by the loss into focus and trigger the grief-related feelings associated with the chronic sorrow. Triggers of chronic sorrow vary depending on the loss experience. For example, the most frequent trigger of chronic sorrow among parents of young children with disabilities is the disparity between their children's development and the expected developmental milestones for nondisabled children, whereas the chronic sorrow experienced by bereaved persons is triggered by situations that magnify the absence of the deceased, such as anniversaries and holidays (Eakes, 2004, p. 167–169).

Management methods within the theory of chronic sorrow refer to personal coping strategies used by persons during the chronic sorrow experience and supportive interventions provided by professionals. Personal coping strategies or self-care management strategies are known as internal management methods; supportive interventions are referred to as external management methods. Effective internal and external management methods lead to increased comfort and may serve to extend the time between episodes of chronic sorrow or to decrease feelings of re-grief (Eakes, 2004, p. 169).

Effective internal management strategies used by persons experiencing chronic sorrow are consistent across various loss situations. Internal management strategies are categorized as action, cognitive, and interpersonal. Action-oriented strategies that increase feelings of control are frequently used to cope with the recurrent grief-related feelings of chronic sorrow. Examples of action-oriented coping strategies include continued involvement in activities, gathering information specific to the loss experience, and seeking out respite opportunities. Cognitive strategies include focusing on the positive elements in one's life. Interpersonal ways of coping include talking with someone close and interacting with others in a similar situation such as via a support group (Eakes, 2004, p. 169).

External management interventions are based on the premise that chronic sorrow is a normal response to a significant loss.

External management interventions are based on the premise that chronic sorrow is a normal response to a significant loss. Thus anticipatory guidance is provided regarding the situations and circumstances that are likely to trigger episodes of chronic sorrow. Personal coping mechanisms (i.e., internal management methods) can be assessed, strengthened, and supported. In addition, specific interventions by healthcare professionals categorized as roles have been shown to be helpful for those experiencing chronic sorrow. For example, family caregivers with chronic sorrow often benefit from interventions with the professional in the role of teacher or expert, in which the professional provides situation-specific information for managing caregiving responsibilities. Those in the caregiver role also benefit from actions associated with the professional in the role of empathetic presence, which is characterized by taking time to listen, offering support, and focusing on feelings. Finally, the role of caring professional in which the professional shows sensitivity, respectfulness, and nonjudgmental acceptance has also been described as beneficial (Eakes, 2004, p. 169–170).

Management methods may be either ineffective or effective. Ineffective management occurs when strategies actually increase the person's discomfort or heighten the feelings of sorrow. Conversely, effective management results from strategies that lead to increased comfort (Schreier & Droes, 2010, p. 661).

MAJOR CONCEPTS OF NURSING BASED ON THE THEORY OF CHRONIC SORROW

IN ADDITION TO THE CONCEPTS already presented, the four metaparadigm concepts of nursing are identified in the theory of chronic sorrow. These concepts are summarized in Table 25-1.

Person

Persons within the context of the theory are humans who—as humans do—have an idealized perception of life processes and health and compare their experiences both with the ideal and with the experiences of others around them. Although each person's experiences

TABLE 25-1 Metaparadigm Concepts as Defined in the Theory of Chronic Sorrow	
Person	A human being with an idealized perception of life processes and health who compares his or her experiences both with the ideal and with others around the person
Environment	The interactions that occur within the social context, which includes family, social, work, and the healthcare environments
Health	A normality of functioning; dependent on adaptation to disparities associated with loss
Nursing	Primary roles of nurses: empathetic presence, teacher-expert, and caring and competent caregiver

with loss and disparity are unique, common and predictable features of the loss experience can be identified (Eakes, Burke, & Hainsworth, 1998).

Environment

The environment includes the interactions that occur within the social context, which includes the family, social, work, and healthcare environments. Persons respond to their assessment of themselves in relation to social norms (Eakes, Burke, & Hainsworth, 1998).

Health

Health is a normality of functioning. A person's health depends on his or her adaptation to the disparities associated with loss. Effective coping results in a normal response to life losses (Eakes, Burke, & Hainsworth, 1998).

Nursing

The scope of nursing practice includes diagnosing chronic sorrow and providing interventions. Nurses provide anticipatory guidance to persons at risk. The primary roles of nurses include empathetic presence, teacher-expert, and caring and competent caregiver (Eakes, Burke, & Hainsworth, 1998).

CRITICAL THINKING

After reading the overview of the theory of chronic sorrow, do you agree that chronic sorrow is a normal response to a significant loss? Why or why not?

ANALYSIS OF THE THEORY OF CHRONIC SORROW

THE ANALYSIS PRESENTED HERE CONSISTS of an examination of assumptions and propositions as well as a brief critique of the theory of chronic sorrow as proposed by Eakes, Burke, and Hainsworth.

Assumptions of the Theory of Chronic Sorrow

Assumptions of the theory of chronic sorrow include the following:

❖ Chronic sorrow is a normal human response related to ongoing disparity created by a loss situation.

❖ Chronic sorrow is cyclic in nature.

❖ Predictable internal and external triggers of heightened grief can be categorized and anticipated.

❖ A human who experiences either a single loss or an ongoing loss will perceive a disparity between the ideal and reality.

❖ The disparity between the real and the ideal leads to feelings of pervasive sadness and grief (Eakes, 2004; 2008; Eakes, Burke, & Hainsworth, 1998).

Propositions of the Theory of Chronic Sorrow

Theoretical relationship statements in the theory include the following:

❖ Humans have inherent and learned coping strategies that may or may not be effective in regaining normal equilibrium when they are experiencing chronic sorrow.

❖ Health professionals' interventions may or may not be effective in assisting the person to regain equilibrium (Eakes, 2004; 2008; Eakes, Burke, & Hainsworth, 1998).

Brief Critique of the Theory of Chronic Sorrow

The theory of chronic sorrow was inductively derived and then evaluated from extensive review of the literature and from data gathered during

10 qualitative research studies (Eakes, 2004, p. 165). The assumptions are inherent in the research data. Key concepts are consistently defined, and the proposed relationships between concepts are clear and logical. Although the theory of chronic sorrow was introduced with a focus on a specific patient population, it has since been expanded and shown to be applicable to a wide range of loss situations. As a result of the rich body of research on this topic, chronic sorrow is a widely accepted phenomenon, as is evident in its inclusion in the list of approved North American Nursing Diagnosis Association (NANDA) diagnoses (Schreier & Droes, 2010, p. 667).

THE THEORY OF CHRONIC SORROW AS A FRAMEWORK FOR NURSING PRACTICE

NURSING PRACTICE FRAMED BY THE theory of chronic sorrow includes supporting personal coping strategies, providing provide anticipatory guidance to persons at risk, and functioning in the primary roles of the nurse. These primary nursing roles include empathetic presence, teacher-expert, and caring and competent caregiver (Eakes, Burke, & Hainsworth, 1998).

THE NURSING PROCESS AND THE THEORY OF CHRONIC SORROW

THE NURSING PROCESS IS NOT specifically addressed in the theory of chronic sorrow. Nevertheless, this theory will be examined in this section within the context of the nursing process for the sake of discussion, consistency, and comparison.

Assessment

If in the course of the nurse–patient relationship, the nursing assessment reveals a significant loss, the nurse will assess the patient specifically for chronic sorrow. The Chronic Sorrow Questionnaire or an interview geared toward identifying the indicators for chronic sorrow may be used during this process. Assessment should also include the internal management strategies already being used by the individual and the effectiveness of those strategies. The scope of nursing practice includes the diagnosis of chronic sorrow.

Planning

Planning will include matching the internal and external management strategies that should be the most beneficial to the person based on the specific loss situation.

Implementation

The nurse will provide anticipatory guidance regarding the situations and circumstances that are likely to trigger episodes of chronic sorrow. Personal coping mechanisms should be strengthened and supported. External management strategies will also include the roles of the nurse that are most appropriate for the loss situation, including the role of teacher or expert, the role of empathetic presence, and the role of caring professional.

Evaluation

Evaluation is based on whether the management methods were ineffective or effective. This determination is contingent on either an increase in the person's discomfort or an increase in the person's comfort.

SCENARIO ILLUSTRATING NURSING CARE FRAMED BY THE THEORY OF CHRONIC SORROW UTILIZING THE NURSING PROCESS

THE FOLLOWING SCENARIO ILLUSTRATES NURSING care of the patient relative to one identified nursing problem framed by the theory of chronic sorrow. This scenario is not intended to cover all aspects of care, but rather to stimulate thinking about how specific care might be approached using this theory as a framework for practice.

Mrs. M. is a 72-year-old Caucasian widow who has presented to the clinic at the request of her daughter. Her daughter reports that her mother seems sad all of the time and she is worried about her. Mrs. M. has been a widow for 3 years; she was married to her husband for 50 years. During the assessment interview, Mrs. M. talks about missing her husband and about the wedding anniversary they would have had the previous month. The nurse suspects a diagnosis of chronic sorrow, so she administers the Chronic Sorrow Questionnaire.

Once the diagnosis is verified, the nurse assesses Mrs. M.'s personal coping strategies by asking about her involvement in activities and her interests. The nurse also asks about the positive things going on in her life, and inquires as to whether she is involved in or interested in joining a support group. The nurse supports Mrs. M.'s current personal coping mechanisms and provides assistance to strengthen the potential for adding more coping mechanisms to her current portfolio. It is also important that the nurse educate the Mrs. M. and her daughter about the concept of chronic sorrow so that they will understand that what Mrs. M. is experiencing is normal after a significant loss.

The nurse also provides Mrs. M. and her daughter with anticipatory guidance regarding the situations and circumstances that are likely to trigger episodes of chronic sorrow. The nurse practices in the professional role of empathetic presence by taking time to listen, offering support, and focusing on the feelings of Mrs. M., and in the role of caring professional by showing sensitivity, respectfulness, and nonjudgmental acceptance of Mrs. M. Evaluation of the care of Mrs. M. will occur over time and will be based on whether nursing interventions increased her discomfort or increased her comfort.

The theory of chronic sorrow is a middle-range theory that has a specific focus. Throughout the nursing process, if other issues arise during the nursing encounter that are outside the focus of this theory, the nurse will intervene to provide nursing care using strategies that are congruent with current best clinical practices.

CLASSROOM ACTIVITY 25-1

Form small groups. Each group should add to the plan of care for Mrs. M. in the preceding scenario based on other potential or actual nursing problems. Each group should then share its plan with the class.

CLASSROOM ACTIVITY 25-2

Form small groups. Using a case study provided by the instructor, develop a plan of care using the theory of chronic sorrow as the basis for practice. Each group should then share its plan of care with the class.

CLASSROOM ACTIVITY 25-3

Form small groups. Using a case study provided by the instructor, develop a plan of care using one of the theories as the basis for practice; each group should select a different nursing theory. Each group should then share its plan of care with the class and discuss the similarities and differences in care.

REFERENCES

Eakes, G. G. (2004). Chronic sorrow. In S. J. Peterson & T. S. Bredow (Eds.), *Middle range theories: Application to nursing research* (pp. 165–175). Philadelphia: Lippincott Williams & Wilkins.

Eakes, G. G. (2008). Chronic sorrow. In S. J. Peterson & T. S. Bredow (Eds.), *Middle range theories: Application to nursing research* (2nd ed., pp. 170–185). Philadelphia: Lippincott Williams & Wilkins.

Eakes, G. G., Burke, M. L., & Hainsworth, M. A. (1998). Middle-range theory of chronic sorrow. *Image: The Journal of Nursing Scholarship, 30*(2), 179–184.

Lazarus, R. S., & Folkman, S. (1984). *Stress, appraisal, and coping.* New York: Springer.

Lindgren, C. L., Burke, M. L., Hainsworth, M. A., & Eakes, G. G. (1992). Chronic sorrow: A lifespan concept. *Scholarly Inquiry for Nursing Practice, 6,* 27–40.

Olshanksy, S. (1962). Chronic sorrow: A response to a mentally defective child. *Social Casework, 43,* 191–193.

Schreier, A. M., & Droes, N. S. (2010). Georgene Gaskill Eakes, Mary Lermann Burke, Margaret A. Hainsworth: Theory of chronic sorrow. In M. R. Alligood & A. M. Tomey (Eds.), *Nursing theorists and their work* (7th ed., pp. 656–672). Maryland Heights, MO: Mosby.

THEORY OF CARING:
Kristen M. Swanson

26

LEARNING OBJECTIVES

After completing this chapter the student should be able to

1. Identify and describe the major concepts as proposed by Swanson in the theory of caring

2. Explain the major concepts important to nursing as defined in Swanson's theory of caring

3. Plan nursing care for a patient scenario utilizing the theory of caring

KEY TERMS

Being with
Caring
Doing for

Enabling
Knowing
Maintaining belief

BACKGROUND

KRISTEN SWANSON EARNED HER BACCA-LAUREATE degree in nursing in 1975 from the University of Rhode Island's College of Nursing. She initially practiced nursing in a cardiac critical care unit at the University of Massachusetts Medical Center, which is where her preparation for studying caring-based therapeutics from a psychosocial perspective began (Swanson, 2006, p. 352). At this point in her career, what mattered most to Swanson in terms of nursing practice was her "emerging technological savvy, understanding of complex pathophysiological processes, and conveying that same information to other nurses" (Swanson, 2006, p. 353).

When Swanson applied to graduate school, she intended to teach nursing and focus on the care of the acutely ill adult. Consequently, she enrolled in the Adult Health and Illness Nursing program at the University of Pennsylvania. During this time, she served as a student representative to the graduate curriculum committee. At a retreat, Swanson heard Dr. Jacqueline Fawcett speak about health, environment, persons, and nursing as the four concepts underlying the nursing profession. Shortly thereafter, in 1978, Swanson graduated with a master's degree in nursing and was hired as a temporary instructor at the University of Pennsylvania to teach undergraduate medical–surgical nursing. In addition, she enrolled as a postmaster's student in Fawcett's course on the conceptual basis of nursing. It was during this time that Swanson began to understand nursing from an experiential, personal, and academic point of view and began to understand her values and abilities as they related to understanding and working with people going through transitions of health, illness, and healing (Swanson, 2006, p. 353).

The next year Swanson enrolled in the PhD nursing program at the University of Colorado in Denver, where her area of study was psychosocial nursing with an emphasis on the concepts of loss, stress, coping, caring, transactions, and person–environment fit. As part of her doctoral study, she participated in cesarean birth support group. The topic for one evening was miscarriage. After the guest speaker had finished the presentation, Swanson observed that the women attending the meeting were more interested in talking about their personal experiences with pregnancy loss. At this point, Swanson decided to learn more about the human experience and responses to miscarriage. Dr. Jean Watson, Swanson's dissertation chair, suggested that she examine caring in the context of miscarriage. Ultimately, caring and miscarriage became the focus of her doctoral dissertation study and her program of research (Swanson, 2006, p. 352)

After her completion of the PhD program, Swanson was awarded a National Research Service postdoctoral fellowship from the National Center for Nursing Research, which she completed under the direction of Dr. Kathryn Barnard at the University of Washington in Seattle. Swanson then joined the faculty at the University of Washington's School of Nursing. In addition to shouldering her teaching and administrative responsibilities, she continues to conduct research, to publish, and to mentor faculty and students; she also serves as a consultant. Swanson has received many honors for her contributions to the discipline of nursing, including induction as a fellow in the American Academy of Nursing (Wojnar, 2010, p. 742).

OVERVIEW OF THE THEORY OF CARING

SWANSON'S THEORY OF CARING (1991; 1993; 1999a) offers an explanation of what it means to practice nursing in a caring manner. In this theory, **caring** is defined as a "nurturing way of relating to a valued other toward whom one feels a personal sense of commitment and responsibility" (Swanson, 1991, p. 162). Swanson (1993) posits caring for a person's biopsychosocial and spiritual well-being as a fundamental and universal component of good nursing care.

Five additional concepts are integral to Swanson's theory of caring and represent the five basic processes of caring: maintaining belief, knowing, being with, doing for, and enabling.

❖ The concept of **maintaining belief** is sustaining faith in the other's capacity to get through an event or transition and face a future with meaning. This includes believing in the other's capacity and holding him or her in high esteem, maintaining a

> Caring is defined as a "nurturing way of relating to a valued other toward whom one feels a personal sense of commitment and responsibility."

hope-filled attitude, offering realistic optimism, helping to find meaning, and standing by the one cared for, no matter what the situation (Swanson, 1991, p. 162).

❖ The concept of **knowing** refers to striving to understand the meaning of an event in the life of the other, avoiding assumptions, focusing on the person cared for, seeking cues, assessing meticulously, and engaging both the one caring and the one cared for in the process of knowing (Swanson, 1991, p. 162).

❖ The concept of **being with** refers to being emotionally present to the other. It includes being present in person, conveying availability, and sharing feelings without burdening the one cared for (Swanson, 1991, p. 162).

❖ The concept of **doing for** refers to doing for others what one would do for oneself, including anticipating needs, comforting, performing skillfully and competently, and protecting the one cared for while preserving his or her dignity (Swanson, 1991, p. 162).

❖ The concept of **enabling** refers to facilitating the other's passage through life transitions and unfamiliar events by focusing on the event, informing, explaining, supporting, validating feelings, generating alternatives, thinking things through, and giving feedback (Swanson, 1991, p. 162).

These caring processes are sequential and overlapping. In fact, they may not exist separate from one another because each is an integral component of the overarching structure of caring (Wojnar, 2010, p. 746). According to Swanson (1999b), knowing, being with, doing for, enabling, and maintaining belief are essential components of the nurse–client relationship, regardless of the context.

> Knowing, being with, doing for, enabling, and maintaining belief are essential components of the nurse–client relationship, regardless of the context.

MAJOR CONCEPTS OF NURSING BASED ON THE THEORY OF CARING

In addition to the concepts already presented, the four metaparadigm concepts of nursing are identified by Swanson in the theory of caring. These concepts are summarized in Table 26-1.

<center>TABLE 26-1 Metaparadigm Concepts as Defined in Swanson's Theory of Caring</center>	
Person	"Unique beings who are in the midst of becoming and whose wholeness is made manifest in thoughts, feelings, and behaviors" (Swanson, 1993, p. 352)
Environment	"Any context that influences or is influenced by the designated client" (Swanson, 1993, p. 353)
Health	Health and well-being is "to live the subjective, meaning-filled experience of wholeness. Wholeness involves a sense of integration and becoming wherein all facets of being are free to be expressed" (Swanson, 1993, p. 353).
Nursing	Informed caring for the well-being of others (Swanson, 1991, 1993)

Person

Persons are defined as "unique beings who are in the midst of becoming and whose wholeness is made manifest in thoughts, feelings, and behaviors" (Swanson, 1993, p. 352). Swanson acknowledges that nursing also serves families, groups, and societies.

According to Swanson, the life experiences of each person are influenced by a complex interplay of a "genetic heritage, spiritual endowment, and the capacity to exercise free will" (p. 352). She goes on to explain that "spiritual endowment connects each being with an eternal and universal source of goodness, mystery, life, creativity, and serenity. The spiritual endowment may be a soul, higher power/Holy Spirit, positive energy, or, simply grace" (p. 352). "Free will [is] equated with the choice and the capacity to decide how to act when confronted with a range of possibilities" (p. 352); however, limitations set by race, class, gender, or access to health care may prevent persons from exercising free will. Acknowledging free will does require that the nurse honor individuality.

Environment

Swanson defines the environment as "any context that influences or is influenced by the designated client" (1993, p. 353). She continues by explaining that the terms "environment" and "person-client" may be view interchangeably; in fact, what is considered an environment in one situation may be considered the client in another. For example, "the lens on

CRITICAL THINKING

Compare Swanson's definition of caring to other theorists' definitions of this concept. What are the similarities? What are the differences? Which of the theorists' definitions of caring best fits your own definition of caring? Explain your answer by comparing what you believe about the concept of caring with the other definitions.

environment/designated client may be specified to the intra-individual level, wherein the 'client' may be at the cellular level and the environment may be the organs, tissues, or body of which the cell is a component" (p. 353).

Consistent with this view of the environment, persons do indeed influence, and they are influenced by their environment. Other influences on the environment include cultural, social, biophysical, political, and economic factors (Wojnar, 2010).

Health

To experience health and well-being is "to live the subjective, meaning-filled experience of wholeness. Wholeness involves a sense of integration and becoming wherein all facets of being are free to be expressed" (Swanson, 1993, p. 353). These facets of being include the many selves that make persons human—for example, the individual's spirituality, thoughts, feelings, intelligence, creativity, relatedness, femininity, masculinity, and sexuality. Consistent with this definition, Swanson views reestablishing well-being as a process of healing that entails "releasing inner pain, establishing new meanings, restoring integration, and emerging into a sense of renewed wholeness" (Swanson, 1993, p. 353).

Nursing

The goal of nursing is to promote the well-being of others (Wojnar, 2010, p. 746). Nursing is defined by Swanson as informed caring for the well-being of others (1991, 1993), where caring refers to "a nurturing way of relating to a valued other toward whom one feels a personal sense of commitment and responsibility" (Swanson, 1991, p. 162). The discipline of nursing is informed by empirical knowledge from nursing and related disciplines, as well as by ethical knowledge, personal knowledge, knowledge derived from the humanities, knowledge derived from clinical experience, and personal and societal values and expectations (Swanson, 1993, p. 352).

T HE ANALYSIS PRESENTED HERE CONSISTS of an examination of assumptions and propositions as well as a brief critique of the theory of caring as proposed by Swanson.

ANALYSIS OF THE THEORY OF CARING

Assumptions of the Theory of Caring

Major assumptions of the theory of caring are included in the definitions of major concepts:

❖ Persons are dynamic and growing.

❖ Persons are self-reflecting.

❖ Persons are spiritual beings who yearn to be connected with others.

❖ Nurses are responsible for taking leadership roles in fighting for human rights, equal access to health care, and other humanitarian causes.

❖ Nurses also direct their caring to self and other nurses.

Propositions of the Theory of Caring

Identified theoretical relationship statements within Swanson's theory of caring include the following:

❖ Applying caring processes in therapeutic communication with clients enhances comfort and accelerates healing.

❖ Well-being is enhanced by the receipt of caring from a nurse who is informed about common human responses to a designated health problem (Swanson, 1993).

Brief Critique of the Theory of Caring

Swanson's theory of caring was empirically derived through an inductive methodology known as phenomenological inquiry (Wojnar, 2010, p. 746). The theory is presented in a clear and logical manner. It is a simple theory with a minimal but appropriate number of concepts for a middle-range theory. The concepts within the theory are consistently defined. The theory of caring is applicable across settings and with diverse populations making it useful in practice. It exemplifies both traditional and contemporary values of the profession of nursing (Wojnar, 2010, p. 748).

THE THEORY OF CARING AS A FRAMEWORK FOR NURSING CARE

THE PRIMARY PURPOSE OF THE theory of caring is to help practitioners deliver nursing care that specifically focuses on the needs of persons in a way that fosters dignity, respect, and empowerment (Wojnar, 2010, p. 748). This goal is accomplished through the set of sequential caring processes that provide the structure of caring. Although maintaining belief, knowing, being with, doing for, and enabling are essential components of the nurse–client relationship regardless of the context, Swanson has identified a difference in the caring therapeutics delivered by novice nurses versus the care provided by more experienced nurses. The novice nurse, according to Swanson (1993), has a more limited repertoire of caring therapeutics due to his or her inexperience; by comparison, the caring techniques and knowledge embedded in the experienced nurse may be so subtle that they go unnoticed.

THE NURSING PROCESS AND THE THEORY OF CARING

ALTHOUGH THE NURSING PROCESS IS not discussed in Swanson's theory of caring, the theory is examined here in the context of the nursing process for the sake of discussion, consistency, and comparison.

Assessment and Planning

Caring is delivered as a set of sequential processes that are created by the nurse's philosophical attitude—also known within the theory as the process of maintaining belief. During the development of the nurse–patient relationship and assessment phase of the nursing process, it is the nurse's role to *maintain belief*. This responsibility includes sustaining faith in the other's capacity to get through an event or transition and face a future with meaning. Maintaining belief also includes holding the other in high esteem and letting the one cared for know that the nurse will stand by that individual. In addition, maintaining belief encompasses having a hope-filled attitude, offering realistic optimism, and helping to find meaning (Swanson, 1991, p. 162).

During the assessment phase of the nursing process, the nurse also engages in understanding or knowing. Knowing comprises focusing on the person cared for and striving to understand the meaning of an event in the life of the other. It includes seeking cues, assessing the other, and avoiding assumptions. Knowing requires engaging both the one caring and the one cared for in the process of knowing (p. 162).

Implementation

During the implementation phase of the nursing process, the nurse conveys to the client, through both verbal and nonverbal messages, that he or she is emotionally present. The "being with" concept includes being present in person, conveying availability, and sharing feelings without burdening the one cared for (Swanson, 1991, p. 162).

During the implementation phase, the nurse also engages in doing for and enabling. Doing for includes those therapeutic actions necessitated by the required care of the client. The "doing for" concept refers to doing for others what one would do for oneself, including anticipating needs, comforting, performing skillfully and competently, and protecting the one cared for while preserving his or her dignity (p. 162). Enabling also includes therapeutic actions, but refers to facilitating the other's passage through life transitions and unfamiliar events by focusing on the event, informing, explaining, supporting, validating feelings, generating alternatives, thinking things through, and giving feedback (p. 162).

Evaluation

The intended client outcome is referred to in Swanson's theory of caring as the consequences of caring. The intended outcome or consequence of the caring process is client well-being or wholeness. As mentioned earlier in this chapter, within the context of this theory, well-being means "to live the subjective, meaning-filled experience of wholeness" (Swanson, 1993, p. 353).

SCENARIO ILLUSTRATING NURSING CARE FRAMED BY THE THEORY OF CARING UTILIZING THE NURSING PROCESS

THE FOLLOWING SCENARIO ILLUSTRATES NURSING care of the patient relative to one identified nursing problem framed by Swanson's theory of caring. This scenario is not intended to cover all aspects of care, but rather to stimulate thinking about how specific care might be approached using this theory as a framework for practice.

Mrs. M. is young woman who experienced the loss of infant daughter several months ago. In the wake of her loss, she continues to experience sadness, loss of appetite, weight loss, and loss of sleep. The nurse has followed Mrs. M. for several weeks in the clinic and has faith in her capacity to get through this event. The nurse has openly expressed to Mrs. M. that she holds her in high esteem and will stand by her through this experience. Throughout her time with Mrs. M., the nurse focuses on Mrs. M., making an effort to understand the meaning of such an event in the life of Mrs. M. The nurse seeks cues and is careful to avoid assumptions.

The nurse conveys to Mrs. M., using both verbal and nonverbal messages, that she is emotionally present and available to listen to Mrs. M. if she needs to express feelings, describe her experiences, or talk about any other issues. The nurse anticipates the needs of Mrs. M. and comforts her. The nurse assists Mrs. M. as she navigates her passage through this life event. Along the way, the nurse facilitates the process of thinking things through and validating Mrs. M.'s feelings—feelings that she may be unable to express in another setting. In addition to supporting Mrs. M., the nurse provides information and explanations of signs and symptoms that Mrs. M. is experiencing. The nurse performs all skills competently, such as nutritional assessment: Mrs. M. has experienced decreased appetite and weight loss. She refers Mrs. M. to an appropriate support group. If the sadness that Mrs. M. is experiencing does not resolve within a reasonable time frame, the nurse will also refer Mrs. M. for consultation with a mental health provider.

Evaluation of the care provided for Mrs. M. is based on the level of well-being experienced by Mrs. M. It is expected that the caring process will provide comfort and enhance well-being and wholeness in Mrs. M.

The theory of caring is a middle-range theory that has a specific focus; however, it also incorporates the therapeutic actions of doing for and enabling. These components make it clear that the nurse is responsible for providing nursing care using strategies that are applicable to all aspects of patient care; all care should be consistent with current best clinical practices and delivered within the context of the caring.

Classroom Activity 26-1

Form small groups. Each group should add to the plan of care for Mrs. M. in the preceding scenario based on other potential or actual nursing problems typical for a patient with the same medical diagnosis or symptoms and demographics. Each group should develop a plan for one additional nursing problem using Swanson's theory of caring as the basis for practice. Each group should then share its plan with the class.

Classroom Activity 26-2

Form small groups. Using a case study provided by the instructor, develop a plan of care using Swanson's theory of caring as the basis for practice. Each group should then share its plan of care with the class.

Classroom Activity 26-3

Form small groups. Using a case study provided by the instructor, develop a plan of care using one of the theories as the basis for practice; each group should select a different nursing theory. Each group should then share its plan of care with the class and discuss the similarities and differences in care.

REFERENCES

Swanson, K. M. (1991). Empirical development of a middle range theory of caring. *Nursing Research, 40*(3), 161–166.

Swanson, K. M. (1993). Nursing as informed caring for the well-being of others. *Image: The Journal of Nursing Scholarship, 25*(4), 352–357.

Swanson, K. M. (1999a). The effects of caring, measurement, and time on miscarriage impact and women's well-being in the first year subsequent to loss. *Nursing Research, 48*(6), 288–298.

Swanson, K. M. (1999b). What's known about caring in nursing: A literary meta-analysis. In A. S. Hinshaw, J. Shaver, & S. Freetham (Eds.), *Handbook of clinical nursing research* (pp. 31–60). Thousand Oaks, CA: Sage.

Swanson, K . M. (2006). Kristen M. Swanson: A program of research on caring. In M. E. Parker (Ed.), *Nursing theories and nursing practice* (2nd ed., pp. 351–259). Philadelphia: F. A. Davis.

Wojnar, D. M. (2010). Kristin M. Swanson: Theory of caring. In M. R. Alligood & A. M. Tomey (Eds.), *Nursing theorists and their work* (7th ed., pp. 741–752). Maryland Heights, MO: Mosby.

THEORY OF COMFORT:
Katharine Kolcaba

LEARNING OBJECTIVES

After completing this chapter the student should be able to

1. Identify and describe the major concepts of the theory of comfort

2. Explain the major concepts important to nursing as defined in the theory of comfort

3. Plan nursing care for a patient scenario utilizing Kolcaba's theory of comfort

KEY TERMS

Comfort

BACKGROUND

KATHARINE KOLCABA ENTERED NURSING PRACTICE after completion of a diploma in nursing in 1965. In 1987, she graduated from the RN to MSN program at the Frances Payne Bolton School of Nursing, Case Western Reserve University, with a specialty in gerontology. Kolcaba's clinical experience prior to returning to school was in medical–surgical nursing, long-term care, and home care. While enrolled in the RN to MSN program, she job-shared in a head nurse position in a dementia unit. During this experience, she began theorizing about the outcome of comfort (Dowd, 2010, p. 706).

Kolcaba accepted a faculty position at the University of Akron's College of Nursing after the completion of her master's degree. She also completed her doctorate at Case Western Reserve University. During the course of her doctoral work, she focused on her interest in the concept of comfort, publishing a concept analysis of comfort (Kolcaba & Kolcaba, 1991), diagramming aspects of comfort (Kolcaba, 1991), operationalizing comfort as an outcome of care (Kolcaba 1992), contextualizing comfort as a middle-range theory (Kolcaba, 1994), and testing the theory in an intervention study (Kolcaba & Fox, 1999). Kolcaba has her own company, known as the Comfort Line, which assists healthcare organizations in implementing the theory of comfort (also known as comfort care). She continues to work with students who are conducting studies related to the concept of comfort and teaches nursing theory part-time at the University of Akron, where she is currently an emeritus associate professor of nursing (Dowd, 2010, p. 706–707).

The ideas of three early nurse theorists were referenced by Kolcaba to postulate the types of comfort: relief, ease, and renewal. Orlando (1961) proposed that nurses relieve the needs expressed by patients. Henderson (1966) described 14 basic functions of human beings to be maintained during nursing care. Renewal was described by Kolcaba as a state in which one rises above problems or pain. Paterson and Zderad (1975) proposed that patients rise above or transcend their difficulties with the help of nurses. Later, the term "renewal" was changed by Kolcaba to "transcendence," as this term was already being used in the nursing literature by Paterson and Zderad (Dowd, 2010, p. 708; Kolcaba, 2004, p. 258).

Historically, prior to the development of medical curative techniques, nurses believed that comfort was their unique and primary mission. Kolcaba (2004) suggests that Florence Nightingale may have been the first nurse to recognize that comfort was essential to patients when she said, "It must never be lost sight of what observation is for. It is not for the sake of piling up miscellaneous information or curious facts, but for the sake of saving life and increasing health and comfort" (Nightingale, 1860/1969, p. 70). Nightingale also claimed that patients who were kept comfortable by nurses would be in a better position to regain health.

Comfort, as described by Kolcaba (2004, p. 255) in the theory of comfort, is the immediate experience of being strengthened by having needs for relief, ease, and transcendence addressed in four contexts—physical, psychospiritual, sociocultural, and environmental; it is much more than simply the absence of pain or other physical discomfort. Physical comfort pertains to bodily sensations and homeostatic mechanisms. Psychospiritual comfort pertains to the internal awareness of self, including esteem, sexuality, meaning in one's life, and one's relationship to a higher order or being. Sociocultural comfort pertains to interpersonal, family, societal relationships, and cultural traditions. Environmental comfort pertains to the external background of the human experience, which includes light, noise, color, temperature, ambience, and natural versus synthetic elements (Kolcaba, 2004, p. 258).

Comfort care encompasses three components: an appropriate and timely intervention to meet the comfort needs of patients, a mode of delivery that projects caring and empathy, and the intent to comfort. Comfort needs include patients' or families' desire for or deficit in either relief, ease, or transcendence in the physical, psychospiritual, sociocultural, or environmental contexts of human experience. Comfort measures—a related concept—refers to interventions that are intentionally designed to enhance patients' or families' comfort (Kolcaba, 2004, p. 255).

The theory of comfort also addresses intervening variables—negative or positive factors over which nurses and institutions have little control, but that affect the direction and success of comfort care plans. Examples

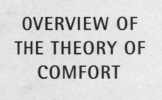

OVERVIEW OF THE THEORY OF COMFORT

Comfort is the immediate experience of being strengthened by having needs for relief, ease, and transcendence addressed in four contexts—physical, psychospiritual, sociocultural, and environmental; it is much more than simply the absence of pain or other physical discomfort.

of intervening variables include the presence or absence of social support, poverty, prognosis, concurrent medical or psychological conditions, and health habits (Kolcaba, 2004, p. 255).

An additional concept within the theory comprises the health-seeking behaviors of patients and families. Health-seeking behaviors are those behaviors that patients and families engage in either consciously or unconsciously while moving toward well-being. Health-seeking behaviors can be either internal or external, and can include dying peacefully. It is posited that enhanced comfort results in engagement in health-seeking behaviors (Kolcaba, 2004, p. 255).

MAJOR CONCEPTS OF NURSING BASED ON THE THEORY OF COMFORT

IN ADDITION TO THE CONCEPTS already presented, the four metaparadigm concepts of nursing are identified in Kolcaba's theory of comfort. These concepts are summarized in Table 27-1.

Person

Recipients of care in the theory of comfort may be individuals, families, institutions, or communities in need of health care. Nurses themselves may be the

TABLE 27-1 Metaparadigm Concepts as Defined in Kolcaba's Theory of Comfort	
Person	Recipients of care may be individuals, families, institutions, or communities in need of health care.
Environment	The environment includes any aspect of the patient, family, or institutional setting that can be manipulated by the nurse, a loved one, or the institution to enhance comfort.
Health	Health is considered optimal functioning of the patient, the family, the healthcare provider, or the community.
Nursing	Nursing is the intentional assessment of comfort needs, design of comfort interventions to address those needs, and reassessment of comfort levels after implementation compared with a baseline.

recipients of comfort—for example, through efforts to improve working conditions (Kolcaba, Tilton, & Drouin, 2006).

Environment

The environment is considered to be any aspect of the patient, family, or institutional setting that can be manipulated by the nurse, manipulated by the loved one, or manipulated by the institution so as to enhance comfort (Dowd, 2010, p. 711).

Health

Health is considered optimal functioning of the patient, the family, the healthcare provider, or the community. Optimal functioning and, therefore, health are defined by the patient or group (Dowd, 2010, p. 711).

Nursing

Within the context of the theory of comfort, nursing is the intentional assessment of comfort needs, the design of comfort interventions to address those needs, and the reassessment of comfort levels after implementation compared with a baseline. Assessment and reassessment of comfort may be achieved through intuitive, subjective, and objective methods (Dowd, 2010, p. 711).

ANALYSIS OF THE THEORY OF COMFORT

THE ANALYSIS PRESENTED HERE CONSISTS of an examination of assumptions and propositions as well as a brief critique of the theory of comfort as proposed by Kolcaba.

Assumptions of the Theory of Comfort

The theory of comfort originally included four assumptions:

❖ Human beings have holistic responses to complex stimuli.

❖ Comfort is a desirable holistic outcome that is germane to the discipline of nursing.

❖ Human beings strive to meet, or to have met, their basic comfort needs.

❖ Comfort is more than the absence of pain, anxiety, or other physical discomfort (Kolcaba, 1994).

Two other assumptions were identified during further explication of the theory:

❖ Patients who are empowered to actively engage in health-seeking behaviors are satisfied with their health care (Kolcaba, 2001).

❖ Institutional integrity is based on a value system oriented to the recipients of care. Of equal importance is an orientation to a health-promoting, holistic setting for families and providers of care (Kolcaba, 2001).

Propositions of the Theory of Comfort

The following are the relational statements within the theory of comfort as identified by Kolcaba (2004, p. 261):

❖ Nurses identify comfort needs of patients and their family members, especially those needs that have not been met by existing support systems.

❖ Nurses design interventions to address needs.

❖ Intervening variables are taken into account in designing the interventions and determining their probability for success.

❖ When interventions are effective and delivered in a caring manner, the immediate outcome of enhanced comfort is attained and the interventions can be called comfort measures. Comfort care entails all of these components.

❖ Patients and nurses agree on desirable and realistic health-seeking behaviors.

❖ If enhanced comfort is achieved, patients and family members are strengthened so that they can engage in health-seeking behaviors, which further enhances comfort.

❖ When patients and family members engage in health-seeking behaviors as a result of being strengthened by comfort care, nurses, families, and patients are more satisfied with health care and demonstrate better health-related outcomes.

❖ When patients, families, and nurses are satisfied with health care in a specific institution, public acknowledgment of the institution's contributions to health in the United State will help those institutions remain viable and flourishing.

Brief Critique of the Theory of Comfort

The concepts of the theory of comfort are described in easy-to-understand language. The theory is simple, incorporating just a few concepts. The concepts are presented at a low level of abstraction, which is appropriate for a middle-range theory. The simplicity of the theory allows students and nurses to easily learn and practice within the context of the theory. Although specific to the concept of comfort, the theory is generalizable across settings, age groups, patient populations, and cultures. The theory of comfort is dedicated to sustaining nursing by bringing the discipline of nursing back to its roots (Dowd, 2010, p. 716).

THE THEORY OF COMFORT AS A FRAMEWORK FOR NURSING CARE

NURSES HAVE TRADITIONALLY PROVIDED COMFORT to patients through interventions that are referred to as comfort measures in Kolcaba's theory. Using the theory of comfort in nursing care assists the nurse to identify and address the comfort needs of patients and families. Assessment and planning account for the intervening variables that might otherwise interfere with the patient care goals of enhanced comfort. In addition to the immediate desired outcome, enhanced comfort is related to other desirable outcomes such as higher patient function, quicker discharge, fewer re-admissions, increased patient satisfaction, and stronger cost–benefit ratios for the institution (Kolcaba, 2004).

THE NURSING PROCESS AND THE THEORY OF COMFORT

THE NURSING PROCESS IS NOT specifically addressed in the theory of comfort. Nevertheless, this theory will be examined within the context of the nursing process here for the sake of discussion, consistency, and comparison.

Assessment

Assessment and reassessment of comfort may be achieved through subjective, intuitive, or objective methods. The nurse may ask if the patient is comfortable, may identify changes in patient behavior that indicate discomfort, or may administer a verbal rating scale to assess the patient's comfort level (Kolcaba, 2003). In clinical practice situations, Kolcaba recommends asking patients to rate their comfort on a scale from zero to ten, with ten being the highest possible comfort in their situation. This verbal rating scale has been shown to be sensitive to changes in comfort over time (Dowd, Kolcaba, Steiner, & Fashinpaur, 2007).

Planning

The assessment data are displayed on a comfort grid, which lists the three comfort needs (relief, ease, and transcendence) across the top horizontal axis and the four contexts of comfort (physical, psychospiritual, sociocultural, and environmental) along the left vertical axis. Based on the assessment data, comfort measures are planned for each area of comfort needs and for each of the context of comfort areas.

Implementation

During the implementation phase of the nursing process, the nurse uses strategies to enhance the comfort of the patient. These strategies will vary depending on the specific context of comfort and needs of the patient, but may include standard comfort interventions, such as patient medications and treatments; coaching interventions, such as emotional support, education, reassurance, listening, and providing access to clergy; and "comfort food for the soul" (Dowd, 2010, p. 718), such as music therapy,

In addition to the immediate desired outcome, enhanced comfort is related to other desirable outcomes such as higher patient function, quicker discharge, fewer re-admissions, increased patient satisfaction, and stronger cost–benefit ratios for the institution.

guided imagery, spending time, reduction of environmental stimuli, personal connections, and energy therapy.

Evaluation

Evaluation focuses on reassessment of comfort, because the goal of any intervention is the enhanced comfort of the patient. To assess for enhanced comfort, the patient may be asked to rate his or her comfort level on a scale from zero to ten. Alternative comfort strategies can be incorporated into the patient's care depending on the level of patient comfort achieved.

T HE FOLLOWING SCENARIO ILLUSTRATES NURSING care of the patient relative to one identified nursing problem framed by Kolcaba's theory of comfort. This scenario is not intended to cover all aspects of care, but rather to stimulate thinking about how specific care might be approached using this theory as a framework for practice.

CRITICAL THINKING

Within the context of the comfort theory, the goal of nursing is to enhance comfort. Is this goal of nursing congruent with your own view of the goal of nursing care?

Mrs. C. is an 87-year-old African American patient who is living in her own home. Her daughter lives next door and is the primary caregiver for her mother. Mrs. C. suffers from pain related to bone cancer metastasis. As the nurse, you have been visiting Mrs. C. for several months. You have noticed behaviors consistent with increasing levels of pain in Mrs. C. During your current visit, you ask Mrs. C. to respond to the verbal rating scale by asking her to rate her level of comfort on a scale from zero to ten, with ten being the highest possible comfort. Mrs. C. rates her comfort level as a two. You question Mrs. C. further to assess the comfort need areas and context. Using these data, you are able to complete the comfort grid. Based on the assessment data, you, Mrs. C., and Mrs. C.'s daughter will plan comfort measures for each area of need and each context area within the comfort grid.

SCENARIO ILLUSTRATING NURSING CARE FRAMED BY THE THEORY OF COMFORT UTILIZING THE NURSING PROCESS

These strategies implemented will vary depending on the specific context of comfort and needs, but may include standard comfort interventions such as the specific medications and treatments that have been ordered for Mrs. C., monitoring vital signs, and assessment for complications. Nursing comfort interventions for Mrs. C. will also include coaching strategies such emotional support, reassurance, and listening. In addition, Mrs. C. may benefit from music therapy or guided imagery, spending time with her family, reduction of environmental stimuli, and having visits and prayer with her pastor.

Evaluation of the effectiveness of nursing interventions for Mrs. C. will focus on reassessment of her comfort. To assess for enhanced comfort, Mrs. C. may be asked to rate her comfort level on a scale from zero to ten again in a few days when you visit her again. You will also observe for behavior indicators of pain versus comfort during the next visit. Strategies will be adjusted based on the level of comfort that Mrs. C. is experiencing during the next visit.

The theory of comfort is a middle-range theory that has a specific focus. At the same time, Kolcaba's theory does include a component that incorporates standard interventions. This element makes it clear that the nurse is responsible for providing nursing care using strategies that are applicable to all aspects of patient care and providing care that is consistent with current best clinical practices; moreover, that it is possible for the nurse to achieve these goals within the context of the comfort.

CLASSROOM ACTIVITY 27-1

Form small groups. Each group should add to the plan of care for Mrs. C. in the preceding scenario based on other potential or actual nursing problems typical for a patient with the same medical diagnosis or symptoms and demographics. Each group should develop a plan for one additional nursing problem using Kolcaba's theory of comfort as the basis for practice. Each group should then share its plan with the class.

CLASSROOM ACTIVITY 27-2

Form small groups. Using a case study provided by the instructor, develop a plan of care using Kolcaba's nursing theory as the basis for practice. Each group should then share its plan of care with the class.

CLASSROOM ACTIVITY 27-3

Form small groups. Using a case study provided by the instructor, develop a plan of care using one of the theories as the basis for practice; each group should select a different nursing theory. Each group should then share its plan of care with the class and discuss the similarities and differences in care.

REFERENCES

Dowd, T. (2010). Katharine Kolcaba: Theory of comfort. In M. R. Alligood & A. M. Tomey (Eds.), *Nursing theorists and their work* (7th ed., pp. 706–721). Maryland Heights, MO: Mosby.

Dowd, T., Kolcaba, K., Steiner, R., & Fashinpur, D. (2007). Comparison of healing touch and coaching on stress and comfort in young college students. *Holistic Nursing Practice, 21*(4), 194–202.

Henderson, V. (1966). *The nature of nursing.* New York: MacMillan.

Kolcaba, K. (1991). A taxonomic structure for the concept of comfort. *Image: The Journal of Nursing Scholarship, 23*(4), 237–240.

Kolcaba, K. (1992). Holistic comfort: Operationalizing the construct as nurse-sensitive outcome. *Advances in Nursing Science, 15*(1), 1–10.

Kolcaba, K. (1994). A theory of holistic comfort for nursing. *Journal of Advanced Nursing, 19,* 1178–1184.

Kolcaba, K. (2001). Evolution of themed range theory of comfort for outcomes research. *Nursing Outlook, 49*(2), 86–92.

Kolcaba, K. (2003). *Comfort theory and practice: A vision for holistic health care and research.* New York: Springer.

Kolcaba, K. (2004). Comfort. In S. J. Peterson & T. S. Bredow (Eds.), *Middle range theories: Application to nursing research* (pp. 255–273). Philadelphia: Lippincott Williams & Wilkins.

Kolcaba, K., & Fox, C. (1999). The effects of guided imagery on comfort in women with early stage breast cancer undergoing radiation therapy. *Oncology Nursing Forum, 26*(1), 67–92.

Kolcaba, K., & Kolcaba, R. (1991). An analysis of the concept of comfort. *Journal of Advanced Nursing, 16,* 1301–1310.

Kolcaba, K., Tilton, C., & Drouin, C. (2006). Comfort the theory: A unifying framework to enhance the practice environment. *Journal of Nursing Administration, 36*(11), 538–544.

Nightingale, F. (1860/1969). *Notes on nursing: What it is and what it is not.* New York: Dover.

Orlando, I. (1961). *The dynamic nurse–patient relationship: Function, process, and principles.* New York: Putnam.

Paterson, J., & Zderad, L. (1975). *Humanistic nursing* (2nd ed.). New York: National League for Nursing.

THEORY OF BUREAUCRATIC CARING:
Marilyn Anne Ray

LEARNING OBJECTIVES

After completing this chapter the student should be able to

1. Identify and describe the major concepts of the theory of bureaucratic caring

2. Explain the major concepts important to nursing as defined in the theory of bureaucratic caring

3. Plan nursing care for a patient scenario utilizing Ray's theory of bureaucratic caring

KEY TERMS

⦂ Caring

BACKGROUND

MARILYN ANNE RAY BEGAN HER nursing career in 1958 after graduating from St. Joseph Hospital School of Nursing in Hamilton, Ontario, Canada. She then worked in a number of units at the University of California, Los Angeles Medical Center. In 1965, she returned to school to earn a bachelor's degree in nursing and subsequently a master's degree in maternal–child nursing from the University of Colorado's School of Nursing. It was during this time that Ray first met Dr. Madeleine Leininger, who profoundly influenced Ray. In the mid-1960s, Ray became a citizen of the United States; she was commissioned as an officer in the United States Air Force Reserve Nurse Corps in 1967. She graduated as a flight nurse from the School of Aerospace Medicine at Brooks Air Force Base, San Antonio, Texas. After earning a second master's degree in cultural anthropology from McMaster University, Ray enrolled in a doctoral program at the University of Utah, where she studied with her mentor Leininger. Ray completed her doctoral studies in 1981 with a dissertation study on caring in the complex hospital organizational culture. It was from her dissertation research that the theory of bureaucratic caring emerged (Coffman, 2010, p. 113–114).

Ray has held nursing faculty positions at the University of California–San Francisco; University of San Francisco; McMaster University in Hamilton, Ontario; and Florida Atlantic University. In addition, she has held visiting professor positions at Virginia Commonwealth University, University of Colorado, and various universities in Australia, New Zealand, and Thailand (Coffman, 2010, p. 113–114).

Ray retired as a colonel after 30 years of service to the United States Air Force Reserve Nurse Corps. As a certified transcultural nurse, she continues to research and publish on the subject of caring in organizational cultures, caring theory and inquiry development, transcultural caring, and transcultural ethics. She remains actively engaged in teaching doctoral students (Ray, 2006, p. 360–361).

THE THEORY OF BUREAUCRATIC CARING origi-
nated as a grounded theory from a qualitative
study of caring in an organizational culture. This
study revealed that nurses struggle with the paradox of
serving the bureaucracy while serving others through
caring. The discovery of bureaucratic caring resulted in
both substantive and formal theories. The substantive
theory, which emerged as differential caring, revealed
that caring in the complex organization of the hospital
is complicated and that caring is differentiated in terms
of meaning by its context. According to differential caring theory, different
units espouse different caring models based on their organizational goals
and values. The formal theory of bureaucratic caring represented a dynamic
structure of caring, which was created from a dialogue between the thesis
of caring as humanistic, social, educational, ethical, and religious/spiritual
and the antithesis of caring as economic, political, legal, and technological.
According to this theory, interactions and symbolic systems of meaning are
formed and reproduced from dominant values in an organization. Nursing
and caring are experiential and contextual and are influenced by the social
structure or the culture in the organization (Ray, 2006, p. 364).

| OVERVIEW OF THE THEORY OF BUREAUCRATIC CARING |

To understand the theory of bureaucratic caring, it is necessary to
review each of the concepts individually. The central concept of the theory is caring. According to Ray, caring occurs within the context of a culture or society, which includes such elements as personal culture, hospital
organizational culture, and societal and global culture. **Caring** is defined
as "a complex, transcultural, relational process grounded in an ethical,
spiritual context" (Coffman, 2010, p. 118). The concept of spiritual–ethical
caring for nurses facilitates the selection of choices for the good of others
that can or should be accomplished (Ray, 1989; 1997).

> Caring is defined as "a complex, transcultural, relational process grounded in an ethical, spiritual context."

Viewing the illustrated model of the theory, the remaining seven concepts are arranged around the central concept of spiritual–ethical caring:

❖ Educational factors include both formal and informal education
  programs as well as other forms of teaching and sharing of information (Ray, 1989).

❖ Physical factors are related to the physical state of being, including both biological and mental patterns. Because the mind and the body are interrelated, each pattern influences the other (Ray, 2006).

❖ Sociocultural factors include ethnicity and family structures, friends and family relationships, communication, social interaction and support, intimacy, and structures of cultural groups, community, and society (Ray, 1989; 2006).

❖ Legal factors include responsibility and accountability, rules and principles to guide behaviors, rights, and the practice of defensive medicine and nursing (Ray, 1989).

❖ Technological factors include nonhuman resources such as machinery used in patient care, diagnostic tests, and pharmaceutical agents, as well as the skill needed to use the resources (Ray, 1989).

❖ Economic factors include budgets, insurance systems, limitations and guidelines imposed by managed care organizations, and allocation of resources as necessary to maintain the economic viability of the organization (Ray, 1989).

❖ Political factors and the structure within healthcare administration influence how nursing is viewed and influence patterns of communication and decision making in the organization (Ray, 1989). An additional issue within the political factor is trust or lack of trust, which can lead to disillusionment and decreased loyalty to the organization (Ray, Turkel, & Marino, 2002).

Within the theory of bureaucratic caring, the seven major concepts are interconnected and everything within the culture is infused with spiritual–ethical caring, which is depicted at the center surrounded by the seven factors.

Within the theory of bureaucratic caring, all of the concepts are interconnected and everything within the culture is infused with spiritual–ethical caring, which is depicted at the center surrounded by the seven factors.

Nursing theorists continue to debate how to best categorize Ray's theory of bureaucratic caring. For example, some have categorized it as a philosophy of nursing. Others have categorized it as a middle-range theory because the scope of the theory is narrower that what is typical of a philosophy of nursing due to the focus on caring in the context organizational culture. Ray has suggested that perhaps it should be considered a holographic theory (Ray, 2006, p. 365–366). Although the theory of bureaucratic caring is grouped with the middle-range theories in this text, we recognize that this issue has not been resolved and that discussion on this front will continue.

IN ADDITION TO THE CONCEPTS already presented, the four metaparadigm concepts of nursing are identified in Ray's theory of bureaucratic caring. These concepts are summarized in Table 28-1.

> **MAJOR CONCEPTS OF NURSING BASED ON THE THEORY OF BUREAUCRATIC CARING**

Person

As viewed within the context of the theory, a person is a spiritual and cultural being. "Persons are created by God, the Mystery of Being, and they engage co-creatively in human organizational and transcultural relationships to find meaning and value" (Coffman, 2010, p. 121).

Environment

The "environment is a complex spiritual, ethical, ecological, and cultural phenomenon" that embodies knowledge and conscience and symbolic systems of patterns of meanings (Coffman, 2010, p. 122). These patterns are preserved or changed through caring values, attitudes, and communication.

TABLE 28-1 Metaparadigm Concepts as Defined in Ray's Theory of Bureaucratic Caring	
Person	A person is a spiritual and cultural being.
Environment	The environment is a complex spiritual, ethical, ecological, and cultural phenomenon.
Health	Health is not simply the consequence of a physical state of being, but rather provides a pattern of meaning for individuals, families, and communities.
Nursing	Nursing is a holistic, relational, spiritual, and ethical caring that seeks the good of self and others in complex community, organizational, and bureaucratic cultures.

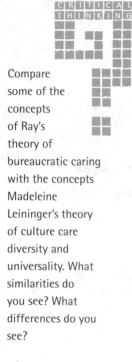

Compare some of the concepts of Ray's theory of bureaucratic caring with the concepts Madeleine Leininger's theory of culture care diversity and universality. What similarities do you see? What differences do you see?

Health

Health is not simply the consequence of a physical state of being, but rather provides a pattern of meaning for individuals, families, and communities. Persons construct their reality of health in terms of biology; mental patterns; image of mind, body, and soul; ethnicity; family structure; societal and community structure; and experiences of caring that give meaning to lives. The social organization of health and illness in society determines the way that people are recognized as sick or well and how health professionals view health and illness. As such, health is related to the way that people in a cultural group, in an organizational culture, or in a bureaucratic system construct reality and give or find meaning (Coffman, 2010, p. 122).

Nursing

"Nursing is a holistic, relational, spiritual, and ethical caring that seeks the good of self and others in complex community, organizational, and bureaucratic cultures" (Coffman, 2010, p. 121). The foundation of spiritual caring is love. Love calls forth a responsible ethical life that enables the expression of actions of caring in the lives of nurses (Coffman, 2010).

ANALYSIS OF THE THEORY OF BUREAUCRATIC CARING

THE ANALYSIS PRESENTED HERE CONSISTS of an examination of assumptions and propositions as well as a brief critique of the theory of bureaucratic caring as proposed by Ray.

Assumptions of the Theory of Bureaucratic Caring

Assumptions within the theory of bureaucratic caring include the following theoretical assertions:

❖ The meaning of caring is highly differential, depending on its structures (i.e., sociocultural, educational, political, economic, physical, technological, and legal).

❖ Caring is bureaucratic as well as spiritual/ethical.

❖ Caring is the primordial construct and consciousness of nursing.

Propositions of the Theory of Bureaucratic Caring

The following theoretical relationship statements exist within the theory:

❖ Nursing and caring are experiential and contextual, and are influenced by the social structure or the culture in the organization.

❖ Caring can positively influence the surrounding structures.

Brief Critique of the Theory of Bureaucratic Caring

The definitions of the major concepts within the theory of bureaucratic caring are clearly stated using terminology that is easily understandable by practicing nurses. The theory is logical, and terminology is used consistently throughout. Considering the complexity of healthcare organizations, the theory incorporates a minimal number of concepts (Coffman, 2010, p. 129). In the current healthcare environment with its sharp focus on the bottom line, the time has never been better for nursing leaders to consider the incorporation of the theory of bureaucratic caring within healthcare organizations (Turkel, 2006).

THE THEORY OF BUREAUCRATIC CARING, while applicable at many levels (including nursing care for individual patients and families), is specific to caring within the context of the healthcare organization, whether at the unit level or considering the entire organization. Nurses typically have a core value of caring, but are all too familiar with the emphasis placed on the bottom line in the current healthcare environment. Studies have confirmed that there is a link between caring and positive patient outcomes. Positive patient outcomes, of course, are necessary for the survival of healthcare organizations (Turkel, 2006). Given the current environment and the available evidence, now is a perfect time for

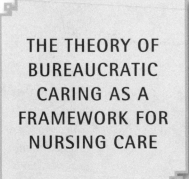

THE THEORY OF BUREAUCRATIC CARING AS A FRAMEWORK FOR NURSING CARE

nurses to proactively embrace the opportunity to transform the cultures within their healthcare organizations by utilizing the theory of bureaucratic caring.

THE NURSING PROCESS AND THE THEORY OF BUREAUCRATIC CARING

WHILE THE THEORY OF BUREAUCRATIC caring does not specifically address the nursing process, it is examined here in terms of this process as adapted for an organizational setting for the sake of discussion, consistency, and comparison.

Assessment

The assessment of a healthcare organization or unit is a complex undertaking that is accomplished through a team effort, although the focus of the assessment depends on which internal or external forces precipitated the assessment. Using the theory of bureaucratic caring as a framework, such an assessment would consider the physical, sociocultural, educational, legal, political, economic, and technological structural factors and their interconnections. The assessment is conducted in a manner that is grounded in caring, with a goal of promoting the good of others within the organization.

Planning

Planning for the implementation occurs within the context of the team, as data are analyzed in each of the structure areas. The process should be one that demonstrates caring and respect for the divergent cultures that exist within different units of the organization and with a readiness to "hear" what the members within organization reveal through the assessment.

Implementation

Strategies for intervention will depend on the results of the assessment and analysis. Although strategies may be directed at specific structural areas, it is important to remember the interconnectedness of those areas as well as the centrality and interconnectedness of spiritual–ethical caring throughout the process. Any changes in any of those areas will affect all other areas due to their intertwined nature.

Evaluation

Health in an organizational culture is related to way that reality is constructed. Because health is viewed as providing a pattern of meaning within Ray's theory, the evaluation of interventions will be based on the patterns of meaning ascribed to the process and outcomes by the members of the organization.

THE FOLLOWING SCENARIO ILLUSTRATES NURSING care relative to one identified problem framed by Ray's theory of bureaucratic caring. This scenario is not intended to cover all aspects of care, but rather to stimulate thinking about how specific care might be approached using this theory as a framework for practice.

> **SCENARIO ILLUSTRATING NURSING CARE FRAMED BY THE THEORY OF BUREAUCRATIC CARING UTILIZING THE NURSING PROCESS**

You are a nurse who is a member of the leadership team at Local Healthcare Organization, which is currently struggling with a high turnover rate among its nursing staff. Aside from the nursing shortages that this trend creates in the patient care units, it is very expensive for the organization to continuously hire and orient new nurses. To address the issue with nursing retention, it will first be necessary to assess the interconnected structural factors for the organization, including the physical, sociocultural, educational, legal, political, economic, and technological structural factors and their interconnections. The assessment should be conducted in a manner that is grounded in caring, with a goal of promoting the good of others within the organization.

Although all of the structural factors are interconnected, the assessment indicates that the political structural factor is a primary problem area for Local Healthcare Organization. Interviews reveal that nurses perceive a lack of communication and a lack of transparency between administration and nursing staff. Members of the nursing staff perceive that they have no input into the decision-making process. These issues have resulted in a lack of trust, growing disillusionment, a decrease in loyalty, and a subsequent decrease in nurse retention rates at Local Healthcare Organization.

In response to these findings, nursing staff are included in the planning process. The strategies implemented will incorporate techniques to increase communication and transparency, maintain visibility, and promote participatory decision making so as to build a caring working environment for nursing staff. A caring culture within Local Healthcare Organization will build trust and increase the retention of the nursing staff. Evaluation of these interventions will be based on the patterns of meaning ascribed to the process and outcomes by the members of Local Healthcare Organization and will ultimately be reflected in trust, loyalty, and nurse retention levels.

The theory of bureaucratic caring is a middle-range theory that has a specific focus. In the scenario presented here, the healthcare organization is the focus of care; however, the theory can be utilized for individuals, families, and communities, as well as for organizations. The nurse is responsible for providing nursing care using strategies that are applicable to all aspects of care and for providing care that is consistent with current best clinical practices even when utilizing a framework with a specific focus.

CLASSROOM ACTIVITY 28-1

Form small groups. Each group should plan additional strategies for incorporation into the preceding scenario. Each group should develop a plan for one additional problem using Ray's theory of bureaucratic caring as the basis for practice. Each group should then share its plan with the class.

REFERENCES

Coffman, S. (2010). Marilyn Anne Ray: Theory of bureaucratic caring. In M. R. Alligood & A. M. Tomey (Eds.), *Nursing theorists and their work* (7th ed., pp. 113–136). Maryland Heights, MO: Mosby.

Ray, M. (1989). The theory of bureaucratic caring for nursing practice in the organizational culture. *Nursing Administration Quarterly, 13*(2), 31–42.

Ray, M. A. (1997). Consciousness and the moral ideal: A transcultural analysis of Watson's theory of transpersonal caring. *Advanced Practice Nursing Quarterly, 3*(1), 25–31.

Ray, M. A. (2006). Part one: Marilyn Anne Ray's theory of bureaucratic caring. In M. E. Parker (Ed.), *Nursing theories and nursing practice* (2nd ed., pp. 360–368). Philadelphia: F. A. Davis.

Ray, M., Turkel, M., & Marino, F. (2002). The transformative process for nursing in workforce redevelopment. *Nursing Administration Quarterly, 26*(2), 1–14.

Turkel, M. C. (2006). Part two: Application of Marilyn Ray's theory of bureaucratic caring. In M. E. Parker (Ed.), *Nursing theories and nursing practice* (2nd ed., pp. 369–379). Philadelphia: F. A. Davis.

SYNERGY MODEL FOR PATIENT CARE: THE AMERICAN ASSOCIATION OF CRITICAL-CARE NURSES

LEARNING OBJECTIVES

After completing this chapter the student should be able to

1. Identify and explain the major concepts of the Synergy Model for Patient Care

2. Describe the major concepts important to nursing as defined by the Synergy Model for Patient Care

3. Plan nursing care for a patient scenario utilizing the Synergy Model for Patient Care

KEY TERMS

Advocacy
Caring practices
Clinical inquiry
Clinical judgment
Collaboration
Complexity
Facilitation of learning
Participation in care

Participation in decision making
Predictability
Resiliency
Resource availability
Response to diversity
Stability
Systems thinking
Vulnerability

BACKGROUND AND OVERVIEW OF THE SYNERGY MODEL FOR PATIENT CARE

THE SYNERGY MODEL FOR PATIENT Care is the result of the American Association of Critical-Care Nurses (AACN) envisioning a new paradigm for clinical practice. In 1993, the AACN Certification Corporation convened a think tank that included nationally recognized experts to develop a conceptual framework for certified practice. The initial work resulted in the description of 13 patient characteristics based on universal needs of patients and 9 characteristics required of nurses to meet patient needs. The patient characteristics identified were compensation, resiliency, margin of error, predictability, complexity, vulnerability, physiological stability, risk of death, independence, self-determination, involvement in care decisions, engagement, and resource availability. The characteristics of nurses were engagement, skilled clinical practice, agency, caring practices, system management, teamwork, diversity responsiveness, experiential learning, and being an innovator-evaluator. The think tank suggested that the synergy emerging from the interaction between the patient needs and the nurse characteristics should results in optimal outcomes for the patient and that these characteristics of the nurse would determine competencies for certified practice (Hardin, 2005a, p. 3–4).

In 1995, the AACN Certification Corporation decided to refine this model, to conduct a study of practice and job analysis of critical care nurses, and to test the validity of the concepts in critical care nurses. The group refined the patient characteristics into eight concepts, merged the nurse characteristics into eight concepts, and delineated a continuum for the characteristics. The eight patient characteristics identified in the current model are resiliency, vulnerability, stability, complexity, resource availability, participation in care, participation in decision making, and predictability. The eight nurse characteristics are clinical judgment, advocacy, caring practices, collaboration, systems thinking, response to diversity, clinical inquiry, and facilitation of learning (Hardin, 2005a, p.4).

While each patient brings a unique set of characteristics to a situation, the eight characteristics identified in the AACN model are consistently seen among patients who experience critical events. These eight characteristics are consistently assessed by nurses and should be assessed in every patient. Each patient characteristic is understood in terms of a scale from one to five, with the level of each patient characteristic being critical in terms of the competency required of the nurse (Hardin, 2005a, p. 4–5, 6–7).

Resiliency is the patient's capacity to return to a restorative level of functioning using compensatory and coping mechanisms (Curley, 1998; Kaplow, 2005a, p. 14). Resiliency can be influenced by factors such as age, comorbidities, and intact compensatory mechanisms (Hardin, 2005a, p. 5), as well as by the patient's history of adaptation to other stressors in the past (Kaplow, 2005a, p. 14). Patients with low level of resiliency include those who are unable to mount a response, those with a failure of compensatory or coping mechanisms, and those who have minimal reserves. These patients are considered to reside at level 1 on the resiliency continuum. A patient who is at level 3 is moderately resilient and is able to mount a moderate response, can initiate some degree of compensation, and has moderate reserves. A level 5 patient is considered highly resilient, is able to mount and maintain a response, and has intact compensatory mechanisms, strong reserves, and endurance (Kaplow, 2005a, p. 14).

Vulnerability refers to the level of susceptibility to actual or potential stressors that may adversely affect patient outcomes (Curley, 1998). A level 1 patient is highly vulnerable, susceptible, unprotected, and fragile, whereas a level 3 patient is moderately vulnerable, somewhat susceptible, and somewhat protected. The level 5 patient is minimally vulnerable, safe, and not fragile (Kaplow, 2005b, p. 20). Vulnerability can be affected by the patient's physiological make-up or health behaviors (Hardin, 2005a, p. 5).

Stability refers to the patient's ability to maintain a steady state of equilibrium (Curley, 1998). A level 1 patient is minimally stable, is labile, is unresponsive to therapies, and has a high risk for death. By comparison, a level 3 patient is moderately stable, is able to maintain a steady state for a limited period of time, and is somewhat responsive to therapy. A level 5 patient is characterized by being highly stable, constant, and responsive to therapies, and is at low risk for death (Kaplow, 2005c, p. 23–24). Response to therapies and nursing interventions can obviously affect the stability of the patient (Hardin, 2005a, p. 5).

Eight characteristics are consistently seen among patients who experience critical events: resiliency, vulnerability, stability, complexity, resource availability, participation in care, participation in decision making, and predictability. These eight characteristics are consistently assessed by nurses and should be assessed in every patient.

Complexity is the intricate entanglement of two or more systems (Curley, 1998). In this case, "systems" refers to either the physiological or emotional state of the body, the family dynamics, or environmental interactions with the patient. The more systems involved, the more complex the patterns displayed by the patient (Hardin, 2005a, p. 5). In the AACN model, a 1 one patient is highly complex and intricate, has complex family dynamics, or has a vague, atypical presentation; in contrast, a level 5 patient is simple and uncomplicated, has a clear-cut presentation, and has routine family dynamics (Kaplow, 2005d, p. 28).

Resource availability is influenced by the extent of resources brought to the situation by the patient, family, and community. These resources may be technical, fiscal, personal, psychological, social, or supportive in nature (Curley, 1998). The level 1 patient has few resources, and the necessary knowledge and skill are not available. Such a patient has minimal personal or psychological supportive resources and few social systems available. A level 3 patient has moderate or limited resources, whereas the level 5 patient has many resources. Specifically, the level 5 patient has extensive knowledge and skills available, has financial resources available, has strong personal and psychological supportive resources, and has access to strong social system resources (Kaplow, 2005e, p. 34). The more resources the person brings to a healthcare situation, the greater the potential for a positive outcome (Hardin, 2005a, p. 5). In contrast, limited availability of resources can hamper a patient's recovery from a critical event (Kaplow, 2005e, p. 34).

Participation in care refers to the participation of the patient and family in terms of being engaged in the delivery of care (Curley, 1998). The level 1 patient and family do not participate in the patient's care; such a patient has no capacity or desire for decision making. The level 3 patient and family have moderate levels of participation. They demonstrate limited capacity and seek advice from others in decision making. The level 5 patient and family have the capacity for decision making and fully participate in decision making. They actively seek information, are open to instruction, and desire an active role in the delivery of care (Kaplow, 2005f, p. 38). Patient and family participation can be influenced by educational background, resource availability, and cultural background (Hardin, 2005a, p. 5).

Participation in decision making refers to the level of engagement of the patient and family in comprehending the information provided by healthcare providers and in acting upon this information to execute informed decisions (Hardin, 2005a, p. 5). A level 1 patient and family have no capacity for decision making and need a surrogate decision maker to act on their behalf. A level 3 patient and family have a limited capacity for decision making and seek advice from others. A level 5 patient and family are able to make decisions for themselves (Kaplow, 2005g, p. 45). Patient and family engagement in clinical decisions can be influenced by the knowledge level of the patient, his or her capacity to make decisions given the disease or injury, the patient's cultural background, and the level of inner strength during a crisis (Hardin, 2005a, p. 5).

Predictability is the characteristic that allows one to expect a certain trajectory (Curley, 1998); in other words, it allows one to expect a certain course of events or course of illness (Hardin, 2005a, p. 5). A level 1 patient is not predictable. He or she may have an uncommon illness, may be part of an uncommon patient population, or may have an uncommon clinical course. This patient does not follow a critical pathway or may have a condition for which no clinical pathway has been developed. By comparison, the level 3 patient is moderately predictable but is wavering. The level 5 patient is highly predictable, is part of a commonly encountered patient population, and follows an expected course or critical pathway (Kaplow, 2005h, p. 51).

The eight nurse characteristics can be considered competencies that are essential for providing care for critically ill patients. All eight competencies reflect an integration of knowledge, skills, and experience of the nurse. Each nurse characteristic is understood on a continuum from one to five (Hardin, 2005a, p. 5–6).

Clinical judgment refers to clinical reasoning that includes decision making, critical thinking, and the global grasp of a situation coupled with the nursing skills acquired through a process of integrating education, experiential knowledge, and evidence-based guidelines (AACN, 2002). Clinical judgment lies at the very heart of nursing. Nurses are accountable for making the best decisions for their patients given the context of the specific situation. This is not a skill that develops overnight; rather, making decisions for and with patients comprises both an art and a science

The eight nurse characteristics—clinical judgment, advocacy, caring practices, collaboration, systems thinking, response to diversity, clinical inquiry, and facilitation of learning—can be considered competencies that are essential for providing care for critically ill patients. All eight competencies reflect an integration of knowledge, skills, and experience of the nurse.

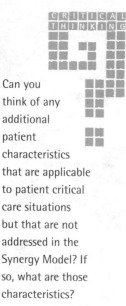

Can you think of any additional patient characteristics that are applicable to patient critical care situations but that are not addressed in the Synergy Model? If so, what are those characteristics?

(Hardin & Stannard, 2005, p. 57), with clinical judgment qualitatively differing depending on where the nurse is located along the skill-acquisition continuum. Nurses at the advanced beginner level of skill acquisition (level 1) are capable of collecting and interpreting basic-level data. Clinical decisions are limited to the nurse's knowledge. At the competent stage of skill acquisition (level 3), nurses can readily care for the usual and customary patients using their experiential knowledge and will seek guidance from more seasoned nurses if they are confronted with something new. The expert nurse (level 5) can synthesize and interpret multiple sources of data, and can understand and respond to the unique needs of patients and family situations (Hardin & Stannard, 2005, p. 59–60).

Advocacy is working on another's behalf when the other person is not capable of advocating for himself or herself. The nurse serves as a moral agent in identifying and helping resolve ethical and clinical concerns (Hardin, 2005a, p. 65). The nurse at level 1 competency works on behalf of the patient and begins to self-assess personal values. Such a nurse is aware of the patient's rights and ethical conflicts that may surface. However, at level 1, the nurse's ethical decisions are made based on guiding principles and the nurse's personal values, and the nurse typically works as an advocate when the patient's framework is consistent with his or her own values. The level 3 nurse considers the patient's values and incorporates these values into care even if the patient's values differ from the nurse's own values. The level 3 nurse is able to deviate from the rules and is able to demonstrate flexibility by allowing the patient and family to represent themselves when possible and is able to identify internal resources when complex decisions are required. The level 5 nurse is capable of advocating for the patient, family, and community even if the nurse's personal values are incongruent with the values of the client. The nurse advocates for the client using internal and external resources and empowers the patient and family to drive moral decision making through mutuality of relationships with providers (AACN, 2002; Stannard & Hardin, 2005, p. 65–66).

Caring practices are the constellation of nursing interventions that create a compassionate, supportive, and therapeutic environment for patients and staff, with the joint aims of promoting comfort and healing and preventing unnecessary suffering (AACN, 2002; Hardin, 2005b, p.

71). Caring behaviors include compassion, vigilance, engagement, and responsiveness to the patient and family (Hardin, 2005a, p. 6).

Collaboration refers to the nurse's ability to work with others to promote optimal outcomes. The patient, family, and members of other healthcare disciplines work toward promoting optimal and realistic patient goals (AACN, 2002; Hardin, 2005a, p. 6). Collaboration is a development process that matures over time. Competency in collaboration requires that the nurse participate fully as a team member (Hardin, 2005c, p. 78)

Systems thinking refers to the tools and knowledge that the nurse utilizes to recognize the interconnected nature within and across the healthcare or non-healthcare system and to manage environmental and system resources for the patient (AACN, 2002). The ability to understand how one decision can affect the whole is integral to systems thinking. The nurse uses a global perspective in clinical decision making and has the ability to negotiate the needs of the patient and family as they navigate through the healthcare system (Hardin, 2005a, p. 6). The nurse at level 1 competency is often unclear on the steps required within a system to resolve a problem. Such a nurse thinks within the focus of the specific nursing unit rather than considering the entire system. The level 3 nurse has the ability to recognize and react to the needs of patients as they move through the healthcare system. The nurse at level 5 is able to recognize the interrelationships that exist within and across healthcare and non-healthcare systems. The nurse at this level of competency utilizes a variety of resources, can anticipate the needs of the patient, knows how to navigate through the system, and is able to use this systems thinking effectively on behalf of the patient (Hardin, 2005d, p. 86).

Response to diversity refers to the sensitivity to recognize, appreciate, and incorporate differences into the provision of care (AACN, 2002). Individuality can be observed in the patient's spiritual beliefs, ethnicity, family configuration, lifestyle values, and use of alternative and complementary therapies. Nurses need to recognize the individuality of each patient while observing them for patterns that respond to nursing interventions (Hardin, 2005a, p. 6). Areas of competency that should be demonstrated by the nurse include recognizing practices based on diversity that have potentially negative outcomes for the patient, incorporating the patient's values into evidence-based practice, understanding the

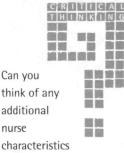

Can you think of any additional nurse characteristics or areas of competency that are not included in the categories of the Synergy Model? If so, what are those characteristics or competencies?

differences in culture between the nurse and the patient, developing skill in working with interpreters, and developing skill in conflict resolution (Hardin, 2005e, p. 93).

Clinical inquiry is the ongoing process of questioning and evaluating practice, providing informed practice, and innovating through research and experiential learning (AACN, 2002). To demonstrate competency in clinical inquiry, the nurse should display knowledge-seeking behaviors such as being open to receiving advice, participating in lifelong learning, and seeking knowledge to address clinical questions. In addition, the nurse needs to be competent in identifying clinical problems and searching for evidence in the literature to validate or change clinical practice; likewise, the nurse should be competent in participating in the research process (Hardin, 2005f, p. 98). Clinical inquiry skills evolve as the nurse moves from novice to expert (Hardin, 2005a, p. 6).

Facilitation of learning refers to the nurse's work in facilitating learning for patients, families, nursing staff, physicians, members of other healthcare disciplines, and community through both formal and information mechanisms (Hardin, 2005a, p. 6). Competency of the nurse should be demonstrated by the ability to assist the patient access health information, interpret meaning, and sort out information that fits the patient's needs. The nurse should demonstrate competency in assessment of patients' readiness to learn as well as in the provision of information to increase patients' knowledge of their diagnosis, illness, treatment, and behaviors to promote health (Hardin, 2005g, p. 104). Education should be provided based on individual strengths and weaknesses of the patient and family, with the educational level of the patient and family being considered in the design of the education to ensure their comprehension and ability to make informed decisions (Hardin, 2005a, p. 6).

Given that the premise for the Synergy Model for Patient Care is that optimal outcomes result from the synergy of a nurse's competencies matching the needs of patients and families (Fontaine & Prevost, 2005, p. xi), it stands to reason that the next step in the process was to articulate optional outcomes. In 1996, the AACN Certification Corporation appointed another think tank for the purpose of articulating optimal outcomes. Six major quality outcome indicators were identified: patient and family satisfaction, rate of adverse incidents, complication rate, adherence to the discharge plan, mortality rate, and patient length of stay (Hardin, 2005a, p. 8).

The Synergy Model delineates three levels of outcomes: outcomes derived from the patient, outcomes derived from the nurse, and outcomes derived from the healthcare system. Outcomes data derived from the patient include functional changes, behavioral changes, trust, satisfaction, comfort, and quality of life. Outcomes data derived from nursing competencies include physiological changes, the presence or absence of complications, and the extent to which treatment objectives are attained (Curley, 1998). Outcomes data derived from the healthcare system include re-admission rates, length of stay, and cost utilization (Hardin, 2005a, p. 8–9).

The premise for the Synergy Model for Patient Care is that optimal outcomes result from the synergy of a nurse's competencies matching the needs of patients and families

I N ADDITION TO THE CONCEPTS already presented, the four metaparadigm concepts of nursing are identified in the Synergy Model for Patient Care. These concepts are summarized in Table 29-1.

MAJOR CONCEPTS OF NURSING BASED ON THE SYNERGY MODEL FOR PATIENT CARE

Person

Persons are viewed in the context of patients who are biological, social, and spiritual entities and who are present at a particular developmental stage. Patients

TABLE 29-1 Metaparadigm Concepts as Defined in the AACN Synergy Model for Patient Care	
Person	Persons are viewed in the context of patients who are biological, social, and spiritual entities who are present at a particular developmental stage.
Environment	The concept of environment is not explicitly defined. However, included in the assumptions is the idea that environment is created by the nurse for the care of the patient.
Health	The concept of health is not explicitly defined. An optimal level of wellness as defined by the patient is mentioned as a goal of nursing care.
Nursing	The purpose of nursing is to meet the needs of patients and families and to provide safe passage through the healthcare system during a time of crisis.

can be described in terms of the eight characteristics previously outlined in this chapter.

Environment

The concept of environment is not explicitly defined. Nevertheless, included in the assumptions is the idea that it is the nurse who creates the environment for the care of the patient. Also included in the assumptions is the notion that the context or environment of care affects what the nurse can do.

Health

The concept of health is not explicitly defined. The assumptions refer to the optimal level of wellness, which is defined by the patient in reference to the goal of nursing.

Nursing

According to Fontaine and Prevost (2005, p. xi), the Synergy Model for Patient Care draws from the often quoted definition of nursing proposed by Virginia Henderson (1966, p. 15): "the unique function of the nurse is to assist the individual, sick or well, in the performance of those activities contributing to health or its recovery (or to a peaceful death) that he would perform unaided if he had the necessary strength, will, or knowledge." In the context of the AACN model, the purposes of nursing are to meet the needs of patients and families and to provide safe passage through the healthcare system during a time of crisis (Hardin, 2005a, p. 8). Nurses are described in terms of the eight characteristics outlined earlier in this chapter.

ANALYSIS OF THE SYNERGY MODEL FOR PATIENT CARE

THE ANALYSIS PRESENTED HERE CONSISTS of an examination of assumptions and propositions as well as a brief critique of the AACN Synergy Model for Patient Care.

Assumptions of the Synergy Model

The Synergy Model for Patient Care was originally based on five assumptions, but the list of assumptions later expanded to include nine assumption statements (AACN, 2000, p. 55; Hardin, 2005a, p. 7–8):

❖ Patients are biological, social, and spiritual entities who are present at a particular developmental stage. The whole patient—body, mind, and spirit—must be considered.

❖ The patient, family, and community all contribute to providing a context for the nurse–patient relationship.

❖ Patients can be described by a number of characteristics. Characteristics are connected and contribute to one another; they cannot be looked at in isolation.

❖ Nurses can be described in terms of a number of dimensions. These interrelated dimensions paint a profile of the nurse.

❖ A goal of nursing is to restore the patient to an optimal level of wellness as defined by the patient. Death can be an acceptable outcome if the goal of nursing care is to move a patient toward a peaceful death.

❖ The nurse creates the environment for the care of the patient. The context/environment of care also affects what the nurse can do.

❖ There is an interrelatedness between impact areas. The nature of the interrelatedness may change as the function of experience, situation, and setting changes.

❖ The nurse may work to optimize outcomes for patients, families, healthcare providers, and the healthcare system or organization.

❖ The nurse brings his or her background to each situation, including various levels of education/knowledge and skills/experience.

Propositions of the Synergy Model

The primary theoretical relationship statement of the Synergy Model is that when patient characteristics and nurse competencies match, patient outcomes are optimized. Research is needed to further validate the link between outcome criteria and certified practice (Hardin, 2005a, p. 9).

Brief Critique of the Synergy Model

The Synergy Model for Patient Care is specific to the context of the critical-care patient situation and, therefore, is classified as a middle-range nursing theory. Nevertheless, this model has a focus that is congruent with nursing practice in the current healthcare environment, which is extremely outcome driven. The language used to describe the model is simple and easy to understand for practicing nurses. The model is logical and uses terms consistently. It also incorporates and builds on established concepts from other frameworks—such as the concepts of movement from novice to expert (Benner, 1984/2001) and Henderson's (1966) definition of nursing—that are familiar to practicing nurses.

Even though the Synergy Model was developed as a blueprint for certified practice, it can also be used as in curriculum development and in conducting research related to the interrelationship of competencies and patient outcomes (Curley, 2007; Hardin, 2005a, p. 8). In addition, Curley (2007) has suggested that the Synergy Model is appropriate for additional settings, including ambulatory patient care, staff development and nursing education.

THE SYNERGY MODEL FOR PATIENT CARE AS A FRAMEWORK FOR NURSING CARE

THE SYNERGY MODEL IS A conceptual framework for designing practice and developing competencies to care for critically ill patients, with a goal of optimizing outcomes for patients and families. Optimal outcomes are realized when the competencies of the nurse match the patient and family needs.

ALTHOUGH THE NURSING PROCESS IS not specifically addressed as a concept within the model, many of the concepts incorporated in the Synergy Model for Patient Care are those that have traditionally been associated with the use of the nursing process in the provision of nursing care. For example, the concept of clinical judgment—one of the identified nursing competencies—has historically been grounded in the nursing process of assessment, planning, intervention, and evaluation (Hardin & Stannard, 2005, p. 57). A brief discussion of each of the components of the nursing process within the context of the Synergy Model follows.

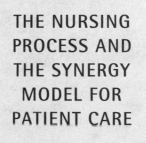

THE NURSING PROCESS AND THE SYNERGY MODEL FOR PATIENT CARE

Assessment

Assessment may be accomplished using various techniques, such as physical assessment, observation, and interview, but will include an assessment of all eight patient characteristics. These eight characteristics are consistently assessed by nurses and should be assessed in every patient. In addition, each patient characteristic must be understood in terms of the patient's status on the continuum from one to five, because the level of each patient characteristic on the continuum is critical in terms of the competency required of the nurse.

Planning

Planning to meet patient needs will involve consideration of each of the eight patient characteristics. Planning will include the patient and family if, considering the patient level, it is possible. Planning should also take into account the need to match the competency level of the nurse with the patient characteristics.

Implementation

Intervention strategies are based on the identified needs related to each of the eight patient characteristics. Implementation must take into account the patient level in regard to the patient characteristics. Interventions will occur in each of the nurse competencies and may vary based on the competency level of the nurse in each of the categories.

Evaluation

Evaluation of nursing care is ultimately based on patient outcomes during the critical event or illness. In the context of the Synergy Model, evaluation also incorporates an evaluation of the outcomes of care from the perspective of the synergy of a nurse's competencies matching the needs of patients and their families.

SCENARIO ILLUSTRATING NURSING CARE FRAMED BY THE SYNERGY MODEL FOR PATIENT CARE UTILIZING THE NURSING PROCESS

THE FOLLOWING SCENARIO ILLUSTRATES NURSING care of the patient relative to one identified nursing problem framed by the Synergy Model for Patient Care. This scenario is not intended to cover all aspects of care, but rather to stimulate thinking about how specific care might be approached using this theory as a framework for practice.

Mrs. M. is an elderly patient who was admitted to the unit with a medical diagnosis of exacerbation of congestive heart failure (CHF). Assessment includes all eight patient characteristics and planning is based on the identified needs. Mrs. M. has been re-admitted to the hospital twice already this month for exacerbation of CHF. Her stability is determined to be a level 3, as she has the ability to maintain stability for some period of time and is moderately responsive to therapy. The level 1 nurse focuses on meeting the basic needs of Mrs. M. and improving disease-specific outcomes based on standards and protocols while maintaining a safe environment. The level 3 nurse is able to sort out extraneous data and see trends, is able to obtain internal resources for Mrs. M., and, during this time of stress, can tailor caring practices to Mrs. M. Evaluation is based on achieving optimal outcomes for Mrs. M. and her family.

The Synergy Model for Patient Care is a middle-range theory that has a specific focus. Throughout the nursing process, if other issues arise during the nursing encounter that are outside of the focus of this theory, the nurse will intervene to provide nursing care using strategies that are congruent with current best clinical practices.

CLASSROOM ACTIVITY 29-1

Form small groups. Each group should add to the plan of care for Mrs. M. in the preceding scenario based on other potential or actual nursing problems typical for a patient with the same medical diagnosis or symptoms and demographics. Each group should develop a plan for one additional nursing problem using the AACN Synergy Model for Patient Care as the basis for practice. Each group should then share its plan with the class.

CLASSROOM ACTIVITY 29-2

Form small groups. Using a case study provided by the instructor, develop a plan of care using the Synergy Model for Patient Care as the basis for practice. Each group should then share its plan of care with the class.

CLASSROOM ACTIVITY 29-3

Form small groups. Using a case study provided by the instructor, develop a plan of care using one of the theories as the basis for practice; each group should select a different nursing theory. Each group should then share its plan of care with the class and discuss the similarities and differences in care.

REFERENCES

American Association of Critical-Care Nurses (AACN). (2000). *Standards for acute and critical care nursing practice* (3rd ed.). Aliso Viejo, CA: AACN Critical Care Publications.

American Association of Critical-Care Nurses (AACN). (2002). *Competency level descriptors for nurse characteristics.* Aliso Viejo, CA: AACN Critical Care Publications.

Benner, P. (1984/2001). *From novice to expert: Excellence and power in clinical nursing practice.* Upper Saddle River, NJ: Prentice-Hall.

Curley, M. A. Q. (1998). Patient–nurse synergy: Optimizing patients' outcomes. *American Journal of Critical Care, 7*(1), 64–72.

Curley, M. A. Q. (2007). *Synergy: The unique relationship between nursing and patients.* Indianapolis, IN: Sigma Theta Tau International.

Fontaine, D. K., & Prevost, S. S. (2005). Foreword. In S. R. Hardin & R. Kaplow (Eds.), *Synergy for clinical excellence: The AACN Synergy Model for Patient Care* (p. xi). Sudbury, MA: Jones and Bartlett.

Hardin, S. R. (2005a). Introduction to the AACN Synergy Model for Patient Care. In S. R. Hardin & R. Kaplow (Eds.), *Synergy for clinical excellence: The AACN Synergy Model for Patient Care* (pp. 3–10). Sudbury, MA: Jones and Bartlett.

Hardin, S. R. (2005b). Caring practices. In S. R. Hardin & R. Kaplow (Eds.), *Synergy for clinical excellence: The AACN Synergy Model for Patient Care* (pp. 69–73). Sudbury, MA: Jones and Bartlett.

Hardin, S. R. (2005c). Collaboration. In S. R. Hardin & R. Kaplow (Eds.), *Synergy for clinical excellence: The AACN Synergy Model for Patient Care* (pp. 75–82). Sudbury, MA: Jones and Bartlett.

Hardin, S. R. (2005d). Systems thinking. In S. R. Hardin & R. Kaplow (Eds.), *Synergy for clinical excellence: The AACN Synergy Model for Patient Care* (pp. 83–89). Sudbury, MA: Jones and Bartlett.

Hardin, S. R. (2005e). Response to diversity. In S. R. Hardin & R. Kaplow (Eds.), *Synergy for clinical excellence: The AACN Synergy Model for Patient Care* (pp. 91–95). Sudbury, MA: Jones and Bartlett.

Hardin, S. R. (2005f). Clinical inquiry. In S. R. Hardin & R. Kaplow (Eds.), *Synergy for clinical excellence: The AACN Synergy Model for Patient Care* (pp. 97–101). Sudbury, MA: Jones and Bartlett.

Hardin, S. R. (2005g). Facilitator of learning. In S. R. Hardin & R. Kaplow (Eds.), *Synergy for clinical excellence: The AACN Synergy Model for Patient Care* (pp. 103–107). Sudbury, MA: Jones and Bartlett.

Hardin, S. R., & Stannard, D. (2005). Clinical judgment. In S. R. Hardin & R. Kaplow (Eds.), *Synergy for clinical excellence: The AACN Synergy Model for Patient Care* (pp. 57–62). Sudbury, MA: Jones and Bartlett.

Henderson, V. (1966). *The nature of nursing.* New York: MacMillan.

Kaplow, R. (2005a). Resiliency. In S. R. Hardin & R. Kaplow (Eds.), *Synergy for clinical excellence: The AACN Synergy Model for Patient Care* (pp. 13–17). Sudbury, MA: Jones and Bartlett.

Kaplow, R. (2005b). Vulnerability. In S. R. Hardin & R. Kaplow (Eds.), *Synergy for clinical excellence: The AACN Synergy Model for Patient Care* (pp. 19–22). Sudbury, MA: Jones and Bartlett.

Kaplow, R. (2005c). Stability. In S. R. Hardin & R. Kaplow (Eds.), *Synergy for clinical excellence: The AACN Synergy Model for Patient Care* (pp. 23–25). Sudbury, MA: Jones and Bartlett.

Kaplow, R. (2005d). Complexity. In S. R. Hardin & R. Kaplow (Eds.), *Synergy for clinical excellence: The AACN Synergy Model for Patient Care* (pp. 27–31). Sudbury, MA: Jones and Bartlett.

Kaplow, R. (2005e). Resource availability. In S. R. Hardin & R. Kaplow (Eds.), *Synergy for clinical excellence: The AACN Synergy Model for Patient Care* (pp. 33–36). Sudbury, MA: Jones and Bartlett.

Kaplow, R. (2005f). Participation in care. In S. R. Hardin & R. Kaplow (Eds.), *Synergy for clinical excellence: The AACN Synergy Model for Patient Care* (pp. 37–41). Sudbury, MA: Jones and Bartlett.

Kaplow, R. (2005g). Participation in decision making. In S. R. Hardin & R. Kaplow (Eds.), *Synergy for clinical excellence: The AACN Synergy Model for Patient Care* (pp. 43–48). Sudbury, MA: Jones and Bartlett.

Kaplow, R. (2005h). Predictability. In S. R. Hardin & R. Kaplow (Eds.), *Synergy for clinical excellence: The AACN Synergy Model for Patient Care* (pp. 49–54). Sudbury, MA: Jones and Bartlett.

Stannard, D., & Hardin, S. R. (2005). Advocacy/moral agency. In S. R. Hardin & R. Kaplow (Eds.), *Synergy for clinical excellence: The AACN Synergy Model for Patient Care* (pp. 63–68). Sudbury, MA: Jones and Bartlett.

GLOSSARY

The names in parentheses at the ends of the definitions indicate the theorist(s) with whom the term/definition is associated.

Achievement subsystem: A subsystem that functions to control or master an aspect of self or environment to achieve a standard and encompasses intellectual, physical, creative, mechanical, and social skills (Johnson).

Activity-related affect: The subjective positive or negative feelings that occur before, during, and following behavior based on the stimulus properties of the behavior (Pender).

Adaptation: The process and outcome whereby thinking and feeling persons, as individuals or in groups, use conscious awareness and choice to create human and environmental integration (Roy).

Adaptive modes: Physiologic–physical mode, self-concept–group identify mode, role function mode, and interdependence mode. It is through these four modes that responses to and interaction with the environment can be carried out and adaptation can be observed (Roy).

Advanced beginner stage of skill acquisition: A stage of development at which the nurse demonstrates a marginally acceptable level of performance after having considerable experience coping with real situations, although he or she is still guided by rules and is oriented toward task completion (Benner).

Advocacy: Working on another's behalf when the other person is not capable of advocating for himself or herself (AACN).

Affiliative or attachment subsystem: A subsystem that forms the basis for social organization and consequences, such as social inclusion, intimacy, and the formation and maintenance of strong social bonds (Johnson).

Agency: One's sense of and ability to act on or influence a situation (Benner).

Aggressive or protective subsystem: A subsystem that functions to protect and preserve the system (Johnson).

Anticipatory stage (for a mother): A time of initial social and psychological adjustment to pregnancy, when expectations of the maternal role are learned by seeking information and visualizing oneself as a mother (Mercer).

Assumptions: Statements accepted as truths that represent the values and beliefs of a theory or conceptual framework.

Behavior-specific cognitions and affect: Variables within the health promotion model that are considered to have motivational significance and are the target of nursing intervention because they are amenable to change. These variables include (1) perceived benefits of action, (2) perceived barriers to action, (3) perceived self-efficacy, and (4) activity-related affect (Pender).

Being with: One of the caring processes; being emotionally present to the other, including being present in person, conveying availability, and sharing feelings without burdening the one cared for (Swanson).

Canon: A rule or principle (Nightingale).

Caring: (1) The intentional and authentic presence of the nurse with another, who is recognized as living in caring and growing in caring (Boykin and Schoenhofer). (2) A complex, transcultural, relational process grounded in an ethical, spiritual context (Ray). (3) A nurturing way of relating to a valued other toward whom one feels a personal sense of commitment and responsibility (Swanson).

Caring practices: The constellation of nursing interventions that creates a compassionate, supportive, and therapeutic environment for patients and staff, with the aim of promoting comfort and healing and preventing unnecessary suffering (AACN).

Caritas: To cherish, to appreciate, to give special attention, and to convey the concept of love (Watson).

Clarity: Consistency in terms of terminology and structure of a theory.

Clinical inquiry: The ongoing process of questioning and evaluating practice, providing informed practice, and innovating through research and experiential learning (AACN).

Clinical judgment: Clinical reasoning—including decision making, critical thinking, and the global grasp of a situation—coupled with the nursing skills acquired through a process of integrating education, experiential knowledge, and evidence-based guidelines (AACN).

Cognator subsystem: An adaptive process that responds through four cognitive–emotional channels: perceptual and information processing, learning, judgment, and emotion (Roy).

Collaboration: The nurse's ability to work with others to promote optimal outcomes (AACN).

Comfort: The immediate experience of being strengthened by having needs for relief, ease, and transcendence addressed in four contexts (physical, psychospiritual, sociocultural, and environmental); it is much more than the absence of pain or other physical discomfort (Kolcaba).

Competent stage of skill acquisition: A stage of development in which the nurse begins to recognize patterns and is able to discern which features of a situation require attention (Benner).

Complexity: The intricate entanglement of two or more systems (AACN).

Components of nursing care: The fundamentals of nursing that include helping others provide for their basic needs (Henderson).

Concept: A term or label that describes a phenomenon or group of phenomena.

Conceptual model: A set of concepts and statements that integrate the concepts into a meaningful configuration.

Consciousness: A system's ability to interact with the environment (Newman).

Conservation: A term derived from the Latin word meaning "to keep together" (Levine).

Conservation of energy: Principle that addresses the requirement of individuals in relation to a balance of energy and a constant renewal of energy to maintain life processes and activities (Levine).

Conservation of personal integrity: A principle that recognizes the sanctity of life that is manifest in all persons (Levine).

Conservation of social integrity: A principle that recognizes life gains meaning through social communities and the meaning of health is socially determined (Levine).

Conservation of structural integrity: A principle that addresses healing as a process of restoring structural and functional integrity through conservation and defense of wholeness, whereas those with permanent effects of illness or loss of structure are guided to a new level of adaptation (Levine).

Created environment: An environment that may be expressed consciously or unconsciously and functions to insulate the client from environmental stressors by providing a mechanism for protective coping (Neuman).

Culture care accommodation or negotiation: Assistive, supportive, facilitative, or enabling professional actions and decisions that help people of a specific culture or subculture adapt to or negotiate with others for meaningful, beneficial, and congruent health outcomes (Leininger).

Culture care preservation or maintenance: Assistive, supportive, facilitative, or enabling professional actions and decisions that help people of a specific culture maintain meaningful care values and lifeways for their well-being, recover from illness, or deal with a handicap or dying (Leininger).

Culture care repatterning or restructuring: Assistive, supportive, facilitative, or enabling professional actions and decisions that help patients reorder, change, or modify their lifeways so as to obtain new, different, and beneficial health outcomes (Leininger).

Deliberative nursing process: The process used to share and validate the nurse's direct and indirect observations (Orlando).

Dependency subsystem: A subsystem that promotes helping or nurturing behaviors, and whose consequences include approval, recognition, and physical assistance (Johnson).

Derivable consequences: The end results of a theory; the key to the theory's importance.

Developmental self-care requisites: Requirements that relate to different stages in the human life cycle, such as marriage or retirement (Orem).

Doing for: One of the caring processes, which refers to doing for others what one would do for self, including anticipating needs, comforting, performing skillfully and competently, and protecting the one cared for while preserving his or her dignity (Swanson).

Eliminative subsystem: A subsystem that addresses when, how, and under what conditions we eliminate wastes from the body (Johnson).

Empirical precision: The testability and the usability of a theory.

Enabling: One of the processes of caring, which refers to facilitating the other's passage through life transitions and unfamiliar events by focusing on the event, informing, explaining, supporting, validating feelings, generating alternatives, thinking things through, and giving feedback (Swanson).

Environment: Human beings' significant others and physical surroundings, as well as local, regional, national, and worldwide cultural, social, political, and economic conditions that are associated with human beings' health.

Expert stage of skill acquisition: A stage of development at which the nurse no longer relies on rules to connect his or her understanding of the situation to the appropriate action, but rather has an intuitive grasp of the situation and has the ability to recognize patterns from his or her deep experiential background (Benner).

Extrapersonal stressors: External environmental interaction forces that occur outside the boundaries of the client system at the distal range (Neuman).

Facilitation of learning: The nurse's ability to bring about learning for patients, families, nursing staff, physicians, members of other healthcare disciplines, and community, using both formal and information mechanisms (AACN).

Flexible line of defense: The outer boundary of the defined client system, which protects the normal line of defense (Neuman).

Formal stage (for a mother): A stage that begins with the birth of the infant and continues through physical restoration of the mother; during this time, maternal behavior is learned from others, including professionals, and the new mother replicates and practices the learned behaviors (Mercer).

Generality: The scope of the concepts and the purpose of a theory.

Health: Human processes of living and dying.

Health-deviation self care requisites: Six categories that are related to deviations in structure or function of a human being (Orem).

Helicy: The unpredictable but continuous, nonlinear evolution of energy fields, as evidenced by a spiral development that is a continuous, non-repeating, and innovative patterning reflecting the nature of change (Rogers).

Homeodynamics: Collectively, the principles of helicy, resonancy, and integrality; it describes the nature of change within human and environmental energy fields (Rogers).

Humanbecoming: Synonym for health (Parse).

Human being (person): Any individual, family, community, or other group who is a participant in nursing.

Informal stage (for a mother): The period from two weeks through approximately four months after the birth of a child, which is characterized by approaching normalization as the mother learns infant cues and develops her own style of mothering (Mercer).

Ingestive subsystem: A subsystem that deals with when, how, what, how much, and under what conditions we eat (Johnson).

Integrality: The continuous mutual process of person and environment (Rogers).

Interaction–transaction process: A nursing process using King's theory in which assessment focuses on perceptions, communication, and interaction. Planning involves making a decision about goals and reaching agreement as to how to attain those goals; implementation focuses on transactions; and evaluation focuses on goals attained.

Interpersonal stressors: External environmental interaction forces that occur outside the boundaries of the client system at the proximal range (Neuman).

Interpersonal systems: Systems that are formed when two or more individuals interact; they include the concepts of communication, interaction, role, stress, and transaction (King).

Intrapersonal stressors: Internal environmental forces that occur within the boundary of the client system (Neuman).

Johnson's nursing diagnostic and treatment process: The nursing process for the behavioral system model. The components of this process include determination of the existence of a problem, diagnostic classification of problems, management of nursing problems, and evaluation of behavioral system balance and stability.

Knowing: One of the processes of caring, which involves striving to understand the meaning of an event in the life of the other, avoiding assumptions, focusing on the person cared for, seeking cues, assessing meticulously, and engaging both the one caring and the one cared for in the process of knowing (Swanson).

Lines of resistance: A series of concentric broken circles surrounding the basic structure that are activated following invasion of the normal line of defense by environmental stressors (Neuman).

Macrosystem (exosystem): A system consisting of the relationships between two or more mesosystem factors (Mercer).

Maintaining belief: One of the processes of caring, which includes sustaining faith in the other's capacity to get through an event or transition and face a future with meaning as well as holding him or her in high esteem, maintaining a hope-filled attitude, offering realistic optimism, helping to find meaning, and standing by the one cared for no matter what the situation (Swanson).

Management methods (in the theory of chronic sorrow): Personal coping strategies (internal management methods) used by persons during the chronic sorrow experience and supportive interventions (external management methods) provided by professionals (Eakes, Burke, and Hainsworth).

Maternal identity: An end point of maternal role attainment, when the mother experiences a sense of harmony, confidence, and competence in how she performs the role of mother (Mercer).

Maternal role attainment: An interactional and developmental process that occurs over time in which the mother becomes attached to her infant, acquires competence in caretaking tasks involved in the maternal role, and expresses pleasure and gratification in the role (Mercer).

Meaning: Linguistic and imagined content and interpretation that one gives to something defined by the concepts of imaging, valuing, and languaging (Parse).

Mesosystem: The extended family, school, work, church, and other systems in a community that influence the microsystem (Mercer).

Metaparadigm: The most global perspective of a discipline; the global concepts that identify the phenomenon of central interest to a discipline, the global propositions that describe the concepts, and the global propositions that state the relations between or among the concepts.

Microsystem: In the maternal context, the system consisting of the mother, the infant, her partner, and close relationships within the family; it is the most influential factor in maternal role attainment (Mercer).

Modeling: The process used by the nurse as he or she develops an image and understanding of the client's world as the client perceives it (Erickson, Tomlin, and Swain).

Moderating–mediating factors: Personal and contextual variables such as age, gender, life experiences, and social environment that can influence the relationships between vulnerability and self-transcendence and between self-transcendence and well-being (Reed).

Movement: A reflection of consciousness that indicates inner organization or disorganization of persons and communicates the harmony or a person's pattern with the environment (Newman).

Neuman systems model nursing process format: A nursing process with three categories (nursing diagnosis, nursing goals, and nursing outcomes) that has been designed for use with the Neuman systems model.

Normal line of defense. A boundary indicating what the client has become or the usual wellness state (Neuman).

Novice stage of skill acquisition: A stage of development in which the person has no background experience of the situation. The novice stage is characterized by the person requiring rules to govern performance; typically, the individual has difficulty distinguishing between the relevant and irrelevant features of a situation (Benner).

Nursing: Actions taken by nurses on behalf of or in conjunction with human beings, the goals or outcomes of nursing actions, and the process that encompasses assessment, diagnosis, planning, intervention, and evaluation activities.

Nursing process discipline: A discipline composed of three elements: the behavior of the patient, the reaction of the nurse, and the nursing actions that are designed for the patient's benefit (Orlando).

Nurturance: The fusing and integrating of cognitive, physiological, and affective processes with the aim of assisting a client to move toward holistic health (Erickson, Tomlin, and Swain).

Orientation phase: The stage at which a health problem has emerged, resulting in a "felt need," and professional assistance is sought (Peplau).

Participation in care: Engagement of the patient and family in the delivery of care (AACN).

Participation in decision making: Engagement of the patient and family in comprehending the information provided by healthcare providers and acting on this information to execute informed decisions (AACN).

Pattern: Information that depicts the whole and understanding of the meaning of all relationships at once; it is constantly moving unidirectionally and evolving and includes the dimensions of movement and time–space (Newman).

Pattern integrations: The identification of patterns of the interpersonal relationship between two or more persons that together link or bind them and enable them to transform energy into patterns of action that bring satisfaction or security in the face of a recurring problem (Peplau).

Perceived barriers to action: The anticipated, imagined, or real blocks or personal costs of a behavior (Pender).

Perceived benefits of action: The anticipated positive outcomes resulting from health behavior (Pender).

Perceived self-efficacy: The judgment of personal capability to organize and execute a health-promoting behavior (Pender).

Perceptual acuity and the skill of involvement: The ability to tune into a situation and hone in on the salient issues by engaging with the problem and the person (Benner).

Person (human being): Any individual, family, community, or other group who is a participant in nursing.

Personal systems: A system that includes the concepts of body image, growth and development, perception, self, space, and time (King).

Philosophies of nursing: Descriptions that set forth the general meaning of nursing and nursing phenomena through reasoning and the logical presentation of ideas contributing to the discipline by providing direction, clarifying values, and forming a foundation for theory development.

Predictability: The characteristic that allows a person to expect a certain trajectory—that is, that allows a person to expect a certain course of events or course of the illness (AACN).

Prevention-as-intervention: A format that identifies the entry point condition of the client system into the healthcare system as well as the general type of intervention or action required (Neuman).

Primary prevention-as-intervention: A strategy used for wellness retention, which seeks to protect the client system's normal line of defense or usual wellness state by strengthening the flexible line of defense (Neuman).

Proficient stage of skill acquisition: A stage of development in which the nurse perceives the situation as a whole, formulates plans intuitively, and recognizes certain features of the situation as important without having to stand back and adopt a perspective or choose a plan (Benner).

Proposition: A statement about a concept or a statement of the relationship between two or more concepts.

Reasoning-in-transition: Practical reasoning in an ongoing clinical situation (Benner).

Reconstitution: The determined energy increase related to the degree of reaction; it is identified as beginning at any point following treatment (Neuman).

Regulator subsystem: An adaptive process that responds through neural, chemical, and endocrine coping channels (Roy).

Resiliency: The patient's capacity to return to a restorative level of functioning using compensatory and coping mechanisms (AACN).

Resolution (termination) phase: The period in which the patient gradually adopts new goals and frees himself or herself from identification with the nurse (Peplau).

Resonancy: A wave frequency; an energy field pattern evolution from lower- to higher-frequency wave patterns that is reflective of the continuous variability of the human energy field (Rogers).

Resource availability: The extent of resources brought to the situation by the patient, family, and community. Resources may be technical, fiscal, personal, psychological, social, or supportive in nature (AACN).

Response-based practice: Adaptation of interventions to meet changing needs and expectations of patients (Benner).

Response to diversity: The sensitivity to recognize, appreciate, and incorporate differences into the provision of care (AACN).

Rhythmicity: The cadent, paradoxical patterning of the human universe mutual process defined by the concepts of revealing–concealing, enabling–limiting, and connecting–separating (Parse).

Role identity (personal) stage (of a mother): A period beginning approximately four months post birth of the infant, when there is an internalization of maternal role identity and the mother views herself as competent (Mercer).

Role-modeling: The facilitation and nurturance of the individual in attaining, maintaining, or promoting health through purposeful interventions (Erickson, Tomlin, and Swain).

Secondary prevention-as-intervention: A strategy for wellness attainment that seeks to protect the basic structure by strengthening the internal lines of resistance so as to provide appropriate treatment of symptoms, thereby attaining optimal client system stability and energy conservation (Neuman).

Self-care agency: An acquired ability of mature and maturing persons to know and meet their requirements for deliberate and purposive action to regulate their own human functioning and development; it includes the dimensions of development, operability, and adequacy (Orem).

Self-care knowledge: Individuals' knowledge of what has altered their health status and what they need to improve and optimize their health status, promote their growth and development, and maximize their quality of life (Erickson, Tomlin, and Swain).

Self-care resources: Internal and external resources that are mobilized through self-care action to help again, maintain, and promote the optimal level of holistic health (Erickson, Tomlin, and Swain).

Self-transcendence: The capacity to expand self-boundaries intrapersonally, interpersonally, temporally, and transpersonally (Reed).

Sexual subsystem: The function of procreation and gratification, which includes development of gender-role identity and gender-role behaviors (Johnson).

Simplicity: Refers to how simple a theory is.

Skilled know-how: Also known as "embodied intelligent performance"; knowing what to do, when to do it, and how to do it (Benner).

Stability: The patient's ability to maintain a steady state of equilibrium (AACN).

Social systems: Collectively, religious systems, educational systems, and healthcare systems. Concepts important to understanding the social system include authority, decision making, organization, power, and status (King).

Sunrise model: An enabler that is a visual guide for the exploration of cultures; it is used to clarify the essential components of the theory of culture care diversity and universality (Leininger).

Systems thinking: The tools and knowledge that the nurse uses to recognize the interconnected nature within and across the healthcare or non-healthcare system and manage environmental and system resources for the patient (AACN).

Tertiary prevention-as-intervention: A strategy for wellness maintenance or return to wellness following treatment, which relies on supporting existing strengths and conserving client system energy. It can begin at any point during client reconstitution after treatment once some degree of client system stability has occurred (Neuman).

Theory: An organized, coherent, and systematic articulation of a set of statements related to significant questions in a discipline that are communicated in a meaningful whole and that are discovered or invented for describing, predicting, or prescribing events, situations, conditions, or relationships.

Therapeutic self-care demand: The summation of care measures necessary to meet all of an individual's known self-care requisites (Orem).

Time: An index of consciousness; consciousness expands space–time and transcends limitations of the linear and physical boundaries to extend beyond the present (Newman).

Transcendence: Reaching beyond what is possible; it is defined by the concepts of powering, originating, and transforming (Parse).

Transcultural nursing: A substantive area of study and practice focused on comparative cultural care (caring) values, beliefs, and practices of individuals or groups of similar or different cultures with the goal of providing culture-specific and universal nursing care practices in promoting health or well-being or helping people face unfavorable human conditions, illness, or death in culturally meaningful ways (Leininger).

Trigger events: Those milestones, situations, or circumstances that bring the disparity created by a loss into focus and trigger the grief-related feelings associated with chronic sorrow (Eakes, Burke, and Hainsworth).

Universal self-care requisites: Requirements found in all human beings that are associated with life processes (Orem).

Vulnerability: The level of susceptibility to actual or potential stressors that may adversely affect patient outcomes (AACN).

Working phase: Events including the exploration of feelings by the patient and the nurse focusing the patient on the achievement of new goals (Peplau).

Worldview: A commitment that can be expressed as a set of presuppositions that a person holds about the basic constitution of reality, and that provides the foundation on which the individual lives and moves and has as his or her being.

INDEX

Tables are indicated by "t" following the page number.